D1563085

Brain-Disabling Treatments in Psychiatry

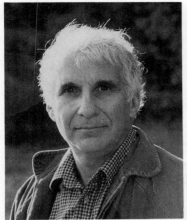 **Peter R. Breggin, MD,** is a psychiatrist in private practice in Bethesda, Maryland, where he works with children, adults, and families. He is also active as a forensic medical expert. In 1971, he founded the Center for the Study of Psychiatry and Psychology, a reform-minded organization that has been called "the conscience of American psychiatry." He is also on the faculty of The Johns Hopkins University Department of Counseling and Human Services. He is noted for his critiques of biological psychiatry and his focus on psychosocial alternatives for healing emotional suffering in children and adults.

Dr. Breggin is the author of many books and articles, including *Toxic Psychiatry* (1991), *Beyond Conflict* (1992), and with Ginger Ross Breggin, *Talking Back to Prozac* (1994) and *The War Against Children* (1994). In addition to *Brain-Disabling Treatments in Psychiatry*, Springer will soon publish his latest book on therapy, *The Heart of Being Helpful: Empathy and the Creation of a Healing Presence.*

Dr. Breggin's work is frequently covered in the media and he gives workshops throughout North America and Europe.

Dr. Breggin and the Center for the Study of Psychiatry and Psychology can be reached at 4628 Chestnut Street, Bethesda, MD 20814, or at their web site, www.breggin.com.

Brain-Disabling Treatments in Psychiatry

DRUGS, ELECTROSHOCK, AND THE ROLE OF THE FDA

Peter R. Breggin, MD

 Springer Publishing Company

The Publisher does not warrant or guarantee any of the procedures described herein and has not performed any independent analysis in connection with any of the information contained herein. The Publisher does not assume, and expressly disclaims, any obligation to obtain and include information other than provided by the author.

The reader is expressly warned to consider and adopt all safety precautions that might be indicated by the activities described herein, and to avoid all potential hazards.

The Publisher shall not be liable for any special, consequential, or exemplary damages resulting, in whole or in part, from the readers' use of, or reliance on, the information contained in this book.

Copyright © 1997 by Springer Publishing Company, Inc.

Springer Publishing Company, Inc.
536 Broadway
New York, NY 10012-3955

Cover design by Margaret Dunin
Acquisitions Editor: Bill Tucker
Production Editor: Jeanne Libby

97 98 99 00 01 / 5 4 3 2 1

Library of Congress Cataloging-in-Publication Data

Breggin, Peter Roger, 1936–
    Brain-disabling treatments in psychiatry : drugs, electroshock, and the role of the FDA / Peter R. Breggin.
        p.   cm.
    Includes bibliographical references and index.
    ISBN 0-8261-9490-7
    1. Psychotropic drugs—Side effects.   2. Brain—Effect of drugs on.
3. Electroconvulsive thearpy—Complications.   4. Iatrogenic diseases.
5. Brain damage—Etiology.   I. Title.
    [DNLM: 1. Mental Disorders—thearpy.   2. Brain Damage, Chronic—
etiology.   3. Psychotropic Drugs—adverse effects   4. Electroconvulsive
Therapy—adverse effects.   5. Drug Industry—United States—legislation.
WM 400 B833b 1997]
    RC483.B726   1997
    616.89'1—dc21
    DNLM/DLC
    for Library of Congress   97-3969
                                                                                                            CIP

NOTICE TO THE READER

A Warning Concerning the Use of Psychiatric Drugs

The psychiatric drugs discussed in this book are far more dangerous to take than many doctors and patients realize, but they can also become hazardous if discontinued too abruptly. Many are addictive, and most can produce withdrawal symptoms that are emotionally and physically distressing and sometimes life-threatening. Stopping or withdrawing from psychiatric drugs should usually be done gradually with the aid of experienced clinical supervision.

A book cannot substitute for individualized medical or psychological care, and this book is not intended as a treatment guide. It provides a critical analysis of biological treatments in psychiatry written from a scientific, ethical, psychological, and social viewpoint.

Peter R. Breggin, MD

BOOKS BY PETER R. BREGGIN, MD

NONFICTION

College Students in a Mental Hospital: An Account of Organized Social Contacts Between College Volunteers and Mental Patients in a Hospital Community (1962) (Jointly authored)

Electroshock: Its Brain-Disabling Effects (1979)

The Psychology of Freedom: Liberty and Love as a Way of Life (1980)

Psychiatric Drugs: Hazards to the Brain (1983)

Toxic Psychiatry: Why Therapy, Empathy and Love Must Replace the Drugs, Electroshock and Biochemical Theories of the 'New Psychiatry' (1991)

Beyond Conflict: From Self-Help and Psychotherapy to Peacemaking (1992)

Talking Back to Prozac: What Doctors Aren't Telling You About Today's Most Controversial Drug (1994) (Co-authored by Ginger Breggin)

The War Against Children: The Government's Intrusion into Schools, Families and Communities in Search of a Medical "Cure" for Violence (1994) (Co-authored by Ginger Ross Breggin)

Psychosocial Approaches to Deeply Disturbed Patients (1996) (Editor) (E. Mark Stern, co-editor)

The Heart of Being Helpful: Empathy and the Creation of a Healing Presence (1997)

FICTION

The Crazy from the Sane (1971)

After the Good War (1972)

How to Contact

Peter R. Breggin, MD

and

The Center for the Study of Psychiatry and Psychology

Founded in 1971, the Center for the Study of Psychiatry and Psychology is a nonprofit international network of individuals concerned about the impact of mental health practices on individual well-being, human values, and community. It has spearheaded reform in psychiatry. The center sends a newsletter to its general membership and periodically offers information packages to the public and the professions on critical issues in mental health. Its web site provides networking, research, and informational materials.

The board of directors and advisory council of the center are composed of more than 100 professionals in the fields of counseling, psychology, social work, neurology, and psychiatry, as well as members of the U. S. Congress and other leading citizens. Dr. Breggin is National Director of the center, which also has eastern and western divisions in the United States and divisions in Canada and Australia.

For further information concerning the Center for the Study of Psychiatry and Psychology, write to 4628 Chestnut Street, Bethesda, Maryland 20814, or contact the web site at www.breggin.com.

Contents

Introduction
and Acknowledgments

When Springer Publishing Company decided to bring out my first two medical books, *Electroshock: Its Brain-Disabling Effects* (1979) and *Psychiatric Drugs: Hazards to the Brain* (1983a), it required courage. The president of the company, Ursula Springer, and the senior editor at the time, Carole Saltz, had to be concerned about publishing a viewpoint so critical of seemingly established concepts of treatment. I am grateful that they found the books of sufficient merit and importance to take the risk, and that they now seem to feel it was well worth it. The opportunity they gave me has helped to encourage a lifetime of work in the field.

While this new book incorporates some features and content of the 1983 book on psychiatric drugs, it is essentially a new book, combining the subjects of drugs and shock treatment, and deleting and adding many chapters. Those few sections that are based on earlier materials have been completely re-edited and updated. The book begins with an entirely new chapter that identifies, for the first time, the principles of brain-disabling treatment in biopsychiatry.

While the subject of electroshock has been added to the book, one chapter cannot do it justice. The interested reader is urged to delve into *Electroshock: Its Brain-Disabling Effects*. Although written in 1979, it remains relevant today.

Psychiatric Drugs: Hazards to the Brain broke new ground with the first extensive review of the subject of neuroleptic-induced dementia. It also took a firm stand that the neuroleptics frequently cause tardive dyskinesia (TD) in young people. TD in children has become an accepted reality and so that section has been reduced in size. Tardive dementia remains controversial—although it should not be—and a much greater mass of evidence now supports my earlier observations.

The focus of this new book has been tightened around the central theme: The brain-disabling effects of the physical treatments in psychiatry. My views on how to help disturbed and disturbing people are readily available elsewhere (Breggin, 1991a, 1992, 1997; Breggin & Breggin, 1994a; Breggin & Stern, 1996). Similarly, my exploration of the wider socioeconomic context in which drugs and shock are prescribed—the psychopharmaceutical complex—has been dealt with in three other books (Breggin, 1991a; Breggin & Breggin, 1994a, 1994b). My criticism of involuntary treatment appears in the original *Psychiatric Drugs* (1983) and elsewhere.

I have acknowledged so many people for so much in my earlier books, it's time to be more parsimonious. First, I want to thank the President of Springer Publishing Company, Ursula Springer, and senior editor Bill Tucker. I want to thank my wife, Ginger, and our former assistant, Melissa Magruder. Ginger created and Melissa helped to maintain the files that made this book possible. They also provided me the daily help and moral support to deal with these often onerous issues. Melissa helped with the editing of this book and with some of the research as well. Ginger continues to help with everything in my life.

A number of my friends and colleagues read portions of the manuscript or, in a few cases, the entire thing. For their editorial efforts, I want to thank Kevin McCready, Thomas J. Moore, John Friedberg, Fred Baughman, Jr., Robert Grimm, Leonard Frank, and Bertram Karon. I am especially grateful to David Cohen who worked extensively on several stages of the project. Of course, I remain wholly responsible for the content.

CHAPTER 1

The Brain-Disabling Principles of Psychiatric Treatment

The last decade has seen escalating reliance upon psychiatric drugs, not only within psychiatry, but throughout medicine, mental health, and even education. Nearly every patient who is psychiatrically hospitalized is encouraged or forced to take medications. There is a movement within psychiatry to make it easier to force clinic outpatients to take long-acting injections of drugs. In private practice psychiatry, it is common to give patients a medication on the first visit and then to instruct them that they will need drugs for their lifetime. Family practitioners, internists, and other physicians liberally dispense antidepressants and minor tranquilizers. Nonmedical professionals, such as psychologists and social workers, feel obliged to refer their patients for drug evaluations. Managed care aggressively pushes drugs to the exclusion of psychotherapy. Adult medications are increasingly prescribed for children.

Laypersons have joined in the enthusiasm for drugs. Because of media support for medication, as well as direct advertising and promotion to the public, patients frequently arrive at the doctor's office with the name of a psychiatric drug already in mind. Teachers often recommend children for drug evaluation or treatment.

As a part of this overall resurgence in biological psychiatry, electroshock has become increasingly popular. Even psychosurgery once again has its vociferous advocates (reviewed in Breggin & Breggin, 1994b).

This "drug revolution" views psychiatric medications as far more helpful than harmful, even as an unmitigated blessing. Much as insulin or penicillin, they are frequently seen as specific treatments for specific illnesses. Often they are said to correct biochemical imbalances in the brain. These beliefs have created an environment in which emphasis upon adverse drug effects is greeted without enthusiasm and criticism of psychiatric medication in principle is uncommon heresy.

This book takes a decidedly different viewpoint—that psychiatric drugs achieve their primary or essential effect by causing brain dysfunction, and that they tend to do far more harm than good. I will show that psychiatric drugs are not specific treatments for any particular "mental disorder." Instead of correcting biochemical imbalances, psychiatric drugs cause them, sometimes permanently.

The critiques in this book coincide with an alternative view that psychological, social, educational, and spiritual approaches are the most effective in helping individuals to overcome their personal problems and to live more fulfilling lives. I have described some of these approaches elsewhere (e.g., Breggin, 1991a, 1992a, 1997; Breggin & Breggin, 1994a; Breggin & Stern, 1996). Many others have continued to voice strong criticism of the biological model and physical treatments from a variety of perspectives (Armstrong, 1993; Breeding, 1996; Caplan, 1995; Cohen, 1990; Colbert, 1995; Fisher & Greenberg, 1989; Grobe, 1995; Jacobs, 1995; Kirk & Kutchins, 1992; Modrow, 1992; Mosher & Burti, 1989; Romme & Escher, 1993; Sharkey, 1994). Here I want to re-evaluate the underlying assumptions used to justify drug and shock treatment in psychiatry, and to document their brain-disabling and brain-damaging effects.

The principles that are introduced in this chapter will be documented and elaborated throughout the book. Therefore, citations will be omitted in chapter 1.

PRINCIPLES OF BRAIN-DISABLING TREATMENT

Modern psychiatric drug treatment gains its credibility from a number of assumptions that professionals and laypersons alike too often accept as scientifically proven. These underlying assumptions qualify as myths: fictions that support a belief system and a set of practices. In contrast to these myths, this book identifies principles of psychopharmacology that are based on scientific and clinical evidence, as well as on common sense.

Together these form the *brain-disabling principles* of psychiatric treatment. While the book in its entirety provides the evidence for these principles, this chapter will summarize them:

I. All biopsychiatric treatments share a common mode of action—the disruption of normal brain function.

Pharmacologists speak of a drug's *therapeutic index*, the dosage ratio between the beneficial effect and the toxic effect. The first brain-disabling principle of psychiatric treatment reveals that the toxic dose *is* the therapeutic dose—that brain disability causes the seemingly therapeutic effect. This same principle applies to electroshock and psychosurgery.

The brain-disabling principle states that as soon as toxicity is reached the drug begins to have a psychoactive effect, that is, it begins to affect the brain and mind. Without toxicity, the drug would have no psychoactive effect.

II. All biopsychiatric interventions cause generalized brain dysfunction.

Although specific treatments do have recognizably different effects on the brain, they share the capacity to produce generalized dysfunction with some degree of impairment across the spectrum of emotional and intellectual function. Because the brain is so highly integrated, it is not possible to disable circumscribed mental functions without impairing a variety of them. For example, even the production of a slight emotional dullness, lethargy, or fatigue is likely to impair cognitive functions such as attention, concentration, alertness, self-concern or self-awareness, and social sensitivity.

Shock treatment and psychosurgery always produce obvious generalized dysfunction. Some medications may not obviously produce these effects in their minimal dose range, but they may also lack any substantial "therapeutic effect" in that range.

III. Biopsychiatric treatments have their "therapeutic" effect by impairing higher human functions, including emotional responsiveness, social sensitivity, self-awareness or self-insight, autonomy, and self-

determination. More drastic effects include apathy, euphoria,[1] and lobotomy-like indifference.

Higher mental, psychological, and spiritual functioning are impaired by biopsychiatric interventions as a result of generalized brain dysfunction, as well as specific effects on the frontal lobes, limbic system, and other structures. Sometimes there is a lobotomy-like indifference to self and to others—a syndrome that I have called deactivation (see chapters 2 and 4 of this volume).

Biopsychiatric treatments are deemed effective when the physician and/or the patient prefer a state of diminished brain function with its narrowed range of mental capacity or emotional expression. If the drugged individual reports feeling more effective and powerful, it is most likely based on an unrealistic appraisal, impaired judgment, or euphoria. When patients on "maintenance doses" do not experience noticeable effects, either the dose is too low to have a clinical effect or the patient is unable to perceive the drug's impact.

IV. Each biopsychiatric treatment produces its essential or primary brain-disabling effect on all people, including normal volunteers and patients with varied psychiatric diagnoses.

Despite the deeply held convictions of drug proponents, there are no specific psychoactive drug treatments for specific mental disorders.

There is, of course, a certain amount of biological and psychological variation in the way people respond to drugs, shock treatment, or even lobotomy or an accidental head injury. However, as a general principle, biopsychiatric interventions have a nonspecific impact that does not depend on the person's mental state or condition. For example, it will be shown that neuroleptics and lithium affect animals and normal volunteers in much the same way as they affect patients.

V. Patients respond to brain-disabling treatments with their own psychological reactions, such as apathy, euphoria, compliance, or resentment.

---

[1]The term euphoria as used in psychiatry indicates an exaggerated, irrational, or unrealistic sense of well-being. It can be psychological in origin but is commonly caused by brain damage or drug toxicity.

There is some variation in the way individuals respond to drugs. For example, the same antidepressant will make one person sleepy and another energized. Ritalin quiets many children but agitates others.

It can be very difficult to separate out drug-induced from psychologically induced responses. For example, nearly all of the antidepressants can cause euphoria and mania.[2] At the same time, some of the people who receive these drugs have their own tendency to develop these mental states. Similarly, a variety of drugs are capable of generating agitation and hostility in patients, yet people can develop these responses without medication. The docility and compliance seen following the administration of neuroleptics can be caused by the drug-induced deactivation syndrome, but can also result from the patient's realization that further resistance is futile or dangerous.

Later in this chapter, I will introduce the concept of iatrogenic helplessness and denial which addresses the combined neurological and psychological impact of biopsychiatric treatment. In chapter 11, I will discuss some of the criteria for determining that a drug can itself cause abnormal mental and emotional responses, including destructive behavior.

VI. The mental and emotional suffering routinely treated with biopsychiatric interventions have no known genetic and biological cause.

Despite more than two hundred years of intensive research, no commonly diagnosed psychiatric disorders have been proven to be either genetic or biological in origin, including schizophrenia, major depression, manic-depressive disorder, the various anxiety disorders, and childhood disorders, such as attention-deficit hyperactivity.

At present, there are no known biochemical imbalances in the brain of typical psychiatric patients—until they are given psychiatric drugs. It is speculative and even naive to assert that antidepressants such as Prozac correct underactive serotonergic neurotransmission (a serotonin biochemical imbalance), or that neuroleptics such as Haldol correct overactive dopaminergic neurotransmission (a dopamine imbalance). The failure to demonstrate the existence of any brain abnormality in psychiatric patients, despite decades of intensive effort, suggests that these defects do not exist.

---

[2]Euphoria is unusual in patients treated with the neuroleptics because of the suppressive effects on the CNS (see chapter 2). It is more common among patients treated with antidepressants, stimulants, and minor tranquilizers.

It seems theoretically possible that some of the problems treated by psychiatrists could eventually be proven to have a biological basis. For example, mental function often improves when certain physical disorders, such as hypothyroidism or Cushing's Syndrome, are adequately treated.

However, the vast majority of problems routinely treated by psychiatrists do not remotely resemble diseases of the brain (see chapters 5 and 9). For example, they do not produce the cognitive deficits in memory or abstract reasoning characteristic of brain disorders. They are not accompanied by fever or laboratory signs of illness. To the contrary, neurological and neuropsychological testing usually indicate normal if not superior brain function, and the body is healthy. There seems little likelihood that any of the routinely treated psychiatric problems are based on brain malfunction rather than on the life experiences of individuals with normal brains.

If some patients diagnosed with major depression or schizophrenia do turn out to have subtle biochemical imbalances, this would not justify current biopsychiatric practice. Since these presumed imbalances have not yet been identified, it makes no sense to give toxic drugs, including the currently available antidepressants and neuroleptics, all of which grossly impair brain function.

To claim that an irrational or emotionally distressed state in itself amounts to impaired brain function is simply false. An analogy to television may illustrate why this is so. If a TV program is offensive or irrational, it does not indicate that anything is wrong with the hardware or electronics of the television set. It makes no sense to attribute the bad programming to bad wiring. Similarly, a person can be very disturbed psychologically without any corresponding defect in the "wiring" of the brain. However, the argument is moot, since no contemporary biopsychiatric interventions can truthfully claim to correct a brain malfunction the way an electronics expert can fix a television set. Instead, we blindly inflict toxic substances on a brain that is far more subtle and vulnerable to harm than a television set. We even shock or mutilate the brain in ways that would appall TV repair persons or their customers, while ruining their television sets.

It is often suggested that persons suffering from extremes of emotional disorder, such as hallucinations and delusions, or suicidal and murderous impulses, are sufficiently abnormal to require a biological explanation. However, the emotional life of human beings has always included a wide spectrum of mental and behavioral activity. That a particular mental state or action is especially irrational or destructive does not, per se, indicate a physical origin. If extremes require biological explanation, then it would be more compelling to ascribe extremely ethical, rational, and loving behaviors to genetic and biological causes, since they are especially rare in human life.

The fact that a drug "works"—that is, influences the brain and mind in a seemingly positive fashion—does not confirm that the individual suffers from an underlying biological disorder. Throughout recorded history, individuals have medicated themselves for a variety of spiritual and psychological reasons, from the quest for a higher state of consciousness to a desire to make life more bearable. Alcoholic beverages, coffee and tea, tobacco, and marijuana are commonly consumed by people to improve their sense of well-being. Yet there's no reason to believe that the results they obtain are due to an underlying biochemical imbalance.

VII. To the extent that a disorder of the brain or mind already afflicts the individual, currently available biopsychiatric interventions will worsen or add to the disorder.

The currently available biopsychiatric treatments are not specific for any known disorder of the brain. One and all, they disrupt normal brain function without correcting any brain abnormality. Therefore, if a patient is suffering from a known physical disorder of the brain, biopsychiatric treatment can only worsen or add to it. A classic example involves giving Haldol to control emotionally upset Alzheimer patients. While subduing their behavior, the drug worsens their dementia.

After psychiatric drugs are developed and marketed by drug companies, attempts are made to justify their use on the basis of correcting presumed biochemical imbalances. For example, it is claimed that Prozac helps by improving serotonergic neurotransmission. Even electroshock and lobotomy are justified on the grounds that they correct biochemical imbalances. There is no likelihood that these intrusions correct a biochemical imbalance. Too wide a variety of brain-disabling agents are used to treat every disorder—everything from Prozac to Xanax to electroshock is prescribed for depression—and each treatment ends up disrupting innumerable brain functions. In reality, all currently available biopsychiatric interventions cause direct harm to the brain and hence to the mind without correcting any known malfunctions.

VIII. Individual biopsychiatric treatments are not specific for particular mental disorders.

It is often said that psychiatry has specific treatments for specific diagnostic categories of patients: for example, neuroleptics for schizophrenia, antidepressants for depression, minor tranquilizers for anxiety, lithium for mania, and stimulants, such as Ritalin, for attention-deficit hyperactivity. In actual practice, many individual patients are given all of the above categories of drugs at one time or another, and even on occasion all at once. Often the recommended use of a drug changes over the years. While there is a general tendency for patients labeled schizophrenic to be initially treated with neuroleptics or for depressed patients to be initially prescribed antidepressants, this is, in part, a matter of convention within the profession.

When a drug seems more effective in a particular disorder, it often depends on whether it has a suppressive or an energizing effect on the CNS. For example, if depressed patients are already emotionally and physically slowed down, giving them a neuroleptic that causes psychomotor retardation would tend to make them look worse. These patients are more likely to seem improved when artificially energized. Conversely, if schizophrenic patients are agitated and difficult to control, it would not make sense to give them stimulants. They are more likely to be judged ''improved'' when taking a neuroleptic that reduces or flattens their overall emotional responsiveness. These gross behavioral effects, however, are a far cry from having a ''magic bullet'' for a specific disease.

IX. The brain attempts to compensate physically for the disabling effects of biopsychiatric interventions, frequently causing additional adverse reactions and withdrawal problems.

The brain does not welcome psychiatric medications as nutrients. Instead, the brain reacts against them as toxic agents and attempts to overcome their disruptive impact. For example, when Prozac induces an excess of serotonin in the synaptic cleft, the brain compensates by reducing the output of serotonin at the nerve endings and by reducing the number of receptors in the synapse that can receive the serotonin. Similarly, when Haldol reduces reactivity in the dopaminergic system, the brain compensates, producing hyperactivity in the same system by increasing the number and sensitivity of dopamine receptors.

It is difficult if not impossible to accurately determine the underlying psychological condition of a person who is taking psychiatric drugs. There are so many complicating factors, including the drug's brain-disabling effect, the brain's compensatory reactions, and the patient's psychological responses to taking the drug.

Because the brain attempts to compensate for the effects of most psychoactive drugs, patients can have difficulty withdrawing from most psychiatric medications. Physically, the brain cannot recover from the drug effect as quickly as the drug is withdrawn, so that the compensatory mechanisms can require weeks or months to recover after the drug has been withdrawn. Sometimes, as in tardive dyskinesia, the brain fails to recover. Psychologically, individuals fear that their emotional suffering will worsen without the medication. They may have been told by psychiatrists that they require the medication for the rest of their lives. This can make withdrawal even more difficult.

X. Patients subjected to biopsychiatric interventions often display poor judgment about the positive and negative effects of the treatment on their functioning.

Generalized brain dysfunction tends to reduce the individual's ability to perceive the dysfunction. Impaired individuals not only tend to minimize their dysfunction, they often see themselves as performing better than ever. Individuals intoxicated with alcohol, for example, often show poor judgment in estimating their capacity to drive an automobile or to carry on a sensible conversation. Many individuals who chronically smoke marijuana believe that it improves their overall psychological and social functioning, but if they withdraw from the drug, it may become apparent to them that their memory, mental alertness, emotional sensitivity, and social skills have been impaired while using the drug. People intoxicated with stimulants, such as amphetamine, may feel they have superior or even superhuman capacities, when they are often seriously impaired. The same is true of all psychiatric drugs. Often the patient will have little appreciation for the degree of mental or emotional impairment until the drug has been stopped for some time and the brain has had time to recover.

In my experience as a clinician and forensic medical expert, I have seen patients remain for years in severe states of intoxication from one or more psychiatric drugs without realizing it. Attributing their condition to their own emotional reactions or to stresses in the environment, they may ask for more medication.

After shock treatment and psychosurgery, patients may also fail to understand the iatrogenic source of their mental dysfunction and instead believe that they need further interventions.

The failure to perceive the extent of treatment-induced impairment can have several interrelated psychological and physiological bases:

Psychological denial. Individuals overcome by emotional suffering are likely to deny the degree of their psychological dysfunction. They don't want to admit to being severely mentally impaired. If they are hoping to feel better with the use of a drug, their denial can be further reinforced.

Placebo effect. Patients have faith that biopsychiatric interventions will be helpful rather than harmful, encouraging them to disregard drug-induced dysfunction or to mistakenly attribute it to their emotional problems.

Compliance. To an extraordinary extent, patients will tell doctors what the doctors want to hear. If a psychiatrist clearly wants to hear that a drug is helpful, and not harmful, many patients will comply by giving false information or by withholding contradictory evidence.

Psychologically induced confusion. Emotionally upset individuals can easily lose their judgment concerning the cause of their worsening condition. They can easily mistake a negative drug effect, such as rebound anxiety from a minor tranquilizer or depression from a neuroleptic, for a worsening of their emotional problems. Typically, they blame themselves rather than the medication. This confusion is abetted when the physician exaggerates the drug's benefits and fails to inform the patient of its potential adverse effects.

Drug-induced confusion. Almost all biopsychiatric interventions can at times induce confusion, impairing the patient's awareness of the drug-induced mental dysfunction.

Drug-induced anosognosia. Anosognosia refers to the capacity of brain damage to cause denial of lost function. Anosognosia is a hallmark of central nervous system (CNS) disability (see below and chapter 5). It has a physical basis in addition to a psychological one.

XI. Physicians who prescribe biopsychiatric interventions often have an unrealistic appraisal of their risks and benefits.

In recent years, doubt has been thrown on the objectivity of controlled clinical trials in which drugs are compared to placebo or to alternative medications (see chapters 6 and 11). Too often the investigators are influenced by their conscious or unconscious biases.

If clinical and scientific studies can be distorted by bias, it is even more likely that routine clinical practice will be affected by the hopes and expectations of the prescribing physician. Physicians in great numbers have prescribed drugs with unbounded enthusiasm for years before the agents have proven to be worthless or unacceptably dangerous. Amphetamines, for example, were freely dispensed for many years to millions of patients for both depression and weight control without regard for their lack of efficacy and addictive potential. Similarly, minor tranquilizers, such as Valium, were given to millions of patients before the profession recognized that they have little or no long-term benefit and can become addictive. Both psychosurgery and electroshock continue to be utilized, despite obviously devastating effects on the mental life of the patients and the absence of proven efficacy.

IATROGENIC HELPLESSNESS AND DENIAL (IHAD)

I have coined the term *iatrogenic helplessness and denial* (IHAD) to designate the guiding principle of biopsychiatric interventions (Breggin, 1983b). It describes how the biological psychiatrist uses authoritarian techniques, enforced by brain-disabling interventions, to produce increased helplessness and dependency on the part of the patient.

Iatrogenic helplessness and denial include the patient's and the doctor's mutual denial of the damaging impact of the treatment, as well as their mutual denial of the patient's underlying psychological and situational problems. Overall, iatrogenic helplessness and denial account for the frequency with which psychiatry has been able to utilize brain-damaging technologies, such as electroshock and psychosurgery, as well as toxic medications.

Before the potential patient encounters a psychiatrist, he or she has usually been feeling helpless for some time. In my formulation, helplessness is the common denominator of all psychological failure. Helplessness is at the core of most self-defeating approaches to life (Breggin, 1992a, 1997). People who feel helpless tend to give up using reason, love, and self-determination to overcome their emotional suffering, inner conflicts, and real-life stresses. They instead seek answers from outside themselves. In modern times, this often means from "experts."

Iatrogenic helplessness and denial go far beyond relatively benign *suggestion* (as used in medicine and psychiatry, for example, to help overcome physical pain or addiction). First, in iatrogenic helplessness and denial the psychiatrist compromises the brain of the patient, enforcing the patient's submission to suggestion through mental and physical dysfunction. Second, in iatrogenic helplessness and denial the psychiatrist denies to himself or herself the damaging effects of the treatment as well as the patient's continuing psychological or situational problems.

Often denial is accompanied by *confabulation*—the patient's use of rationalizations and various "cover stories" to hide the extent of mental dysfunction. Confabulation is well understood in psychiatry and neurology, but is generally ignored in regard to treatment-induced effects. Many patients confabulate good results from drug therapy when they are obviously impaired by it.

Denial is closely linked to indifference. Sometimes it is difficult to tell if the patient doesn't care, or if the patient cares so much that he cannot bear to face up to his mental and physical dysfunction. Denial is also related to euphoria. After lobotomy or shock treatment, and sometimes during drug treatment, the patient can develop an unrealistic "high."[3]

Denial is one of the most primitive ways of responding to threats. The person avoids facing problems and thereby becomes unable to make headway with them. Denial as a basic defense tends to result in ineffective, impotent lives.

Brain damage and dysfunction from any cause, including accidents and illness, frequently produces helplessness and denial; but only in psychiatry is damage and dysfunction used as "treatment" to produce these disabling effects.

CONCLUSION

As I have discussed in earlier books (1991a, 1994a, 1994b), I believe that the concepts of "mental illness" and "mental disorder" are misleading, and that none of the problems commonly treated by psychiatrists are genetic or biological in origin. The terms "schizophrenia" and "major depression," for example, are based on concepts whose validity can easily be challenged. However, the brain-disabling principles remain valid even if some of the mental phenomena that are being treated turn out to have

---

[3]See footnote 2, page 5.

a genetic or biological basis. All of the currently available biopsychiatric treatments—drugs, electroshock, and psychosurgery—have their primary or therapeutic effect by impairing or disabling normal brain function.

CHAPTER 2

Deactivation Syndrome (Chemical Lobotomy) Caused by Neuroleptics

One of the great myths within psychiatry is the specificity of neuroleptics such as Thorazine, Mellaril, Haldol, Navane, and Prolixin for the treatment of schizophrenia. Despite a lack of confirmatory studies (reviewed in Breggin, 1983a, 1991a), many clinicians and researchers postulate a specific antipsychotic and even antischizophrenic effect for these drugs. The concept is used to justify neuroleptic treatment as a legitimate medical approach. Instead, the neuroleptics produce what can be called a deactivation syndrome or effect, a central aspect of the lobotomy syndrome.

THE DEACTIVATION SYNDROME

In order to help organize the clinical material that follows, it may be helpful to begin with a closer look at the concept of deactivation (Breggin, 1993):

> The term deactivation will be used to designate a continuum of phenomena variously described as disinterest, indifference, diminished concern, blunting, lack of spontaneity, reduced emotional reactivity, reduced motivation or will, apathy, and, in the extreme, a rousable stupor.

The deactivation effect is the essence of what is euphemistically called the antipsychotic effect. Consistent with the brain-disabling principles of psychiatric treatment, this lobotomy-like impact is the sought-after, primary, and supposedly therapeutic effect. Any specific antipsychotic effect is very speculative compared to the obvious and almost unvarying deactivation effect.

We will find that nearly all psychiatric drugs can produce this effect to some degree. Even stimulants, such as Ritalin, can cause sufficient apathy or indifference in a child to enable adults to more easily control or direct the child (see chapter 9). However, deactivation appears in its purest form in neuroleptic treatment.

Deactivation is closely related to the frontal lobe syndrome; it focuses on the affective or emotional component. Adams and Victor (1989) divide the manifestations of frontal lobe syndrome into (a) cognitive and intellectual changes, such as loss of abstract reasoning and planning, (b) personality deterioration, and (c) "impairment or lack of initiative and spontaneity" (p. 333). The impairment of initiative and spontaneity is deactivation, which Adams and Victor call the most common effect of frontal lobe disease.

Similarly, Stuss and Benson (1987) ascribe two basic functions to the anterior portion of the frontal lobes: "sequence, set, and integration," and "drive, motivation, and will" (p. 241). The "most common alteration is apathy" (p. 242).

Much of what we know about the frontal lobe syndrome comes from studying the effects of psychosurgery, whose primary clinical effect is the production of deactivation or what Kalinowsky (1973, p. 20) called "diminished concern." My clinical experience and reviews of the literature (Breggin, 1975, 1980, 1981b), as well as neuropsychological research (Hansen, Andersen, Theilgaard, & Lunn, 1982), indicate that the newer stereotactic procedures, such as cingulotomy, amydalotomy, and thalamotomy, continue to produce a frontal lobe syndrome, especially deactivation. Hansen et al. (1982) describe the impact of modern psychosurgery in a way that is indistinguishable from neuroleptic effects:

> The patient's options for action are reduced by a weakening of initiative and ability to structure his situation; emotionality fades, is organized more shallowly and is more dependent upon the immediate situation. Contact with other people becomes more flattened and the immediate bearing more mechanical. (p. 115)

As we shall see, pioneers in the use of neuroleptics almost uniformly cited deactivation as the main clinical effect of neuroleptics. Because of this, clinicians often referred to the neuroleptics as a chemical lobotomy (Haase, 1959, p. 206). Bleuler (1978) observed that long-term neuroleptic use "also often dampens the vitality and the initiative of the person" (p. 301). He concluded: "So we see that long-term maintenance with neuroleptics is fraught with some of the same disadvantages that are ascribed to lobotomies" (p. 301). Chapter 5 will discuss permanent cognitive impairment and dementia from these drugs.

The Anatomy of Deactivation

Deactivation can result from dysfunction in either the frontal lobes and limbic system (as an aspect of frontal lobe syndrome) or the basal ganglia (as an aspect of subcortical dementia). The neuroleptics impair the dopaminergic pathways to all of these regions. The neuroleptics can also produce deactivation through suppression of the reticular activating system which has rich interconnections with the basal ganglia (see chapter 5 for more details).

The neuroleptic deactivation effect so closely resembles psychosurgery in its clinical impact because it disrupts the same regions of the brain. Classical lobotomy, for example, cuts the descending fibers from the frontal lobes to deeper brain structures, while the neuroleptics tend to impair the ascending dopaminergic fibers.

THE CLASS OF PHARMACOLOGIC SUBSTANCES

More than a dozen drugs, almost all of them in use for many years, can be classed as neuroleptics. The phenothiazine derivatives were originally the most commonly used class of neuroleptic drugs. Chlorpromazine is the prototype, developed in France and introduced into North America in 1953 by Heinz Lehmann. Its brand name in Canada and England is Largactil, and in the United States, Thorazine.

Other neuroleptics include haloperidol (Haldol), thiothixene (Navane), chlorprothixene (Taractan), perphenazine (Trilafon), pimozide (Orap), droperidol (Inapsine), thioridazine (Mellaril), molindone (Moban), trifluoperazine (Stelazine), mesoridazine (Serentil), fluphenazine (Prolixin, Permitil), triflupromazine (Vesprin), piperacetazine (Quide), and loxapine (Loxitane). Triavil or Etrafon is a neuroleptic (Trilafon) combined with an antidepressant (Elavil). Reserpine (Serpasil) is a neuroleptic that is more often used to suppress the symptoms of tardive dyskinesia (chapter 4). Prochlorperazine (Compazine) is used as an antiemetic and rarely as a neuroleptic. The antidepressant amoxapine (Asendin) is metabolized into a neuroleptic and has similar effects and, more importantly, adverse effects, such as tardive dyskinesia.

More recently, clozapine (Clozaril), risperidone (Risperdal), and olanzapine (Zyprexa) have been approved in the United States and other "novel" antipsychotics are on their way through the Food and Drug Administration (FDA) approval process, including remoxipride and raclopride.

Different neuroleptics require different doses for similar effects and may exaggerate one or another toxic effect. They also vary in the length of time they remain active in the body. With some exceptions, most of these drugs can be described as a single group sharing the same characteristics and side effects. There is no evidence that any of these drugs has a substantially different impact on mental functioning, other than the tendency for some to produce more sedation. Two of the drugs, Haldol and Prolixin, also come in long-acting injectable preparations.

Two newer atypical neuroleptics, including Risperdal and Clozaril, have a somewhat different profile of effects; but they share the lobotomizing impact, sometimes to a more intense degree than other neuroleptics.

Various neuroleptics are also used for nonpsychiatric purposes, usually in smaller doses over shorter durations. However, severe effects can sometimes develop from these limited uses. Nonpsychiatric preparations include some antihistamines, such as methdilazine (Tacaryl) and trimeprazine (Temaril); some antinausea drugs, such as thiethylperazine (Torecan); and adjuncts to anesthesia, such as propiomazine (Largon) and promethazine (Phenergan), which is also used as an antinausea, antimotion sickness agent. Metoclopramide (Reglan) is used in gastroesophageal reflux, diabetic gastric stasis, and as an anti-emetic. It is well established that Reglan can cause irreversible neurological effects identical to the routinely used neuroleptics. Some researchers estimate the prevalence to be 100 times more than the 0.2% reported in the *Physicians' Desk Reference* ("Metoclopramide-induced," 1992).

THE LOBOTOMY-LIKE EFFECT
IN HISTORICAL PERSPECTIVE

The very first report on the psychiatric use of chlorpromazine was published in 1952 in France by Delay and Deniker (1952; also see Jarvik, 1970). Their article described the actual state of the patient for a medical world which as yet had no familiarity with the drug:

> Sitting or lying, the patient is motionless in his bed, often pale and with eyelids lowered. He remains silent most of the time. If he is questioned, he answers slowly and deliberately in a monotonous, indifferent voice; he expresses himself in a few words and becomes silent. (cited in Jarvik, 1970)

They also described the patient as "fairly appropriate and adaptable. . . . But he rarely initiates a question and he does not express his anxieties, desires or preferences."

Notice the nonspecific nature of these effects. Not only symptoms such as anxiety, but also desires and preferences are aborted or buried beneath indifference or apathy. As Delay and Deniker put it, there is an "apparent indifference or the slowing of responses to external stimuli" and "the diminution of initiative and anxiety."

Heinz Lehmann introduced chlorpromazine into North America via Montreal in May, 1953. Lehmann and Hanrahan (1954) published the first article in English promoting its psychiatric use. They stated:

> The aim is to produce a state of motor retardation, emotional indifference, and somnolence, and the dose must be increased accordingly as tolerance develops.

The doses required to achieve "retardation," "emotional indifference," and "lethargy" rarely exceeded 800 mg/day, and sometimes did not exceed 100 mg/day. Much larger doses—sometimes thousands of milligrams—are used in contemporary treatment by psychiatrists.

Writing with that burst of honesty so characteristic of pioneers, Lehmann and Hanrahan go on to say:

> The patients under treatment display a lack of spontaneous interest in the environment . . . they tend to remain silent and immobile when left alone and to reply to questions in a slow monotone. . . . Some patients dislike

the treatment and complain of their drowsiness and weakness. Some state they feel "washed out," as after an exhausting illness, a complaint which is indeed in keeping with their appearance.

Lehmann and Hanrahan recognized that they were suppressing their patients without specifically affecting symptoms such as hallucinations and delusions: "We have not observed a direct influence of the drug on delusional symptoms or hallucinatory phenomena."

The following year Lehmann (1955) published his second article on chlorpromazine. With relatively small doses, he found the primary disabling effect: "Many patients dislike the 'empty feeling' resulting from the reduction of drive and spontaneity which is apparently one of the most characteristic effects of this substance." He also speaks of "lassitude" and compares the effects to lobotomy: "In the management of pain in terminal cancer cases, chlorpromazine may prove to be a pharmacological substitute for lobotomy."

The first British report concerning chlorpromazine as a psychiatric treatment (Anton-Stephens, 1954) confirms the impact of the drug using small doses (200 mg/day). Anton-Stephens calls it "psychic indifference" and compares it to lobotomy.

Throughout the 1950s some psychiatric texts continued to accurately describe the impact of the neuroleptics on the mind. Here, for example, is the lobotomy-like clinical picture of *maximum benefit* described by Noyes and Kolb in the 1958 edition of *Modern Clinical Psychiatry*:

> If the patient responds well to the drug, he develops an attitude of *indifference* both to his surroundings and to his symptoms. He shows *decreased interest* in and response to his hallucinatory experiences and a *less assertive* expression of his delusional ideas. [italics added] (p. 654)

In recent times, it has been unfashionable in psychiatry to recognize the primary lobotomizing effects of the neuroleptics, but occasionally recognition can be found in the literature. In a 1991 editorial in *Biological Psychiatry*, entitled "Neuroleptic Dysphoria," Emerich and Sanberg describe various adverse emotional reactions to Haldol and other neuroleptics, including "cognitive blunting." The editorial describes the self-administration of Haldol by Belmaker and Wald (1977) in which each of these "normal experimental subjects" "complained of a paralysis of volition, lack of physical and psychic energy. The subjects felt unable to

read, telephone or perform household tasks of their will, but could perform
these tasks if demanded to do so.'' The editorial also mentions reports
of other mind-subduing effects, including ''chemical straightjacketing,''
''lack of motivation,'' and a feeling ''like a shade coming down.'' The
editorial fails to make the obvious comparison to lobotomy.

In clinical discussions, the lobotomy effect is now sometimes subsumed
under ''neuroleptic-induced deficit syndrome'' (NIDS). Malcolm Lader
(1993), chairperson of an international symposium on the subject, wrote:

> The benefits of treatment with classical neuroleptics are, however, obtained
> at the expense of a number of side effects, and many patients frequently
> complain of feeling ''drugged'' or drowsy and of being unable to concen-
> trate; they lack motivation and are emotionally unresponsive: they also
> appear slow-moving and physically rigid. Some patients have complained
> of ''feeling like a zombie.'' (p. 493)

At the symposium (Lader, 1993), Wolfgang Straus described a related
neuroleptic-induced ''dyscognitive syndrome'' characterized by ''aphasia,
thought disturbances, emotional withdrawal, difficulties in directing
thought by will, ambivalence, thought deprivation, and reduced creativity''
(p. 495–496). Noting that early studies tried to demonstrate improved
cognitive functioning on neuroleptics, Straus observed that more rigorous
recent studies confirmed a detrimental effect.

ATYPICAL NEUROLEPTICS

More recently marketed atypical neuroleptics, such as clozapine (Clozaril)
and risperidone (Risperdal), affect not only the dopaminergic neurotransmitter system but others as well. Regardless of the mechanism, all produce
lobotomy-like indifference or deactivation. This is the primary effect of all
drugs thus far developed for the control of patients labeled schizophrenic or
acutely manic. If the medications failed to produce a deactivation effect,
they would probably not be found useful for the control of very difficult
or disturbed individuals. We shall find that these drugs produce all of the
more severe CNS impairments caused by other neuroleptics. They also
have their own particular hazards. A general summary of the adverse
effects of the atypical neuroleptics will be provided in chapter 5.

SOCIAL CONTROL WITH NEUROLEPTICS

Suppression of Nursing Home Inmates

Neuroleptics are routinely used in every institution in which social control and behavioral suppression are a top priority, and in which drugs can replace human services (see Breggin, 1983a, for details). For decades, the suppression of elderly nursing home inmates with neuroleptics has been a national scandal (Hughes & Brewin, 1979; Rogers, 1971). A study of nursing home residents in Tennessee found that 44% were being given the drugs (studies summarized in Bishop, 1989). A 1989 Massachusetts study (Avorn, Dreyer, Connelly, & Soumerai, 1989) found that 39% of patients were receiving neuroleptics. According to the report, ''In most cases, the prescriptions had been written in the remote past and were refilled automatically.''

When public scandal did not substantially improve nursing homes over the years (Kolata, 1991), Congress passed regulations limiting the use of restraints and medications in nursing homes. These statutes went into effect in 1991, too often with spotty enforcement and therefore incomplete success (Spiegel, 1991). However, when actually applied, the new regulations have reduced the use of neuroleptics in nursing home settings (Semla, Palla, Poddig, & Brauner, 1994).

There has been a growing awareness of the inappropriateness and harmfulness of prescribing neuroleptics to elderly patients (''Antipsychotic drug therapy poses hazards for elderly patients,'' 1988; Gomez & Gomez, 1990; Sherman, 1987). The use of neuroleptics for the behavioral control of the elderly produces toxicity even more readily than in younger patients and it cannot substitute for needed human services. Sherman (1987) calls into question the pharmaceutical company practice of placing advertisements for neuroleptics like Haldol and Navane in journals with a geriatric-practice orientation.

Deactivating People and Animals in Varied Settings

In *Psychiatric Drugs: Hazards to the Brain* I devoted considerable time to confirming the brain-disabling principle of neuroleptic treatment by pointing to its effects on a variety of diverse populations. I also discussed other confirmatory sources in the literature. The material in this section that draws on older citations is presented at greater length in my earlier book.

The deactivation syndrome produced by neuroleptics is confirmed by their use in state mental hospitals for the control of patients regardless of their diagnoses and in psychoprisons in the former U.S.S.R. for the control of political dissidents (Block & Reddaway, 1977; "Excerpts from statement," 1976; Fireside, 1979; " 'Madhouse' Brainwashing," 1976; Podrabinek, 1979). They have been used in prisons for the suppression of difficult inmates (Booth, 1993; Breggin & Breggin, 1974; Coleman, 1974; Greenhouse, 1979; Kaufman, 1980; McDonald, 1979; Mitford, 1973; Morgan, 1974; Oregon State Prisoner, 1971; "Prison Drug Bill," 1977). Convicted prisoners have recently reported that the brain-numbing effects rendered them unable to make a proper defense in court (Espinosa, 1993; Ogilvie, 1992; Pund, 1993).

Neuroleptics are commonly used in institutions for the developmentally disabled for the control of children and adults (Clements, 1975; Kuehnel & Slama, 1984; Plotkin & Rigling, 1979). Kuehnel and Slama warn that the neuroleptics can further compromise the learning abilities of the developmentally disabled and cause "the sedative 'snowed' effect, which can reduce a client's positive response to learning cues" (p. 94).

Many critical books have decried the use of neuroleptics and other drugs in the suppression of children in hospitals and other settings (Armstrong, 1993; Hughes & Brewin, 1979; Sharkey, 1994; Shrag & Divoky, 1974; Wooden, 1976). The control of children with neuroleptics will also be discussed in chapter 9 of this book.

The use of neuroleptics in veterinary medicine to control wild and domestic animals provides another illustration of the deactivation effect and its independence from any presumed mental illness in the individual being treated (Booth, 1977; Hall, 1971; Rossoff, 1974). Hartlage (1965) found that Thorazine dampened the emotional responses of animals, "thereby perhaps providing some clue to the widespread acceptance of the drug as effective in psychiatric settings" (also see Kostowski, 1978; Mirsky, 1970; Slikker, Brocco, & Killam, 1976). Jarvik (1970) pointed out that the neuroleptics produce diminished spontaneous activity and emotional indifference in all animal species, including man; but he nonetheless argued for a specific antipsychotic effect.

Not surprisingly, a variety of studies on human beings, including normals, have also shown impairment of mental functioning, including memory and learning (DiMascio & Shader, 1970; Fischman & Smith, 1976; Gillis, 1975; Seppala, Saario, & Mattila, 1976; Tecce, Cole, & Savignana-Bowman, 1975).

Many former psychiatric patients and inmates have described the brain- and mind-numbing effects of the neuroleptics (Burstow & Weitz, 1988; Chamberlin, 1978; Frank, 1980; Grobe, 1995; Hudson, 1980; Millett, 1990; Modrow, 1992).

I am not the first to suggest that neuroleptic medications are highly toxic. In fact, it was considered common knowledge in the first decades of their use (Hunter, Earl, & Thornicroft, 1964; Hunter, Blackwood, Smith, & Cumings, 1968). In support of the use of lithium, a number of investigators have criticized the neuroleptics for their stupefying effects. Fieve (cited in Shah, 1973), for example, said that neuroleptics "zonk a person out" and put them in a "mental straight jacket." Fieve (1989) also refers to the "zombielike appearance" (p. 4) produced by neuroleptics. A National Institute of Mental Health (1970) brochure compared the drugs unfavorably to lithium because of their effect of "wrapping the patient's entire mind in a cocoon of stupefaction." In the same vein, as an advocate of lithium, Schou observed that the neuroleptics cause a "suppression" of symptoms and "bring the patients into what is in most cases clearly a drug-produced state of quietude," while the underlying problem persists. Similarly, Prien, Caffey, and Klett (1972) found that "most patients receiving chlorpromazine were sluggish or fatigued." Wittrig and Coopwood (1970) confirmed the lobotomy-like effect of impaired "initiative and planning" which they called "the chemical straightjacket" (p. 488). Robitscher (1980) noted that patients frequently feel "dead or 'like a zombie' " (p. 90).

In recent times, psychiatrists have become much more reluctant to publish criticism of any treatments or to mention their brain-disabling effects.

THE UNIQUE FUNCTION OF THE BRAIN

Some proponents of brain disability as therapy assume that a little toxicity is helpful and that only excessive toxicity is harmful. They bring up precedents in medicine for drugs that reduce function of one organ or another in order to improve its effectiveness. Thus some cardiac medications actually weaken heart muscle function in the interest of preventing arrhythmias. But the analogy falls short when dealing with the brain. When the strength of the heart muscle is reduced, nothing substantial is done to the mind or personality of the person—unless of course the patient goes into heart failure. But when brain function is reduced, the individual's capacities as a sentient being are directly and proportionally reduced. He or she becomes less able to think, to feel, to choose, and to initiate activities.

Beyond this, one must also look at the purposes of medical and psychiatric interventions. The medical intervention that disrupts one kind of heart function is intended to improve overall heart function. The psychiatric intervention that disables the brain is aimed at controlling certain thoughts, emotions, or behaviors at the cost of reducing overall mental function. In doing so, it renders the individual less self-aware and less self-determining, more helpless, and more manageable. The individual may appear to be less emotionally disturbed when he or she is in reality less emotionally aware or vital.

In summary, the neuroleptics have been shown to produce a lobotomy-like deactivation syndrome characterized by indifference or apathy, reduced spontaneity, and docility. This is clinically obvious in the great majority of patients, and is confirmed in studies of animals, normal human beings, political dissenters, and rebellious children, as well as in studies of the inmates of mental hospitals, institutions for the developmentally disabled, nursing homes, and prisons. These observations contradict the notion that the neuroleptics have their clinical impact through a specific antischizophrenic or antipsychotic effect. The overriding clinical effect of these drugs is to render any and all individuals (and animals) more emotionally flat and indifferent, more apathetic and docile, less autonomous and self-directed, and hence more manageable.

CHAPTER 3

Neuroleptic-Induced Anguish, Including Agitation, Despair, and Depression

Despite the lobotomy-like indifference to suffering produced by neuroleptic-induced deactivation described in chapter 2, many patients experience varying degrees of physical and mental pain and torment in response to these drugs. The deactivation itself is often experienced as dreadful, a kind of living death or an imprisonment within one's own brain.

This chapter will describe the most common, reversible, drug-induced neurological reactions: acute dystonia, acute akathisia, parkinsonism, and a broad, ill-defined category called dysphoria. All of them tend to begin early in treatment, but can start later on as well. Chapters 4 and 5 will review the sometimes delayed and often irreversible adverse reactions, including irreversible forms of akathisia and dystonia.

Most of the neurological disorders associated with the neuroleptics fall into the category of extrapyramidal reactions. The extrapyramidal system of the brain is an extensive, complex network that moderates and adjusts motor control. Abnormalities in the system cause a variety of dysfunctions, including tremors, muscular rigidity and spasms, and various involuntary movements.

Casey (1993) reported that acute extrapyramidal syndromes occur in up to 90% of patients receiving neuroleptics, often causing physical and mental impairment. Unfortunately, physicians too often continue or increase the patient's medication, despite the discomfort and suffering, because they have mistaken the toxic drug reaction for a psychiatric disorder. A young male patient, for several months after termination of neuroleptic treatment, suffered from a dystonia that caused one arm to rise above his shoulders. In family sessions, his parents persisted in viewing the disorder as a willful and defiant act. These acute symptoms may linger a considerable time after drug termination, even in regard to newer neuroleptics thought to produce them less frequently or intensively (Kane et al., 1994). Sometimes they become permanent.

It has been known for some time that the neurotoxic effects described in this and the following chapters become even more frequent and disabling in the elderly (Gomez & Gomez, 1990; Simpson, 1977; see chapter 4).

NEUROLEPTIC-INDUCED ANGUISH
AS A CAUSE OF RESISTANCE TO TREATMENT

Van Putten (1974) evaluated the attitudes of 85 patients toward a variety of neuroleptics. "Dysphoric responders" were defined as individuals who "habitually complained about the drug effect" and who felt "miserable" and "continually pleaded to have the drug stopped or the dosage reduced." A remarkable 38% of the patients fell into this extreme category of drug resistance. When the criteria for drug resistance were broadened to include anyone who had "to be pressured" into taking medication, 46% were found to display "drug reluctance."

The study most likely underestimates the actual percentage of drug reluctance among the total population of patients on the ward. Some, and perhaps many, patients almost surely disguised their reluctance to avoid angering the staff, while quietly throwing away their pills.

How easy it is to feign taking medication in typical psychiatric hospitals is indicated by Rosenhan's (1973) study in which normal individuals had themselves admitted to various mental hospitals by faking symptoms. "All told, the pseudopatients were administered nearly 2,100 pills, including Elavil, Stelazine, Compazine, and Thorazine, to name but a few. . . . Only two were swallowed. The rest were either pocketed or deposited in the toilet." This is a remarkable figure indeed: Less than 1 out of 1,000 doses were taken, and none of the hospital staff were aware of it. The Rosenhan study also disclosed that regular patients were routinely disposing of their medications in the same manner. Rosenhan believes that the failure of the staff to detect what was happening reflects their tendency to ignore everything done by the patients unless it causes obvious trouble.

ACUTE DYSTONIC REACTIONS

Very little has been written about the suffering associated with acute dystonia, a drug-induced neurological disorder that causes painful muscle spasms, most commonly but not exclusively in the head and neck, and sometimes bending the entire back in a rigid arc. Similarly, insufficient attention has been paid to the anguish of undergoing an oculogyric crisis, in which the eyes roll up in their sockets and become locked in place.

The spasms can affect any voluntary muscles, including those involved with speech, swallowing, and breathing, as well as gait. Simpson (1977) observes, "The masseter muscles may be tightly contracted so that the mouth cannot be opened and, on rare occasions, this can lead to damage to the teeth, tongue, or even the mandible. The possibility that such reactions can be fatal does exist, particularly if they occur during eating."

Patients who have suffered these experiences may remember them with pain, fear, and resentment for the rest of their lives. Needless to say, if their doctors originally blamed the reactions on the patient's psychiatric problems, the patient can feel enormously betrayed. Often the attacks can be aborted with proper medical intervention, but they can go on endlessly if untreated or if they develop into tardive dystonia (chapter 4).

Silver, Yudofsky, and Hurowitz (1994) underscore the devastating impact of these disorders:

> The most common feature of this syndrome includes uncontrollable tightening of the face and neck, and spasm and distortions of the patient's head and/or back (i.e., opisthotonos). If the extraocular muscles are involved, an oculogyric crisis may occur, wherein the eyes are elevated and "locked" in this position. Laryngeal involvement [spasm] may lead to respiratory and ventilatory difficulties. These reactions are often terrifying to the patient who has no prior experience with these problems or knowledge of this side effect. When a patient with psychosis experiences a dystonic reaction, the fragile trust developed between psychiatrist and patient may be irrevocably damaged. (pp. 909–910)

Too often these reactions are mistakenly attributed to the diagnosis of mental illness. Simpson (1977) observed, "Acute dystonic reactions are of sudden onset and consist of bizarre muscular spasms that have been misdiagnosed as tetany or hysteria (particularly because emotional reactions can contribute to their precipitation and because patients can occasionally be talked out of them)."

The ability of psychiatrists to diagnose dystonia has not improved in recent times. In a survey of 1,114 dystonia patients, only 1% of the 279 who saw a psychiatrist were correctly diagnosed ("Survey shows most psychiatrists . . . ," 1992). Neurologists did considerably better, correctly diagnosing 44% of the cases who came to them.

DESPAIR IN ASSOCIATION
WITH NEUROLEPTIC-INDUCED PARKINSONISM

Parkinson's disease tends to develop spontaneously in the middle and later years of life. Its symptoms include a masklike or rigid face; a tremor of the extremities at rest; intermittent rigidity or spasms of the limbs, and a cog-wheeling, ratcheting of the arms when passively moved; a shuffling, stooped gait; and overall retardation of muscular or motor activities. In its initial or more subtle forms the disease may be manifested by a slowness of motions, or motor retardation, called *bradykinesia*. In its extreme form, *akinesia*, it is grossly crippling. Mental depression, lobotomy-like disinterest, and some degree of dementia frequently accompany it.

The neuroleptics commonly produce a reversible parkinsonism syndrome. They can also cause separate aspects of the syndrome, such as bradykinesia.

Van Putten (1974) describes the following reaction:

> After seven days she complained of unbearable "fatigue" . . . "I have slowed down. I talk slower and move slower (objectively this was apparent only after she called our attention to it). I feel like an old lady. I get tired from walking around the block. I feel discouraged about the future. I have no enthusiasm. I can't type nearly as fast at my job (clerk typist) . . . I want my own personality back." [ellipses in original]

Drug-induced parkinsonism is sometimes confused with schizophrenic apathy. Davis and Cole (1975) warned that psychiatrists should " . . . be aware that patients who appear apathetic, lacking in spontaneity, relatively unable to participate in social activities, lifeless, zombielike, or drowsy may have subtle extrapyramidal side effects.'' As Lavin and Rifkin (1992) confirm, clinicians can mistakenly attribute these symptoms to the patient's mental disorder and either increase the dose of neuroleptic or add an antidepressant or stimulant to the regimen, worsening the patient's condition.

Typically, the parkinsonism remains for the duration of the drug therapy, and takes days, weeks, or even months to clear after discontinuation of the drug. Klawans (in Goetz, Dysken, & Klawans, 1980) attributes the delayed clearing to the persistence of the drug in the patient's body.

Van Putten and May (1978) found bradykinesia and akinesia, an aspect of parkinsonism, in 47% of their patients treated with relatively moderate doses of the drugs. Including relatively mild cases, Korcyzn and Goldberg (1976) found parkinsonism in 61% of 66 patients receiving a variety of neuroleptics. Klawans (Goetz et al., 1980) notes that rates of affliction vary in the literature from 5% to 60% of all patients treated, and offers his own figure of 10% to 15% for "clear parkinsonian features." Klawans also notes that some drugs produce parkinsonism more readily than others, and that one of the most frequently used, haloperidol (Haldol), may produce parkinsonism in more than 90% of patients when sensitive detection methods are used.

I have talked with neurologists who find that neuroleptic-induced parkinsonism does sometimes become permanent. This is consistent with the lessons of lethargic encephalitis in which patients developed irreversible parkinsonism from damage to the same regions of the brain that are damaged by the neuroleptics (see chapters 4 and 5). While some concern about permanent drug-induced parkinsonism was voiced in the first few decades of neuroleptic use (Crane, 1977; Hall, Jackson, & Swain, 1956; Hornykiewicz, 1967; Klawans in Goetz, Dysken, & Klawans, 1980; Korczyn & Goldberg, 1976; Merritt, 1979; Simpson, 1977), little has been expressed in recent times.

Parkinsonism As an Aspect of Brain-Disabling Therapy

Many psychiatrists have connected the parkinsonism syndrome to the therapeutic effect of neuroleptics (described in Davis & Cole, 1975; Paulson, 1959). Cole (1960) said in some cases, the use of drug-induced parkinsonism to control the patient was the equivalent of using toxicity as therapy. Cole goes so far as to use the phrase "pharmacologic strait jacket" to describe the drug effect.

ANGUISH AND PSYCHOSIS
IN ASSOCIATION WITH AKATHISIA

Akathisia is a drug-induced reaction characterized by compelling feelings of restlessness, tension, or anxiety that drive a person to move his or her body (Jeste, Wisniewski, & Wyatt, 1986; Weiner & Luby, 1983). People with akathisia find it difficult to sit or to keep their feet still. Some will walk in place, pace frantically, or search out activities that keep them on the move. I have evaluated patients with permanent akathisia (tardive akathisia, see chapter 4) who, for their entire lives, are trapped in perpetual suffering.

In more subtle cases of akathisia there's no obvious external movement, but the patient experiences an inner irritation that can feel like being tortured from inside out. Doctors, however, are sometimes too reluctant to acknowledge the disorder as akathisia if the patient isn't frantically moving about. A report on "Using Antipsychotics" (1989) summarized the clinical observations of several experts and concluded:

> While it is commonly believed that akathisia is characterized by obvious signs of motor restlessness, it should be noted that behavioral symptoms may be limited to expressions of anxiety, impatience, and hostility. Too often, this manifestation is misdiagnosed as recurrence of psychotic symptomatology. (p. 2)

Van Putten, Mutalipassi, and Malkin (1974) found that 35% of their patients decompensated after one injection of intramuscular fluphenazine, usually as a result of akathisia. Often even the patient wanted to blame the problem on his mental condition:

> The drug-induced regressions resemble the original psychoses so precisely, that at the beginning of the study the treatment team (including the ward director) always explained the decompensation in plausible dynamic terms. Often, the patient himself agreed with the dynamic formulation . . . . Thought processes again became fragmented, and several complained of abject terror, the likes of which they had never experienced. . . . State-

ments such as "It's a horrible feeling," "I can't describe it" or "If this feeling continues, I'd rather be dead" were not unusual.

These anguished responses were rapid in onset. Van Putten, May, and Marder (1980) have also described frequent severe dysphoric reactions to single doses of chlorpromazine and thiothixene.

Van Putten (1975b) found an extraordinarily high rate of akathisia, 45%, on close examination of a ward population. He describes the distress in graphic terms, while demonstrating concern for the patients' suffering. He concludes:

> Since many of life's activities require sitting, a sustained akathisia is a severe hardship. The subtler akathisias often go unrecognized by the physician—but not by the patient! Even a mild akathisia can preclude sitting through the dinner hour, a movie, a therapy session, or a sedentary job.

Akathisia can literally drive a person crazy. Barnes (1992) points to studies indicating that akathisia can induce psychosis. He cites literature confirming that it can cause aggression and violence or suicide. (See also Breggin & Breggin, 1994a, for discussion of akathisia and suicide.) Van Putten and Marder (1987) reviewed the literature and concluded that akathisia "in the extreme case, can drive people to suicide or to homicide." Too often, doctors are likely to mistake the akathisia for the patient's mental disorder and increase the medication, creating a vicious cycle.

Mayerhoff and Lieberman (1992) observe:

> One of the more troublesome side effects of the neuroleptics cited by many authors is a syndrome involving restlessness, excitement and aggressive behavior that may or may not be due to akathisia. . . . There is some evidence to suggest that violent behavior may be more frequent on moderately high-dose haloperidol than on moderate doses of low potency neuroleptics.

Haloperidol (Haldol) is among the most frequently used drugs in emergency attempts to control aggressive and violent behavior. Once again we confront the tragic irony of treating patients with drugs that can worsen their condition.

As already noted in regard to dystonia, drug-induced neurological abnormalities are often subject to some degree of self-control. They can sometimes be partially relieved by sedatives and may worsen in reaction to emotional stress. Sachdev and Kruk (1994) found that the movements in most patients would lessen when they were distracted by something.

Neuroleptic-induced akathisia and anguish continue to be extremely common. Sachdev and Kruk (1994) evaluated 100 patients admitted to two inpatient psychiatric units in teaching hospitals affiliated with the University of New South Wales in Australia. Mild akathisia developed in 41% of patients and moderate-to-severe akathisia in 21%. A number of studies have indicated rates as high as 90% with high-potency neuroleptics, such as Haldol and Prolixin (reviewed in Sachdev & Kruk, 1994).

The rates of akathisia with some of the newer atypical antipsychotics may be lower, but the disorder remains a problem. A single case report (Byerly, Greer, & Evans, 1995) indicates that risperidone can produce severe akathisia, described as behavioral stimulation with anxiety and agitation. In a recent study of clozapine, 2 of 29 patients developed akathisia, one mild and the other moderate in intensity (Chengappa et al., 1994).

DRUG-INDUCED DYSPHORIA, INCLUDING DEPRESSION AND SUICIDE

In *Psychiatric Drugs: Hazards to the Brain* (1983), I reviewed and evaluated earlier studies at some length to document the frequency with which neuroleptics can cause dysphoric and psychotic responses, including schizophrenic-like reactions and depression, with or without accompanying akathisia (e.g., DiMascio, 1970; Marsden & Parkes, 1977; Rifkin, Quitkin, & Klein, 1975; Singh, 1976; Van Putten & May, 1978). The studies typically involved drugs that are still commonly in use, including Haldol. More recently, clozapine has been reported to cause toxic delirium, especially in the elderly (Pitner, Mintzer, Pennypacker, & Jackson, 1995).

Van Putten and May found that 47% of their patients developed akinesia and that most of these became depressed. Confirming the brain-disabling principle, as these patients became depressed, they were rated as improved in their schizophrenia, probably because they became relatively inactive, retarded, withdrawn, and even mute.

Depression is an especially serious reaction to neuroleptic treatment (Aubree & Lader, 1980; Quitkin, Rifkin, & Klein, 1975; Van Putten & May, 1978). Simonson (1964) described how his mother became despairing and hopeless after one small dose of Compazine for nausea. Ayd (1975) disclosed "There is now general agreement that mild to severe depressions that may lead to suicide may happen during treatment with any depot [long-acting intramuscular] neuroleptic, just as they may occur during treatment with any oral neuroleptic."

Small and Kellams (1974) noted reports of patients becoming suicidal as a result of treatment with the long-acting injectable form of Prolixin. Others have confirmed that suicide can result from neuroleptic-induced depression (Alarcon & Carney, 1969; Hogan & Awad, 1983).

Neuroleptic-induced depression continues to be recognized as a problem. Mayerhoff and Lieberman (1992) point out that reported incidence rates of neuroleptic-induced "akinetic depression" reach as high as 50%, with an average of 25%. Frequency probably increases with the long-acting intramuscular neuroleptics.

Emerich and Sanberg (1991) wrote an editorial in *Biological Psychiatry* that examined dysphoric reactions to neuroleptics (see chapter 2 for their description of lobotomy-like effects). They describe an array of anguished reactions, including dysphoria, anxiety, agitation, and panic. Two volunteer normals experienced "severe anxiety" as well as loss of willpower. They describe a study in which relatively small doses of Haldol, 2.5 mg/day, produced "mood swings, crying, sadness, depression and despondence" as well as "lack of motivation." Further lowering of the dose reduced the reactions. They summarize: "Agitation, anxiety attacks, panic attacks, work avoidance, school phobia, separation anxiety and delusions are all antipsychotic side effects that have been reported following neuroleptic treatment."

Chapter 5 will examine evidence indicating that neuroleptic-induced psychoses can become permanent in the form of tardive psychosis and tardive dementia, leading to a tragic situation in which worsening symptoms require greater doses of the offending medication.

The Issue of Coercion

None of the studies reviewed in this chapter considers whether the patients wanted to be in treatment or whether they were being coerced. None mentions whether the patients were legally voluntary or involuntary, let alone whether ostensibly voluntary patients were undergoing treatment under duress, as frequently happens. The absence of such considerations is particularly startling in studies in which drug resistance is the issue under investigation. Psychiatrists too often seem to believe that resistance is wholly a matter of mental illness so that it doesn't matter if the patient resents being forcibly subjected to hospitalization or to therapy. Nor do these studies take into account the reality that patients warn each other against complaining about treatment on the grounds that complaints lead to increased doses of drugs or other punishing results. More than three decades later, my 1964 study, "Coercion of Voluntary Patients in an Open Hospital," remains the only one to systematically investigate the various threats and outright forms of coercion used to control mental patients, including drugs, electroshock, and commitment.

In conclusion, the neuroleptics cause an enormous amount of physical and emotional suffering, including anguish and psychosis. Frequently, the drugs produce a feeling of "deadness" and depression, and they can cause suicide. Often the suffering is associated with extrapyramidal reactions, such as parkinsonism, dystonia, and akathisia.

CHAPTER 4

Neuroleptic Malignant Syndrome, Tardive Dyskinesia, Tardive Dystonia, and Tardive Akathisia

This chapter focuses on two well-known neurological disorders caused by the neuroleptics—tardive dyskinesia (TD) and neuroleptic malignant syndrome (NMS), with emphasis on their frequency and their destructive impact on the physical and emotional life of the individual. It also discusses neuroleptic withdrawal syndrome. The next chapter will explore irreversible damage to the brain that primarily affects mental functioning, including tardive psychosis and tardive dementia. However, as products of neuroleptic neurotoxicity, all these drug-induced abnormalities are clinically and neurologically interrelated.

TARDIVE DYSKINESIA

Within a few years after the development of the first neuroleptic, it became obvious that many patients were not recovering from their drug-induced neurologic disorders even after termination of the therapy. Reports were made in the late 1950s. Delay and Deniker (1968) date their awareness of irreversible neurological syndromes to 1959. By 1968 they were able to provide a vivid review of several varieties, including buccolingual, truncal, and variable choreic movements. In 1964 Faurbye (Faurbye, Rasch, Petersen, & Brandborg, 1964) named the disorder tardive dyskinesia.

As if governed by one mind, psychiatry as a profession refused to give any official recognition to this potential tragedy. Then Crane made it a personal crusade to gain the profession's recognition of the problem (1973). The American College of Neuropsychopharmacology/Food and Drug Administration Task Force (1973) described the syndrome in a special report. Following 1973, everyone in the profession should have been alerted to the dangers of TD; but too many psychiatrists have continued to act as if it hardly exists.

In 1980, the American Psychiatric Association (APA) published a task force report on TD. In 1985 the FDA took the unusual step of setting specifically worded requirements for a class warning in association with all neuroleptic labeling and advertising ("Neuroleptics," 1985). In a wholly unprecedented move, in the same year the APA sent out a warning letter about the dangers of tardive dyskinesia to its entire membership (see chapter 11 for further discussion of the FDA's role).

TD often begins with uncontrolled movements of the face, including the eyes (blinking), tongue, lips, mouth, and cheeks; but it can start with almost any group of muscles. The most common early sign is a quivering or curling of the tongue. Tongue protrusions and chewing movements are also common, and can become serious enough to harm teeth and impair chewing and swallowing. The hands and feet, arms and legs, neck, back, and torso can be involved.

The movements displayed are highly variable, and include writhing contortions, tics, spasms, and tremors. The person's gait can be badly impaired. More subtle functions can be affected and are easily overlooked: respiration (involving the diaphragm), swallowing (involving the pharyngeal and esophageal musculature), the gag reflex, and speech (Yassa & Jones, 1985).

The movements usually disappear during sleep, although I have seen exceptions. They sometimes can be partially suppressed by willpower; frequently are made worse by anxiety; and can vary from time to time (see below).

Many cases of TD appear to be relatively mild, often limited to movements of the tongue, mouth, jaw, face, or eyelids. Nonetheless, they are frequently disfiguring and often embarrassing. Patients have been known to commit suicide (Yassa & Jones, 1985).

The abnormal movements can sometimes become totally disabling. Turner (1971) describes patients who cannot eat and must have their teeth removed in order to facilitate the entry of food into their mouths. He also describes patients who cannot keep shoes on their feet because they wear them out while sitting with the constant foot-shuffling activity. I have evaluated a number of cases in which the tardive dyskinesia was wholly disabling, including massive distortions of the position of the neck or body, rocking and swaying, shoulder shrugging, and rotary or thrusting movements of the pelvis, as well as disturbances of respiration, such as periodic rapid breathing, irregular breathing, and grunting.

Ironically, the disease makes the patient look "very crazy" because of the seemingly bizarre facial and bodily movements. Tragically, this has often led to patients being treated more vigorously with neuroleptics, ultimately worsening their TD.

As in other neurological disorders, the patient may attempt to hide the disorder by adding voluntary movements to the involuntary ones in order to disguise them. For example, to cover up a tendency to move the arms continually, the patient may make grooming movements around the face and hair. This can make it seem as if the individual suffers from a psychological compulsion instead of a neurological disorder. Or the patient may clasp his arms together in order to control the movements, making it seem as if he is trying to psychologically "hold onto himself."

All the neuroleptics (see chapter 2 for a list) can cause tardive dyskinesia, including the atypical neuroleptics clozapine (Weller & Kornhuber, 1993) and risperidone (Addington, Toews, & Addington, 1995). The overall adverse effects of the atypical neuroleptics are summarized in chapter 5.

Masking the Symptoms of TD
with Continued Neuroleptic Treatment

The symptoms of tardive dyskinesia are masked or suppressed by these drugs, so that the disease symptoms do not fully appear until the patient has been removed from the treatment. For this reason, in addition to using the smallest possible dose for the shortest possible time, whenever possible patients should periodically be removed from their neuroleptics, if only for a short period, to determine if they are developing tardive dyskinesia. Permanent removal from the neuroleptics is a more difficult matter, often requiring many months of gradual withdrawal for the brain to adjust to the drug-free environment.

Harold Klawans has discussed the dangerousness of trying to control or treat TD with the causative agent. He asserts (in the discussion following Goetz et al., 1980): "Treatment of tardive dyskinesia with neuroleptics themselves is clearly treatment with the presumed offending agent and should be avoided." He calls it "short-sighted" to use the neuroleptics in the treatment of tardive dyskinesia, and concludes that the therapy "serves to aggravate its pathogenesis." Unhappily, Klawans himself in the same article too readily recommends reserpine as a helpful agent in the treatment of TD, when it too can cause the disorder.

Nonetheless, I have seen cases of TD that were so disabling that the only recourse seemed to be treatment with a neuroleptic. But two points must be borne in mind about these cases. First, in each instance, the case became so severe because physicians failed to detect the disorder when it first appeared and continued neuroleptic treatment long after it should have been terminated. This has been true in nearly all the most disabling cases I have examined. Second, the individuals in question were overcome with suffering and rendered wholly unable to function by the TD. They and their families made informed decisions to continue the offending agent because the TD was making life unbearable for the patient.

The anticholinergic drugs typically used to ameliorate the symptoms of drug-induced parkinsonism also may aggravate the symptoms of TD (Yassa et al., 1992). They include benztropine (Cogentin), biperiden (Akineton), and trihexyphenidyl (Artane, Tremin). These agents are known to worsen similar symptoms in Huntington's chorea (Hunter, Blackwood, Smith, & Cumings, 1968; Klawans, 1973). At present the role of these drugs in the development or exacerbation of tardive dyskinesia is controversial and undetermined, but caution is required in giving them to patients on neuroleptics. Their adverse effects are discussed in chapter 2. These agents are often used to treat acute extrapyramidal symptoms and may be mistakenly prescribed for TD.

Rates of TD

In 1980 the APA produced a detailed analysis of the disease in its *Task Force Report: Tardive Dyskinesia*. It made clear that TD is a serious, usually irreversible, untreatable, and highly prevalent disease resulting from therapy with the neuroleptics. The task force estimated the prevalence rate for TD in routine treatment (several months to 2 years) as *at least* 10%–20% for *more than minimal* disease. For long-term exposure to neuroleptics, the rate was at least 40% for more than minimal disease.

Even after the publication of the 1980 task force report and a mountain of confirmatory evidence, some biologically oriented psychiatrists, such as Nancy Andreasen (1984), in *The Broken Brain: The Biological Revolution in Psychiatry*, continued to misinform the public that tardive dyskinesia is "infrequent" (p. 210) and occurs in "a few patients" (p. 211).

The more recent APA task force (1992) report cites a rate of 5% per year, cumulative over the first several years of treatment. Jeste and Caligiuri (1993) estimate the annual incidence rate among young adults at 4%–5%.

In a recent prospective project emanating from Yale, Glazer, Morgenstern, and Doucette (1993) reported a long-term evaluation of 362 outpatient psychiatric patients who were free of TD at baseline and who were being maintained on neuroleptics. For patients who are starting neuroleptics, according to projections from their data, the risk of tardive dyskinesia will be 31.8% after 5 years of exposure—a rate of slightly over 6% per year. The risk is 49.4% after 10 years, 56.7% after 15 years, 64.7% after 20 years, and 68.4% after 25 years.

Chouinard, Annable, Mercier, & Ross-Chouinard (1986) followed a group of 136 persons who had already been receiving neuroleptics but had not yet manifested TD. Over 5 years, 35%—a rate of 7% per year— developed the disorder.

Overall, in relatively young and healthy patients, the cumulative risk of contracting TD when exposed to neuroleptics ranges from 4%–7% per year during the first several years of treatment. Approximately one-third of the patients will develop this largely irreversible disorder within the first five years of treatment. This represents an astronomical risk for patients and should become part of the awareness of all mental health professionals, their patients, and their patients' families. Furthermore, we shall find that TD brings with it the additional risk of irreversible cognitive dysfunction and dementia (chapter 5).

There is evidence that rates for tardive dyskinesia are increasing. It may be caused by the growing tendency to use drugs with seemingly more toxic effects on the extrapyramidal system, such as Haldol and Prolixin (see Jeste & Wyatt, 1981). These drugs also come in long-acting intramuscular preparations that do not permit patients to independently lower their own dosages by taking fewer pills than prescribed.

It is unusual for TD to develop in less than 3–6 months' treatment and standard texts suggest that TD which develops earlier requires special investigation. However, it is not possible to place too much emphasis on one point that has been mentioned by Tepper and Haas (1979) and others (for example, Hollister, 1976): tardive dyskinesia can develop in low-dose, short-term treatment. DeVeaugh-Geiss (1979) has seen cases develop in a matter of weeks. I have seen several cases develop at around 3 months of treatment. One patient developed tardive dyskinesia after 1 month of recent exposure, with a history of 2 months' prior exposure several years earlier. One case which developed in 3 months of constant exposure had a probable history of prior head injury from childhood. In the elderly, many cases may develop within a few weeks (see below).

THE ELDERLY AND
OTHER VULNERABLE POPULATIONS

It is important to remember that medications in general are more likely to cause dysfunction in the elderly (Nolan & O'Malley, 1988). Nowhere is this demonstrated more tragically than in regard to TD.

A study of elderly nursing home patients by Yassa, Nastase, Camille, and Belzile (1988) found that 41% developed tardive dyskinesia over a period of only 24 months and that none fully recovered. While long-term studies have found a spontaneous dyskinesia prevalence of 1%–5% in the elderly, none of the non-drug-treated controls developed spontaneous dyskinesias during the 2 years. Yassa, Iskander, and Ally (1988) found TD in 45% of an outpatient clinic population with a mean age of 60.

In a more recent study, Yassa, Nastase, Dupont, and Thibeau (1992) followed up patients from a geriatric psychiatric unit who had received neuroleptics for the first time during the hospitalization. Out of 99 patients, 35 (35.4%) had developed TD after a mean exposure of 20.7 months. Of these 35, 21 had moderate TD and 3 had severe. Some had tardive dystonia (see below).

Saltz and his colleagues (1991) found the incidence of TD was 31% following 43 weeks of cumulative neuroleptic treatment in the elderly. The incidence was higher among patients who had previous electroshock treatment. Patients with early signs of parkinsonism developed TD at a faster rate. Of great importance, in this older population, the mean cumulative time while taking neuroleptics was very brief, a mere 22.7 weeks. One patient developed TD at 2 weeks.

Jeste, Lacro, Gilbert, Kline, and Kline (1993), in an ongoing prospective study, found that 26% of middle-aged and elderly patients developed TD after 12 months. The authors also reviewed the literature on neuroleptic withdrawal and found "that almost 60 percent of the patients withdrawn from neuroleptics did not relapse over a mean period of 6 months." They concluded, "it seems feasible to discontinue neuroleptic medication from a select population of older schizophrenic patients, if it is done carefully with adequate monitoring and follow up." They also experimented with brief 2-week placebo-substituted withdrawal in their own group of patients, both younger and older subjects, and found it relatively benign: none relapsed or required resumption of neuroleptics. They concluded, "Given the heightened risk of TD in older patients, it seems that a trial of neuroleptic withdrawal is warranted in this population."

Jeste et al. (1993) emphasize that "The potential seriousness of neuroleptic-induced TD warrants obtaining competent, informed consent to treatment from patients or guardians." They recommended that consent be periodically renewed and cited other sources to confirm their position.

In addition to age, prior brain damage probably increases the risk of TD (Breggin, 1983; Chouinard, Annable, Ross-Chouinard, & Nestoros, 1979), although studies are contradictory and not conclusive. McKeith, Fairbairn, Perry, Thompson, and Perry (1992) found that 13 of 16 patients with Lewy body type dementia showed deterioration on neuroleptics, including the development of extrapyramidal features. The authors conclude, "Severe, and often fatal, neuroleptic sensitivity may occur in elderly patients with confusion, dementia, or behavioral disturbance. Its occurrence may indicate senile dementia of the Lewy body type . . . " Pourcher, Cohen, Cohen, Baruch, and Bouchard (1993) found a correlation between TD and prior organic brain disorder.

Relapse, Exacerbation, and Delayed Onset after Termination

TD typically waxes and wanes, both in the course of a day and in the course of weeks or months. Especially in the elderly, both partial remissions and relapses are common (Lacro et al., 1994).

As in many neurological disorders, the manifestations of TD can worsen during stress and can be somewhat calmed with sedation (Jeste & Caligiuri, 1993). In my experience, anxiety, exhaustion, and other general stresses to the mind and body can temporarily exacerbate the symptoms, while relaxation, when possible, can temporarily reduce them.

With great effort, patients can sometimes suppress some of their symptoms for a short time. They can also integrate their movements into more natural-looking actions, such as grooming or smiling, in order to disguise them. One patient with whom I consulted would hide her involuntary facial grimaces by trying to smile. The effect was to make her look even more strange to the casual observer.

Neither the fact that TD waxes and wanes, sometimes in response to stress, nor the patient's ability to partially suppress it with an exertion of will, should mislead observers into believing that it is psychological or emotional in origin. Too often the early signs of TD are overlooked, denied, or dismissed by physicians on these mistaken grounds.

Christensen, Moller, and Faurbye (1970) have documented that a significant percentage of TD cases may not show up at all until many months or even several years after discontinuation of the treatment. They believe that the symptoms are brought on by the interaction between the damage caused by the drugs and by the aging process. If this is true, then a tragic reality may develop as we observe the evolution of TD in aging populations. I have on occasion seen cases that did not become apparent until several months or more after termination of treatment.

Reversibility Is Rare

In the vast majority of cases, TD is irreversible and there is no effective treatment. One report indicates that among patients with persistent TD, followed for a period of 5 years, 82% showed no overall significant change, 11% improved, and 7% became worse (Bergen et al., 1989).

Another study followed 49 outpatient tardive dyskinesia cases for a mean of 40 weeks (range 1–59 months) after discontinuation of medication (Glazer, Morgenstern, Schooler, Berkman, & Moore, 1990). Many patients showed noticeable improvement in their movements within the first year after stopping neuroleptics, but only 2% showed complete and persistent recovery. The authors conclude, ''A major finding of this study is that complete reversal of TD following neuroleptic discontinuation in chronically treated patients was rare.''

Physician and Patient Denial of TD

Physicians understandably find it painful to face the damaging effects of their treatments. Sometimes it is difficult for them to confront the damage done to patients by other physicians as well. In addition, physicians may consciously seek to protect themselves or their colleagues by failing to acknowledge or to record obvious symptoms of tardive dyskinesia. I have seen many hospital and outpatient records in which obvious, severe cases of tardive dyskinesia have gone either unrecognized or undocumented, sometimes by several physicians in succession. For example, the nurse's notes may make clear that the patient is in constant motion, yet the doctor's physical examination or progress notes will give no indication of the disorder. Even official discharge summaries may fail to record TD in patients who have been demonstrating the disorder throughout the period of hospital or clinic treatment. This denial of the obvious is mirrored within the profession itself, which has been very remiss in recognizing or emphasizing the seriousness of the problem (for an analysis of this history, see Breggin, 1983a; Brown & Funk, 1986; Cohen & McCubbin, 1990; Wolf & Brown, 1987).

Psychiatrists sometimes accuse patients of exaggerating their tardive dyskinesia. In reality, most patients tend to deny the existence or severity of their TD. As discussed in detail in chapter 5, patient denial is caused in part by neuroleptic-induced lobotomy effects and in part by denial associated with brain damage. The mutual denial of TD by physician and patient is an aspect of iatrogenic helplessness and denial—the use of brain-disabling treatments in psychiatry to enforce the patient's denial of both his personal problems and his iatrogenic brain dysfunction and damage (chapter 1).

The Size of the Epidemic

It is difficult to determine the total number of TD cases. Van Putten (see Lund, 1989) estimated 400,000–1,000,000 in the United States. My own earlier estimate is higher, ranging in the several millions (Breggin, 1983). It is no exaggeration to call tardive dyskinesia a widespread epidemic and possibly the worst medically induced catastrophe in history.

Children and TD

When I reviewed the subject in 1983, I was among the first to state that the rate and severity of tardive dyskinesia in children was being vastly underestimated. I therefore reviewed the subject in detail. Fortunately, this is no longer necessary, since it is now well-recognized that children are susceptible to TD at rates no less than adults, and that the disorder is often more virulent in children, because it frequently affects the torso, including posture and locomotion (Breggin, 1983a; Gualtieri & Barnhill, 1988; Gualtieri, Quade, Hicks, Mayo, & Schroeder, 1984; Gualtieri, Schroeder, Hicks, & Quade, 1986). A high percentage of neuroleptic-treated children also develop a permanent worsening of their emotional and behavioral problems, psychoses, or dementia (see chapter 5). Physicians should not use neuroleptics for behavioral control in children.

TARDIVE DYSTONIA

It is now apparent that there are at least two related variants of TD, tardive dystonia and tardive akathisia. In a 1988 review of tardive dystonia, Burke and Kang found 21 reports describing 131 patients (for reviews, also see Greenberg & Gujavarty, 1985, and Kane & Lieberman, 1992).

Tardive dystonia involves ''sustained involuntary twisting movements, generally slow, which may affect the limbs, trunk, neck, or face'' (Burke et al., 1982, p. 1335). The face and neck are by far the most frequently affected areas of the body. Severe deformities of the neck (torticollis) can cause extreme pain and disability. I have seen several cases affecting the orbital muscles of the eyes (blepharospasm) to the degree that the individual's vision was impaired, requiring botulin injections to paralyze the muscles. I've also seen respiratory and abdominal muscles affected in a painful and debilitating manner.

Tardive dystonia can produce cramplike, painful spasms that temporarily prevent the individual from carrying out normal activities. Sometimes the spasms are so continuous that the individual is largely disabled. Damage to the joint and skeleton system, including fractures, can occur (Burke & Kang, 1988). The pain and muscle tension, as well as the effort to compensate for the spasms, can be exhausting and demoralizing.

The torsions can be worsened by other bodily movements, such as attempts to write or to walk. Sometimes they can be relieved by particular movements, such as touching the chin to relieve torticollis or touching the brow to relieve blepharospasm.

As Burke and Kang (1988) point out, tardive dystonia can be mistakenly dismissed as a manifestation of hysteria, psychological in origin: "In this regard it is important to realize that dystonia, like many other neurological disorders, can be influenced transiently by suggestion, placebo, or sedation (e.g., during an amobarbital interview) and such maneuvers cannot exclude a true dystonia." Also, like many other neurological disorders, it can sometimes be partially controlled by extreme exertions of will.

Tardive dystonia can make an individual appear unsympathetic or bizarre, especially to the uninformed observer who equates the facial grimaces or neck distortions with being "crazy." As in all the drug-induced dyskinesias, the individual may try to cover up for the disorder with additional movements that make the disorder seem voluntary, and therefore not a product of mental illness. The result can be very confusing or distressing to the observer.

TARDIVE AKATHISIA

Tardive akathisia involves a feeling of inner tension or anxiety that drives the individual into restless activity, such as pacing (see chapter 3 for details). The first report of tardive akathisia I have located in the literature was published by Walter Kruse in 1960. He described three cases of muscular restlessness that persisted at least 3 months after discontinuation of treatment with fluphenazine and triflupromazine. The "akathisic syndrome . . . consisted of inability to sit still, pacing the floor all day, jerky movements of arms and shoulders." Once again Delay and Deniker (1968) were also among the first clinicians to notice the disorder. In discussing "syndromes persisting after cessation of medication," they mention "hyperkinetic" ones. As early as 1977, Simpson more definitively made an association between tardive dyskinesia and akathisia that would not respond to treatment.

Gualtieri and Sovner (1989) reviewed the subject of tardive akathisia, cited studies with prevalence rates of 13%–18%, and called it "a significant public health issue." Nonetheless, the drug companies have ignored it in the labeling of their products.

The anguish associated with akathisia should not be minimized. Consider Van Putten's (1974) description of a mild, temporary akathisia or hyperkinesia: "Patient feels 'all nerved up,' 'squirmy inside,' 'uptight,' 'nervous,' 'tense,' 'uncomfortable,' 'impatient'. . . . Subjective feeling of ill-being may be accompanied by restless changes in posture.''

One reason that so little attention has been given to the mental disruption associated with the dyskinesias is the tendency to blame the mental component on the mental illness of the patient. Indeed, it has been commonplace to blame the obvious motor disturbances on the mental illness as well, often resulting in increased treatment, and a worsening of the symptoms, until immobility sets in, masking the entire process.

It takes no great imagination to grasp the suffering of a patient condemned to a relatively mild tardive akathisia for a lifetime. I have seen cases of this kind that were previously mistaken for severe anxiety or agitated depression. Chapter 3 reviewed research indicating that acute akathisia can drive a patient into psychosis, and to violence and/or suicide. Considering the millions of patients subjected to this torment, the problem takes on epidemic proportions.

Tardive akathisia can be subtle. A woman in her mid-sixties consulted me because of seemingly bizarre feelings that other doctors attributed to her depression and to somatic delusions or hallucinations. She had a feeling of ''electricity'' going in periodic bursts throughout her body. Although she sat quietly in the office, she spoke of feeling fidgety and driven to move about.

Her hospital and clinic charts disclosed that 2 years earlier she had been treated for approximately 6 months with neuroleptics. The sensation she was describing had first been noted while she was taking the medication. I concluded that she probably had tardive akathisia, a subtle case that did not actually force her to move about. However, because she didn't show external signs of the disorder, other physicians were reluctant to make the diagnosis. The patient felt ''driven to distraction'' and even to suicide by the disorder; but after my probable diagnosis, she actually felt somewhat relieved. At least she was being taken seriously.

In 1993, Gualtieri wrote:

> In terms of clinical treatment and the public health, however, TDAK [tardive akathisia] is a fact, not a question. It is one more serious side effect of neuroleptic treatment, like TD and the Neuroleptic Malignant Syndrome. Taken together, they define neuroleptic treatment as a necessary evil, a treatment that should be administered with care and caution, and reserved for patients who have no other recourse.

RESPONSES TO TARDIVE DISORDERS

Physical Exhaustion

Fatigue to the point of exhaustion almost always accompanies tardive disorders of any severity. The patient can be exhausted by the movements themselves, by the effort to hide them, and by increased effort required to carry out daily activities. The primary impact on the brain itself may also produce fatigue. Although the disorders tend to disappear in sleep, they can make it difficult to fall asleep, adding to the exhaustion. Having to contend with the physical pain associated with tardive akathisia (inner torment) and with tardive dystonia (muscle spasms) can also wear a person down.

Psychological Suffering

Commonly, patients experience shame and humiliation, often leading to social withdrawal. Even a seemingly mild dyskinesia that affects facial expression can be sufficiently humiliating to cause a person to withdraw from society. So can a speech abnormality that makes a person seem to "talk funny."

The experience of constant pain from dystonia or inner torture from akathisia can drive a person to suicidal despair. The physical disabilities associated with disorders can also become very depressing to patients.

In a clinical report from the Mayo Clinic by Rosenbaum (1979), depression was found closely linked to tardive dyskinesia. Rosenbaum states, "Almost all patients in our series had depressive symptoms accompanying the onset of tardive dyskinesia," and he cites other studies confirming his observation.

Tardive dyskinesia patients often feel very betrayed by the doctors who prescribed the medication or who later failed to detect the disorder or to tell the patient about it. Too frequently, perhaps in a self-protective stance toward their colleagues, several psychiatrists in a row will fail to inform the patient or family about the obvious iatrogenic disorder. This can leave patients feeling that they cannot trust psychiatrists. In the extreme, it can create an understandable distrust of doctors in general.

Even a slight or minimal degree of tardive disorder can end up seriously impairing an individual's quality of life.

NEUROLEPTIC WITHDRAWAL SYNDROME

Withdrawal frequently causes a worsening mental state, including tension and anxiety. With those drugs that produce potent anticholinergic effects, such as Thorazine and Mellaril, a cholinergic withdrawal syndrome (cholinergic rebound) may develop that mimics the flu, including emotional upset, insomnia, nausea and vomiting, diarrhea, anorexia and weight loss, and muscle aches.

Withdrawal symptoms can also include a temporary worsening of dyskinetic effects, both painful and frightening.

While classic addiction to these substances has not been demonstrated, the drugs should be considered addictive in the sense that withdrawal symptoms can make it impossible for patients to stop taking them. For this reason, I have suggested viewing these drugs as addictive (Breggin, 1989a, 1989b).

Because of the withdrawal symptoms, it is often necessary to reduce these drugs at a very slow rate. Sometimes withdrawal seems to be impossible. I have described the principles of withdrawing from psychiatric drugs in *Talking Back to Prozac.*

NEUROLEPTIC-INDUCED PSYCHOSIS AND DEMENTIA

The following chapter will describe irreversible psychosis and dementia associated with the neuroleptics. These may first become obvious as withdrawal effects that make it seemingly impossible to stop the drug therapy.

OTHER NEUROLEPTIC-INDUCED
NEUROLOGICAL IMPAIRMENTS

The neuroleptics can produce a variety of other symptoms of central nervous system dysfunction, including abnormal electroencephalogram (EEG) findings, an increased frequency of seizures, respiratory depression, and disturbances of body temperature control (Davis, 1980; Davis & Cole,

1975). Endocrine disorders, especially in females, may also be of central nervous system origin (Davis, 1980). There is some evidence that autonomic dysfunction can become irreversible (tardive autonomic disorders).

NEUROLEPTIC MALIGNANT SYNDROME (NMS)

This devastating disorder was seemingly so bizarre, unexpected, and inexplicable that physicians for years literally refused to believe their eyes. Seven years after the introduction of the drugs into North America, Leo Hollister (1961) reviewed their side effects for "Medical Intelligence" in the *New England Journal of Medicine.* In two separate places, he referred to syndromes that probably were NMS. He described a "bizarre" dystonic syndrome that can be "confused with hysteria, tetanus, encephalitis or other acute nervous-system disorders; a rare fatality may occur." Later he mentioned that "other clinical syndromes attributed to central-nervous-system effects of these drugs have resembled acute encephalitis, myasthenia gravis, bulbar palsy or pseudotabes."

Although NMS was identified in an English-language publication by Delay and Deniker as early as 1968, physicians continued to be reluctant to recognize the syndrome. Delay and Deniker declared it was caused by the neuroleptics, specifically including haloperidol (Haldol) and fluphenazine (Prolixin). Any neuroleptic can cause NMS. However, clinicians have found an increased danger with long-acting injectable neuroleptics.

Delay and Deniker were already able to identify many of the components of NMS, including pallor, hyperthermia, a severe psychomotor syndrome with akinesia and stupor or hypertonicity with varying dyskinesias. They warn that, at the first suspicion, "one must stop medication *immediately and completely.*" They were already aware of fatalities. That the syndrome was named and definitively identified in English in 1968 is most remarkable in light of the failure of drug companies to give it formal recognition until compelled to do so by the FDA almost 20 years later (see chapter 11 for further discussion).

Neuroleptic malignant syndrome is characterized by "such symptoms as severe dyskinesia or akinesia, temperature elevation, tachycardia, blood pressure fluctuations, diaphoresis, dyspnea, dysphagia, and urinary incontinence" (Coons, Hillman, & Marshall, 1982). If unrecognized, as too often happens, it can be fatal in more than 20% of cases. The syndrome frequently leaves the patient with permanent dyskinesias and dementia (see chapter 5).

Most cases develop within the first few weeks of treatment (even within 45 minutes!), but some develop after months or years, or after increased dosage (Gratz, Levinson, & Simpson, 1992).

Estimates for rates of neuroleptic malignant syndrome vary widely but studies indicate that they are very high. Pope, Keck, and McElroy (1986) surveyed 500 patients admitted during a 1-year period to a large psychiatric hospital and found a rate of 1.4%. The cumulative rate for patients would be much higher. Addonizio, Susman, and Roth (1986) carried out a retrospective review of 82 charts of male inpatients and found that prevalence for the diagnosed syndrome was 2.4%. Again, the cumulative rate over repeated hospitalizations or years of treatment would be much higher.

Although it is sometimes called "rare," NMS should be described as common or frequent (1/100 is common by FDA standards).

The rates for neuroleptic malignant syndrome, as well as its potential severity and lethality, make it an extreme risk for patients receiving antipsychotic drugs. A risk of this size would probably result in most drugs in general medicine being removed from the market.

I have reviewed cases in which several physicians at a time missed making the correct diagnosis in what seemed, from my retrospective analysis, like an obvious case of NMS. The failure to stop the neuroleptic and to institute proper treatment resulted in severe, permanent impairments, or death. The mistaken idea that NMS is rare may contribute to these errors in judgment.

After reviewing episodes of NMS in 20 patients, Rosebush and Stewart (1989) found that most cases fit the following cluster of symptoms: delirium, a high fever with diaphoresis, unstable cardiovascular signs, an elevated respiratory rate, and an array of dyskinesias, including tremors, rigidity, dystonia, and chorea.

Patients spoke little during the acute illness and later reported that they had found themselves unable to express their anxiety and feelings of doom. Almost all patients were agitated shortly before developing NMS, suggesting to the authors that they were undergoing akathisia. The white blood cell count was elevated in all cases, dehydration was common, and lab tests showed a broad spectrum of enzymatic abnormalities, including indications of muscle breakdown.

There is little or nothing about acute NMS to distinguish it from an acute, severe episode of encephalitis, especially lethargic encephalitis (also called von Economo's disease), except for the fact of exposure to neuroleptic therapy. I have previously compared neuroleptic toxicity and lethargic encephalitis in detail (Breggin, 1993; also see chapter 5).

Although Rosebush and Stewart provide insufficient data to draw exact parallels, their NMS patients also suffered chronic impairments similar to those reported in lethargic encephalitis patients. Of the 20 patients, 14 continued to have "extrapyramidal symptoms or mild abnormalities of vitals signs and muscle enzymes at the time of discharge" (p. 721); but we are not told how many of the 14 specifically had persistent extrapyramidal signs. In a striking parallel with lethargic encephalitis, three patients displayed persistent parkinsonian symptoms until they were lost to follow-up. One patient, who had mild cognitive impairment prior to NMS, developed a persistent worsening of her dementia.

Neuroleptic malignant syndrome has also been reported with the atypical neuroleptics, clozapine (Anderson & Powers, 1991; DasGupta & Young, 1991) and risperidone (Dave, 1995; Mahendra, 1995; Raitasuo, Vataga, & Elomaa, 1994; Singer, Colette, & Boland, 1995).

NEUROLOGICAL MECHANISMS
OF PARKINSONISM AND TD

Drug-induced parkinsonism apparently develops in part, but not wholly, from blockade of dopamine receptors in the basal ganglia, specifically the striatal region or striatum (the caudate and putamen), producing motor retardation, rigidity, and other symptoms. Damage and degeneration in the pigmented neurons of the substantia nigra play a key role. These neurons terminate in the striatum, where, when they are functioning normally, they release dopamine to act on striatal dopamine receptors.

Tardive dyskinesia is a more delayed reaction, probably based on the development of reactive supersensitivity or hyperactivity in these same striatal dopamine receptors following continuous blockade (see American Psychiatric Association, 1980; Fann, Smith, Davis, & Domino, 1980; Klawans, 1973; and chapter 5 in this volume). This supersensitivity of the dopamine receptors becomes most obvious when the drug is reduced or eliminated, terminating the blockade. The overactive, unblocked receptors produce the tardive dyskinesia symptoms. Undoubtedly a great deal more must be learned about the neuropathology of both these drug-induced diseases, which probably involve multiple neurotransmitter system abnor-malities.

CONCLUSION

The widespread use of neuroleptics has unleashed an epidemic of neuro-logic disease on the world. Even if tardive dyskinesia were the only permanent disability produced by these drugs, this would be among the worst medically induced disasters in history. Meltzer (1995) has urged that attempts be made to remove long-term patients from neuroleptics and has attempted to demonstrate its feasibility. Gualtieri (1993), warning about the extreme dangers, has suggested neuroleptics be viewed as a therapy of last resort. I believe the profession should make every possible effort to avoid prescribing them. Although beyond the scope of this book, it is worth ending with a reminder that there is strong evidence that psychosocial alternatives can be more effective in the treatment of both acute and chronic patients labeled schizophrenic (Breggin, 1991a; Breg-gin & Stern, 1996; Karon & Vandenbos, 1981; McCready, 1995; Mosher & Burti, 1989).

Neuroleptic-Induced Brain Damage, Persistent Cognitive Deficits, Dementia, and Psychosis*

Since I first voiced my concerns and reviewed the subject (Breggin, 1983a, pp. 110–146), much more evidence has been accumulating that the neuroleptics can cause persistent damage or dysfunction to the highest centers of the brain, including cerebral atrophy. The results are irreversible intellectual and emotional impairments, including tardive dementia and tardive psychosis (for a compendium of recent articles, see Cohen & Cohen, 1993; for detailed reviews, see Breggin 1983a, 1990, & 1993). These effects may be viewed as the cognitive or mental equivalent to tardive dyskinesia.

The subjects will be dealt with in the following order: (a) clinical evidence, (b) brain scans, (c) human and animal autopsies, (d) the lessons of lethargic encephalitis (LE), (e) the underlying biological mechanisms of neuroleptic-induced brain damage, and (f) schizophrenia as a possible cause of dementia.

---

*A portion of this chapter covers similar material to my 1990 review in *Mind and Behavior*. Some of it also draws upon my 1993 review in *Brain and Cognition*. I wish to express my gratitude to those journals for providing me the original opportunity to publish these concepts.

The term *dementia* will be defined as a syndrome of organically based multiple cognitive deficits, including memory impairment, as well as other brain dysfunctions, such as emotional lability, personality change, or impairments in abstract thinking, judgment, and other higher cortical or executive functions (see American Psychiatric Association, 1987, 1994). The chapter focuses on gradually evolving persistent brain damage and dysfunction associated with chronic exposure to neuroleptics.

CLINICAL EVIDENCE

Evidence from several different clinical sources confirms that the neuroleptics can permanently impair mental functioning.

Early Correlations between Tardive Dyskinesia and Cognitive Dysfunction

An earlier review (Breggin, 1983a) disclosed that many patients with TD are also suffering from severe cognitive dysfunction (e.g., Edwards, 1970; Hunter et al., 1964; Iunik, 1979; Rosenbaum, 1979). Often the data had to be culled from charts and footnotes because most of the studies relegated this correlation to obscurity within the article. Other studies concluded, without evidence, that the brain damage must have predated the TD.

Tardive Dysmentia and Tardive Dementia

Many clinical studies have now confirmed the existence of dementia in association with neuroleptic use. A clinical study of hospitalized drug-treated patients found many suffering from mental deterioration typical of a chronic organic brain syndrome that they label *dysmentia* (Wilson et al., 1983). Tardive dysmentia consists of "unstable mood, loud speech, and [inappropriately close] approach to the examiner." It is probably a variant of hypomanic dementia.[1] The mental abnormalities in the study

---

[1]Euphoria, as well as apathy, can result from frontal lobe damage and dysfunction (Bradley, Daroff, Fenichel, & Marsden, 1991, p. 84).

by Wilson et al. (1983) correlated positively with TD symptoms measured on the Abnormal Involuntary Movement Scale (AIMS). In addition, length of neuroleptic treatment correlated with three measures of dementia: unstable mood, loud speech, and euphoria. The authors stated: "It is our hypothesis that certain of the behavioral changes observed in schizophrenic patients over time represent a behavioral equivalent of tardive dyskinesia, which we will call tardive dysmentia" (p. 188). The tendency in the literature, perhaps in search of a euphemism, has been to use the term tardive dysmentia even when a full-blown dementing syndrome is described.

A variety of studies have confirmed the existence of tardive dysmentia (dementia) (Goldberg, 1985; Jones, 1985; Mukherjee, 1984; Mukherjee & Bilder, 1985; Myslobodsky, 1986). More recently, Myslobodsky (1993) summarized the triad of features of tardive dysmentia as "occasional excessive emotional reactivity, enhanced responsiveness to environmental stimuli, and indifferent or reduced awareness of abnormal involuntary movements." He reviewed a study indicating that schizophrenic patients with TD score significantly higher on measures of aggression and tension. He pointed out that some of these patients suffer from typical frontal lobe signs. He also warned that routine neuropsychological testing may miss the frontal lobe syndrome associated with TD.[2]

In addition to Wilson et al. (1983), several other studies have reported an association between TD symptoms and generalized mental dysfunction (Baribeau, Laurent, & Décary, 1993; DeWolfe, Ryan, & Wolf, 1988; Itil, Reisberg, Huque, & Mehta, 1981; Spohn & Coyne, 1993; Struve & Willner, 1983; Waddington & Youssef, 1986; Wolf, Ryan, & Mosnaim, 1982; many reviewed in Breggin, 1993). After eliminating schizophrenia as a causative factor, Waddington and Youssef (1988) also found increased cognitive deficits in neuroleptic-treated bipolar patients with TD in comparison to those without the disorder.

Wade, Taylor, Kasprisin, Rosenberg, and Fiducia (1987) pointed out that Huntington's and Parkinson's diseases provide a related model for tardive dyskinesia, including the development of cognitive impairments (see Koshino, Hiramatsu, Isaki, & Yamaguchi, 1986; and Breggin, 1993, for similar discussions). They studied 54 manic or schizophrenic patients

---

[2]What is really required is the kind of research that demonstrated subtle yet devastating psychological changes in lobotomy (Tow, 1955) and psychosurgery (Hansen et al., 1982) patients.

with tardive dyskinesia, and concluded tardive dyskinesia is one expression of a larger "chronic neuroleptic-induced neurotoxic process" (Wade et al., 1987, p. 395).

Recently Paulsen, Heaton, and Jeste (1994) reviewed the literature and found "TD was generally reported to be associated with cognitive impairment." Their own study confirmed the literature. From this and other studies, there seems little doubt that tardive dyskinesia is associated with cognitive deficits.

Since the rates of TD are so high (see chapter 4), affecting a large proportion of neuroleptic-treated patients, its association with cognitive dysfunction and dementia is especially ominous. This data by itself provides sufficient evidence to conclude that neuroleptics frequently and irreversibly impair mental function.

A Serendipitous Finding
of Neuroleptic-Induced Generalized Cognitive Dysfunction

A multisite national research project evaluated brain dysfunction caused by polydrug abuse, including street drugs (for a more detailed analysis, see Breggin, 1983a). Using the Halstead-Reitan Neuropsychological Battery, the study unexpectedly uncovered a significant correlation between generalized brain dysfunction and total lifetime psychiatric drug consumption in schizophrenics (Grant, Adams, Carlin, Rennick, Judd, Schooff, & Reed, 1978; Grant, Adams, Carlin, Rennick, Lewis, & Schooff, 1978). More than one quarter of the neuroleptic-treated patients had persistent brain dysfunction. The chronic brain dysfunction was related more to the lifetime neuroleptic intake than to the schizophrenia: "Neuropsychological abnormality was associated with greater antipsychotic drug experience" (Grant, Adams, Carlin, Rennick, Lewis, & Schooff, 1978, p. 1069). Indeed, schizophrenic patients who abused street drugs rather than taking neuroleptics showed no correlation between schizophrenia and increased brain dysfunction. None of the patients had been exposed to neuroleptics for more than 5 years.

In an unpublished version of the paper presented at a professional meeting (Grant, Adams, Carlin, Rennick, Judd, & Schooff, 1978), the authors underscored the connection between tardive dyskinesia and cognitive deficits, and warned in their concluding sentence, "It is also clear that the antipsychotic drugs must continue to be scrutinized for the possibility that their extensive consumption might cause general cerebral dysfunction'' (p. 31). The version published in the *Archives of General Psychiatry* (Grant, Adams, Carlin, Rennick, Lewis, & Schooff, 1978) warned of the possibility of long-term cognitive deficits associated with neuroleptic use, but in somewhat less threatening language.[3]

NEUROLEPTIC-INDUCED
MENTAL DETERIORATION IN CHILDREN

Reports by Gualtieri and his colleagues (Gualtieri & Barnhill, 1988; Gualtieri et al., 1984; Gualtieri et al., 1986) indicated that many institutionalized children and young adults go through a period of worsening of their psychiatric symptoms after withdrawal from neuroleptics. This occurs in developmentally disabled patients in whom there is no complicating schizophrenic process. The researchers attribute the withdrawal-emergent problems to a drug-induced dementing process. Some patients stabilized or improved if kept medication free, but others seemed permanently worsened by the medications. They required increased medication to control their drug-induced symptoms.

Gualtieri and Barnhill (1988) pointed out that ''In virtually every clinical survey that has addressed the question, it is found that TD patients, compared to non-TD patients, have more in the way of dementia'' (p. 149). They believe that the dementia results from damage to the basal ganglia that is also associated with TD (see below).[4]

Denial of Symptoms in TD Patients
As a Symptom of Cognitive Dysfunction

Clinical reports of denial or anosognosia among TD patients also confirm that they are suffering cognitive dysfunction and most probably a dementing process. Anosognosia involves denial of lost function following neuro-

---

[3]The danger of neuroleptic-induced chronic brain dysfunction was expurgated from the *American Journal of Psychiatry* version (Grant, Adams, Carlin, Rennick, Judd, Schooff, & Reed, 1978). The misleading correlation with schizophrenia was highlighted.

[4]They declare that ''neuroleptic treatment is considered by enlightened practitioners in the field to be an extraordinary intervention'' (p. 137) requiring serious justification.

logical injury. It is said to be usually associated with damage to the parietal lobe of the nondominant hemisphere. However, patients with generalized brain disease, such as neurosyphilis and chronic alcoholism or Korsakoff's syndrome, will often deny their impairments and confabulate. My experience coincides with that of Fisher (1989) who states that anosognosia "may qualify as one of the general rules of cerebral dysfunction" (p. 128). Thus, the presence of anosognosia in tardive dyskinesia patients tends to confirm the existence of generalized cerebral dysfunction.

Multiple publications confirm that most tardive dyskinesia patients do not complain about their symptoms and will even refuse to admit their existence when confronted with them (Alexopoulos, 1979; Breggin, 1983a, 1993; Chard, Sharon, & Myslobodsky, 1986; DeVeaugh-Geiss, 1979; Smith, Kuchorski, Oswald, & Waterman, 1979; Wojcik, Gelenberg, La-Brie, & Mieske, 1980).

Patients with tardive dyskinesia not only display indifference toward their symptoms, they sometimes confabulate about them. J. M. Smith and colleagues (1979) cite several studies showing that tardive dyskinesia patients typically refuse to recognize their symptoms. They observe:

> We were so convinced that many patients were aware of their symptoms but unwilling to report them that toward the end of the project we started to ask patients at the completion of the examination if they noticed any abnormal movements in other patients. Several of the patients described the symptoms of tardive dyskinesia in other patients in great detail. Although it is conceivable that these patients might have been unaware of their own tongue or mouth movements, it is difficult to see how they could not have observed their own hand, feet, or leg movements.

DeVeaugh-Geiss (1979) has confirmed denial of symptoms, as well as lobotomy-like indifference in tardive dyskinesia patients. Despite repeated inquiries,

> Seven of these [fifteen TD] patients consistently and repeatedly denied that they had abnormal or involuntary movements, despite the fact that most of them had symptoms that were severe enough to cause some difficulty with speech, ambulation, or coordination of ordinary motor movements such as those used in eating or dressing.

Wojcik et al. (1980) found that 44% of patients with tardive dyskinesia denied awareness of their abnormal movements. Joyce Kobayashi (cited in "Patient May Not Be Cognizant," 1982) described the lack of awareness or concern about their symptoms found in more than half the TD patients selected from four wards at the Bronx Veterans Administration Medical Center.

Myslobodsky, Tomer, Holden, Kempler, and Sigol (1985) found that 88% of the TD patients "showed complete lack of concern or anosognosia with regard to their involuntary movement" (p. 156). The study also found other indications for cognitive deficits in these patients. Myslobodsky (1986) reported "emotional indifference or frank anosognosia of abnormal movements" in 95% of TD patients. He theorized that the most probable cause was "some form of cognitive decline associated with dementia disorder, probably owing to some neuroleptic-induced deficiency within the dopaminergic circuitry" (p. 4). In 1993, Myslobodsky pointed out that patients suffer from denial of TD even while they remain able to voice complaints about their other medical problems and symptoms. He postulated at that time: "TD patients lose the motor part of their 'road map of consciousness.' "

These studies of denial in TD patients strongly confirm the association between TD and cognitive dysfunction.

Permanent Lobotomy or Deactivation

In chapter 2, the primary lobotomizing or deactivating effect of the neuroleptics was described and documented. The anosognosia or denial exhibited by so many tardive dyskinesia cases probably reflects a permanent deactivation phenomenon as well as a more specific anosognosia.

Bleuler (1978, pp. 300–301) suggests that long-term exposure to neuroleptics can produce an irreversible frontal lobe syndrome with apathy and indifference. The syndrome would seem an inevitable consequence of the permanent dysfunction of dopaminergic neurons that frequently results from neuroleptic treatment. Some of these neurons (originating in the ventral tegmentum) project to the limbic system and frontal lobes. Others (from the substantia nigra) project to the striatum where they also interconnect with the limbic system as well as with the reticular activating system (Alheid, Heimer, & Switzer, 1990).

Tardive Psychosis in Neuroleptic-Treated Patients

Chapter 3 documented that the neuroleptics can produce acute depression and psychosis. There is further evidence that the neuroleptics can produce *irreversible*, schizophrenic-like psychoses (tardive psychoses). Chouinard and Jones announced this possibility at the annual meeting of the Canadian Psychiatric Association (see Jancin, 1979). One psychiatrist in the audience protested:

> I put my patients on neuroleptic drugs because they're psychotic. Now you're saying that the same drug that controls their schizophrenia also causes a psychosis and that on top of that the drug causes tardive dyskinesia one third of the time. It's a Hobson's choice. My patients are going to lose in the end either way.

One of the panelists, Barry D. Jones, warned, "Some patients who seem to require lifelong neuroleptics may actually do so because of this therapy."

In the published version (Chouinard & Jones, 1980), the authors suggested that the irreversible "supersensitivity psychosis" results from rebound hyperactivity of the blockaded dopamine receptors in the limbic system. They compare the mechanism of supersensitivity psychosis to that of tardive dyskinesia.

Chouinard and Jones note that both the tardive dyskinesia and the supersensitivity psychosis are "masked" or hidden when the patient is taking drugs. They further state that continuous taking of the drugs tends to worsen both diseases. Neuroleptic-treated patients developed tardive psychoses that became more severe than their original psychiatric disorders (Chouinard & Jones, 1980; Chouinard & Jones, 1982; Chouinard, Jones, & Annable, 1978; Csernansky & Hollister, 1982; Hunt, Singh, & Simpson, 1988; Mayerhoff & Lieberman, 1992; also see news reports by Jancin, 1979 and "Supersensitivity Psychosis," 1983). Tragically, patients can require lifetime medication for a disorder that could have had a much shorter and more benign natural history.

The frequency of tardive psychosis remains controversial within psychiatry. Although Chouinard and Jones have found a prevalence of 30%–40%, Hunt, Singh, and Simpson (1988) reviewed the charts of 265 patients and located 12 probable and no definite cases of tardive psychosis. Kirkpatrick, Alphs, and Buchanan (1992) have cast a critical eye on the existence of tardive psychosis.

Withdrawal Problems and Tardive Psychosis

Clinicians have become increasingly aware of the difficulty of removing patients from neuroleptics, partly because of what appears to be tardive psychosis. Withdrawal from the drugs also can produce transient or persistent dyskinesias, dysphoria, and autonomic imbalances, resulting in nausea and weight loss. As already noted, the difficulties of neuroleptic withdrawal have led me to raise the issue of their addictiveness (Breggin, 1989a, 1989b).

Clozapine may have an especially marked withdrawal syndrome characterized by a worsening psychosis, angry or abusive language, hyperactivity, agitation and restlessness, dyskinesia, confusion, and aggressive or suicidal behavior. It can develop during therapy and result in adverse reactions to the drug ("Clozapine," 1994).

Tardive Akathisia and Cognitive Deficits

Gualtieri (1993) has observed that the anxiety and emotional tension suffered by tardive akathisia patients are primary emotional and cognitive components of the disease. After reviewing the functional neuroanatomy, Gualtieri concluded:

> One is entitled to surmise, therefore, that affective instability and intellectual impairment may be the consequence of neuropathology at the level of the basal ganglia. . . . TDAK [tardive akathisia] is one manifestation of that effect. There are probably others.

In other words, the existence of the syndrome of tardive akathisia demonstrates that the neuroleptics can produce irreversible damage to the mental life of the individual.

BRAIN SCANS

I have reviewed the brain scan literature elsewhere (Breggin, 1990, 1993) and will summarize some of the highlights. Overall, the literature confirms that neuroleptics can and do cause permanent damage to the higher centers of the brain and to the mind.

CT Scans and Neuropsychological Correlations

Many studies involving computerized axial tomography (CT) scans of psychiatric patients, most but not all of whom were diagnosed schizophrenic, have found enlarged lateral ventricles and sometimes enlarged sulci, indicating shrinkage or atrophy of the brain. Nearly all these studies involve patients heavily treated with neuroleptics. A number of the CT scan studies have found a correlation between atrophy and persistent cognitive deficits or frank dementia in these neuroleptic-treated patients (DeMeyer, Gilmore, Hendrie et al., 1984; Famuyiwa, Eccleston, Donaldson, & Garside, 1979; Golden et al., 1980; Johnstone, Crow, Frith, Husband, & Kreel, 1976; Lawson, Waldman, & Weinberger, 1988). Some of these studies used the Nebraska and Halstead-Reitan batteries, considered among the most sensitive for detecting brain damage and dysfunction.

While some of the studies claim that drugs could not have caused the brain abnormalities, they do not provide evidence that confirms this viewpoint (e.g., Johnstone et al., 1976; Johnstone et al., 1978; Lawson et al., 1988; Shelton et al., 1988; Weinberger, Cannon-Spoor, Potkin, & Wyatt, 1980; Weinberger, Torrey, Neophytides, & Wyatt, 1979).

Two studies that have evaluated relatively young and relatively untreated patients have found enlarged ventricles (Schulz et al., 1983; Weinberger, DeLisi, Perman, Targum, & Wyatt, 1982; reviewed in detail in Breggin, 1990). Very small numbers of patients were involved and other studies have not confirmed their findings (Benes et al., 1982; Iacono et al., 1988; Jernigan, Zatz, Moses, & Cardellino, 1982; Tanaka, Hazama, Kawahara, & Kobayashi, 1981).

MRI Scans and Neuropsychological Testing

Magnetic resonance imaging (MRI) studies have begun to replace the CT scan in studies of psychiatric patients. A 1988 MRI study by Kelso, Cadet, Pickar, and Weinberger confirms the general findings on many CT studies. So does an unpublished study by Andreasen and her colleagues (cited in Andreasen, 1988). In the eight studies reviewed by Kelsoe et al. (1988), a few showed no abnormalities, and the majority showed a variety of somewhat inconsistent abnormalities. However, the weight of the studies leans toward a finding of atrophy in the brains of neuroleptic-treated schizophrenic patients. More recently, researchers (Breier et al., 1992) found several areas of reduced volume in the limbic system of the brain of neuroleptic-treated chronic schizophrenic patients.

An MRI twin study, published in the *New England Journal of Medicine* by Suddath, Christison, Torrey, Casanova, and Weinberger (1990), received enormous attention in the general and professional press as demonstrating a causal relationship between schizophrenia and brain atrophy. In reality, it disclosed a much more probable connection between neuroleptic exposure and brain damage. (I have discussed the misleading promotion of this study in *Toxic Psychiatry* [Breggin, 1991a, p. 113].) The project examined the brains of 15 sets of twins, each pair with one member who was diagnosed and treated for schizophrenia, and one member who was not. In 12 pairs, there was evidence of brain shrinkage in the form of reduced hippocampus size and enlarged lateral and third ventricles in the schizophrenic twin.

Suddath's group assumes that schizophrenia is the source of difference in the brains of the schizophrenic twins, but tucked toward the end of the article is the admission that they ''cannot rule out'' treatment as the primary cause of the atrophy. Two patients had been given shock treatment, and all the patients had enormous, long-term exposure to neuroleptics. Most of these patients probably suffered from tardive dyskinesia and yet the authors fail to report, to discuss, or even to mention, TD in their paper. Failure to carefully evaluate each patient for TD and correlate TD with the brain shrinkage renders this study without merit. Several studies, reviewed in this chapter, have shown a correlation between TD, brain shrinkage, and dementia (see below).

I asked Michigan State University psychologist Bertram Karon to review the statistical data in Suddath et al. He responded, ''The conclusion most consistent with the presented data is that the authors have found strong evidence that neuroleptic medication is brain-damaging'' (see Breggin, 1991a, p. 114).

PET Scans

Recently positron emission tomography (PET) scanning has been used to measure the metabolic rate and blood flow of various parts of the brain. This instrument can detect dysfunction that does not necessarily manifest as gross pathology. It can also measure functional changes that have no pathological origin.

From the earliest studies, there has been a somewhat consistent finding of hypoactivity in the frontal lobes and frontal cortex of neuroleptic-treated schizophrenics (Buchsbaum et al., 1982; Farkas et al., 1984; Wolkin et al., 1988 [reviewed in Andreasen, 1988]; Wolkin et al., 1985). However, not all reports confirm the finding of frontal hypoactivity (Gur, Resnick, Alavi et al., 1987; Gur, Resnick, Gur et al., 1987). In most studies, the patients had long histories of neuroleptic treatment prior to being removed temporarily for the PET scans.

The PET scan has been used to study specific parts of the brain in which the neuroleptics are known to produce dysfunction by blockade of the dopamine neurotransmitter system, including the basal ganglia. A variety of studies show that the basal ganglia of neuroleptic-treated patients can develop abnormalities (Farde, Wiesel, Halldin, & Sedvall, 1988). However, there are also many negative PET studies (see Buchsbaum et al., 1992, and a lengthy summary table in Andreasen et al., 1992; also Andreasen, 1988).

One PET study involving unmedicated patients found no frontal hypoactivity (Sheppard et al., 1983). Another with unmedicated patients showed increased frontal metabolism (Cleghorn et al., 1989). Recently, Buchsbaum et al. (1992) found hypofrontality in never-medicated schizophrenic patients. However, the results were not definitive: "The hypofrontality effect was modestly sensitive and not strongly specific."

Some PET studies have measured cerebral blood flow in neuroleptic-naive schizophrenic patients while the subjects were asked to perform a task intended to activate the frontal lobes. Andreasen et al. (1992) found "decreased activation occurred only in the patients with high scores for negative symptoms. These results suggest that hypofrontality is related to negative symptoms and is not a long-term effect of neuroleptic treatment or of chronicity of illness." The conclusion has an obvious flaw: High scores for negative symptoms means that the patients almost surely would have been less cooperative, therefore putting less energy into the task that was supposed to elicit frontal lobe activity.

Overall, the finding of subtle differences in energy usage in the brains of any individuals, schizophrenic or not, could have a psychological origin. It is well known, for example, that different states of consciousness affect the amplitude and frequency of electrical waves. Biofeedback experiments have shown that a person can consciously control these changes.

Correlating TD with Brain Damage and Dementia

Surprisingly few studies have attempted to correlate brain scan findings with the presence of TD. Bartels and Themelis (1983) found abnormalities in the basal ganglia of TD patients; but overall the results have been mixed and inconclusive (Besson, Corrigan, Cherryman, & Smith, 1987; Goetz & van Kammen, 1986; Jeste, Wagner, Weinberger, Reith, & Wyatt, 1980; Koshino, Hiramatsu, Isaki, & Yamaguchi, 1986).

Summary of Brain Scan Data

Mounting radiological evidence from PET, MRI, and CT scans confirms the presence of chronic brain dysfunction (PET scans) and brain atrophy (MRI and CT scans) in neuroleptic-treated schizophrenic patients. The total number of relevant CT scan studies is estimated to be over 90 (Kelso et al., 1988), most of which show damage. Some studies implicate the total lifetime amount of neuroleptic intake (DeMeyer, Gilmore, DeMeyer et al., 1984; Lyon et al., 1981). A number of researchers try to attribute the findings to schizophrenia, but there is little justification for this (see below).

Rates of Tardive Dementia Based on Brain Scans

Studies indicate that the percentage of drug-treated schizophrenic patients with atrophy on CT scans varies from 0% to over 50%. If treatment has been lengthy and intensive, as in Suddath et al. (1990), *most* patients may show brain atrophy. Reported rates are substantial, typically in a range of 10%–40%. Coming to a similar conclusion, Andreasen (1988) reviewed the literature and found a range of 6%–40%. Andreasen noted that higher rates were reported with increasing severity and length of illness. This would also correlate with length and intensity of treatment with neuroleptics.

HUMAN AND ANIMAL AUTOPSY STUDIES

Animal autopsy data strongly confirm that the neuroleptics frequently cause brain damage. Human autopsy studies are too few and contradictory to lead to a definite conclusion.

Animal Autopsy Studies of Neuroleptic-Induced Brain Damage

Multiple controlled animal studies indicate that long-term, and sometimes short-term, neuroleptic treatment causes brain damage. Evidence of structural damage, including cell degeneration and death in the basal ganglia, is especially consistent after chronic administration of neuroleptics (Coln, 1975; Jeste, Lohr, & Manley, 1992; Mackiewicz & Gershon, 1964; Nielsen & Lyon, 1978; Pakkenberg, Fog, & Nilakantan, 1973; Popova, 1967; Romasenko & Jacobson, 1969; reviewed in Breggin, 1983a). Far fewer studies have been negative (Fog et al., 1976; Gerlach, 1975).

After one "comparatively low" dose of chlorpromazine, 0.5 to 5 mg/kg, Popova (1967) found structural changes in rat brains, including "swelling, chromatolysis and vacuolization of the nerve cell bodies" (p. 87) in many regions, including the sensory-motor cortex, midbrain, hypothalamus, thalamus, and reticular formation. In 1992 Jeste, Lohr, and Manley reviewed the literature and published the results of exposing rats to fluphenazine decanoate (5 mg/kg, intramuscular) every 2 weeks for 4, 8, or 12 months. The density of large neurons in the striatum was measured after sacrifice by a computerized image-analysis system. This team found a reduced density by 8 months of treatment.

Most animal studies report irreversible neuronal damage, including cell death, after relatively brief exposure to neuroleptics. Of great importance, animal studies with longer durations of exposure to neuroleptics—1 year (Pakkenberg et al., 1973): 8 months (Jeste et al., 1992); and 36 weeks (Nielsen & Lyon, 1978)—show the expected neuronal deterioration in the basal ganglia.

Animal research provides definitive and apparently incontrovertible evidence that neuroleptics often cause irreversible brain damage.

Human Autopsy Evidence
for Neuroleptic-Induced Brain Damage

There are surprisingly few human autopsy reports related to chronic neuroleptic therapy. They have been reviewed by Bracha and Kleinman (1986); Brown, Colter, et al. (1986); Jeste, Iager, and Wyatt (1986); and Rupniak, Jenner, and Marsden (1983). Although somewhat inconclusive, autopsy evidence does suggest that the neuroleptics can damage the basal ganglia, areas potentially critical in the production of both TD and tardive dementia. The literature, overall, is contradictory and not conclusive. The studies of Arai et al. (1987); Brown et al. (1986); Christensen et al. (1970); Forrest, Forrest, and Roizin (1963); Gross and Kaltenback (1968); Hunter, Blackwood, Smith, and Cumings (1968); Jellinger (1977); Roizin, True, and Knight (1959); and Wildi, Linder, and Costoulas (1967) are reviewed in more detail in Breggin (1990).

Mechanisms of Neuroleptic-Induced Cell Death

Neuroleptics can damage or destroy brain cells through a variety of mechanisms. They not only suppress the gross function of dopaminergic neurons, they disrupt a variety of metabolic functions within neurons and other cells throughout the body. It has been known for many years that these drugs inhibit most enzyme systems in the mitochondria (Teller & Denber, 1970), which are the principal sites for many of the most important metabolic processes in the cell. Recent research by Inuwa, Horobin, and Williams (1994) demonstrates that neuroleptics are absorbed into human cell mitochondria where they interfere with metabolic processes and cause structural abnormalities. The authors suggest ''It is possible that such interaction may be cytopathic leading to premature cell death'' (p. 1091).

I examined several of the major psychiatric and psychopharmacological textbooks and was unable to locate a single mention or reference concerning these important, well-documented cytotoxic processes.

THE LESSONS OF LETHARGIC ENCEPHALITIS[5]

Chapter 3 discussed the similarity between neuroleptic malignant syndrome and an acute episode of the viral disorder, lethargic encephalitis (encephalitis lethargica or von Economo's disease). The parallel suggests that the neuroleptics, in their primary impact, produce a controlled ''chemical encephalitis'' which, when out of control, becomes neuroleptic malignant syndrome, indistinguishable from a fulminating viral encephalitis (Breggin, 1993).

There are many other ways in which neuroleptic drug effects closely mimic those of lethargic encephalitis as reported during and after World War I (Breggin, 1993). Both the neuroleptics and the viral disease produce mental apathy and indifference. In a 1970 retrospective, Deniker observed:

---

[5]This subject fascinated me sufficiently for me to devote an entire paper to it (Breggin, 1993).

It was found that neuroleptics could experimentally reproduce almost all symptoms of lethargic encephalitis. In fact, it would be possible to cause true encephalitis epidemics with the new drugs.

The parallel between lethargic encephalitis and neuroleptic toxicity is remarkable in several respects. Both groups of patients initially display apathy or disinterest, followed by the onset of various dyskinesias. After a delay, the dyskinesias sometimes become permanent in both groups. Many lethargic encephalitis patients seemed to recover, only to relapse into devastating neurological disorders years later. While a Parkinson-like disorder was the most common "tardive," or delayed, motor disorder associated with lethargic encephalitis, other dyskinesias more similar to drug-induced TD were also known to develop.

After an apparent recovery, many of the encephalitis victims later went on to develop severe psychoses and dementia (Abrahamson, 1935; Matheson Commission, 1939). Thus, the completion of the parallel between lethargic encephalitis and neuroleptic effects awaited the discovery that in addition to TD, tardive psychosis and tardive dementia could follow the exposure to neuroleptics.

The parallel between the medication effects and the viral encephalo-pathic effects sounded a warning that similar mechanisms—and, hence, similar adverse outcomes—were possible. This concern was raised early by Paulson (1959), who wrote:

> The sequelae of encephalitis include many muscular, psychic and autonomic responses; and most of the neurologic complications from the phenothi-azines are within the range of post-encephalitic parkinsonism. (p. 800)

Other investigators also noticed comparisons between neuroleptic toxicity and lethargic encephalitis (Brill, 1959; Hunter et al., 1964). Brill documented that the hardest hit areas in lethargic encephalitis are the cells of the basal ganglia and the substantia nigra, the areas most affected by the neuroleptic medications in the production of TD (see Breggin, 1993, for a further discussion of the anatomic pathways). There are multiple interconnections between the basal ganglia, reticular activating system, limbic system, and cerebral cortex, involving the basal ganglia directly and indirectly with mental functions (e.g., Adams & Victor, 1989; Alheid, Heimer, & Switzer, 1990; Brodal, 1969). Neuroleptic-induced damage to the basal ganglia, if severe enough, would be expected to produce persistent cognitive deficits and dementia.

The association of mental deterioration with diseases of the basal ganglia and substantia nigra led to the concept of subcortical dementia (Huber & Paulson, 1985), that is, dementia arising from damage to the basal ganglia and surrounding structures. Patients with subcortical dementia tend to be more depressed and apathetic, without as much evidence of gross impairment to higher cortical functions.

Marsden (1976) observed, "If long-term neuroleptic therapy can cause an apparently permanent change in striatal dopamine-receptor action, then one must assume that the same can occur in the mesolimbic cortical dopamine receptors" (p. 1079). More recently, Marsden and Obeso (1994) have pointed out the complex interconnections between the basal ganglia and the frontal lobes, and their possible role in higher mental functioning.

Animal research has confirmed that supersensitivity of dopamine receptors develops in the mesolimbic and cerebral cortical areas, much as it does in the striatum (Chiodo & Bunney, 1983; White & Wang, 1983) and that it can become chronic after termination of neuroleptic treatment (Jenner & Marsden, 1983; Rupniak et al., 1983). While tardive dyskinesia is difficult to reproduce in animals, Gunne and Haggstrom (1985) have been able to create both acute and irreversible dyskinesias in monkeys and rats. With persistent dyskinesias, they found evidence of irreversible biochemical changes in the basal ganglia and related areas (substantia nigra, medial globus pallidus, and nucleus subthalamicus).

Many researchers have remarked on the relationship between inhibition in the mesolimbic and cortical dopamine system and the clinical production of blunting or apathy (Lehman, 1975; White & Wang, 1983). Irreversible changes in these systems account for many findings of permanent cognitive dysfunction.

Gualtieri and Barnhill (1988) have confirmed these observations:

> Persistent TD is probably the consequence of irreversible striatal damage. But the corpus striatum is responsible for more than motor control; it is a complex organ that influences a wide range of complex human behaviors. No disease that afflicts striatal tissue is known to have only motor consequences; Parkinson's disease and Huntington's disease are only two examples. [citations omitted] (p. 150)

SCHIZOPHRENIA AS A POSSIBLE CAUSE OF DEMENTIA

There is a very cogent reason to believe that the atrophy found on CT scans cannot be the product of schizophrenia. Brain atrophy is far more accurately and definitively evaluated by a direct postmortem pathological examination than on a CT scan. The actual pathology, if it exists, can more easily be identified and accurately measured by direct observation and microscopic studies.

The CT scan and the MRI scan capture images in the range of the human eye. The MRI scan, for example, examines a slice of brain approximately 1–3 mm thick (Innis & Malison, 1995). That's the width of 1–3 pencil leads. Furthermore, the images are limited to black and white. The best MRI resolution only begins to approximate what can be seen with the naked eye on autopsy (Innis & Malison, 1995, pp. 89–90).

An autopsy can also obtain tissue slices for examination with a light microscope or an electron microscope. Furthermore, on gross examination of the brain, instead of estimating tissue loss from MRI pictures, an autopsy can actually weigh and measure the brain, and examine cell density under the microscope. As a result, many diseases of the brain, such as Alzheimer's, require an autopsy rather than an MRI or CT scan to make the definitive diagnosis (Caine, Grossman, & Lyness, 1995, p. 726).

Despite the greater usefulness and relevance of autopsy data, no consistent finding of brain atrophy or any other pathology was made in hundreds of autopsy studies performed on schizophrenics prior to the use of neuroleptics (e.g., Bleuler, 1978, p. 451; Nicholi, 1978; Noyes & Kolb, 1958, pp. 387–389). Arieti (1959) found that hopes for a neuropathology of schizophrenia "have remained unfulfilled" (p. 488). Weinberger and Kleinman (1986) estimated that by 1950 more than 250 studies had claimed to find a gross pathological defect in schizophrenia and "the overwhelming majority of these claims were either never replicated, unreplicable, or shown to be artifacts." The task proved so frustrating that "the effort stalled in the 1950s" (p. 52). When the Task Force on Tardive Dyskinesia (American Psychiatric Association, 1980) made a brief reference to the initial CT scan findings of brain atrophy in neuroleptic-treated patients, it remarked, "this observation is quite surprising as it is not consistent with earlier neurologic evaluations of chronic schizophrenics; it requires further critical evaluation" (p. 59).

Furthermore, prior to the neuroleptics there was no consistent dementia syndrome found in association with schizophrenia. That is why schizophrenia became known as a "functional" rather than an "organic" disorder, and why a diagnosis of schizophrenia in fact requires first ruling out an underlying organic disorder.

In reply to the question "do schizophrenic patients have cerebral atrophy, dilated ventricles, neurological deficits, dementia," Lidz (1981) observed that "for 100 years investigators have reported a neuropathological or physiopathological cause of schizophrenia. The trouble is that no such findings have been replicated. If the patient suffers from dementia, the diagnosis is not schizophrenia" (p. 854). Lidz recommended taking into account the impact of medications and shock treatment on the brain.

The failure to obtain consistent findings of cerebral pathology on postmortem examination prior to the drug era strongly indicates that recent findings of atrophy on brain scans are the result, not of schizophrenia, but of some new threat to the brain of these patients. The new threat is the widespread use of the neuroleptic drugs which are already known to cause brain diseases, including TD and NMS.

Other reasons to doubt that schizophrenics have a deteriorating brain disorder have been reviewed by Manfred Bleuler (1978). First, unless they are caused by a toxic agent which is then removed, organic disorders characterized by brain atrophy and dementia are usually progressive. Yet it is well-documented by Bleuler and others that many schizophrenic patients improve over time; up to one third or one half show significant recovery over the years. They do not tend to show the physical signs of deterioration usually associated with progressive neurological losses, such as premature aging, infirmity, seizures, or neurological signs and symptoms. They die of the same diseases that afflict normal people. In following 208 patients for decades, Bleuler found that most of them remained in generally good health "in spite of advanced age" (p. 450).

Second, a dementing disorder, once it has progressed, would rarely if ever clear up spontaneously. Yet there are many examples, even before the advent of medications, of patients abruptly and spontaneously improving for years at a time or for a lifetime. Similarly, many patients wax and wane, showing great clarity at one moment and extreme irrationality at another (see E. Bleuler, 1924; M. Bleuler, 1978).

Sometimes an emergency will temporarily arouse a seemingly chronic and incapacitated patient into a state of acute awareness and rational behavior. As a resident, I was the admitting doctor for a patient diagnosed paranoid schizophrenic. She refused to let me perform a routine physical examination as a part of her admission to the psychiatric ward, until I noticed from her breathing that she had signs of pneumonia. When I told her, in effect, "You're really sick; I need to examine you," she stopped behaving irrationally and allowed me to listen to her lungs, confirming my suspicion of pneumonia. When the exam was over, she reverted to her previous nearly catatonic behavior.

Third, schizophrenic patients do not suffer from the typical signs of the earlier stages of a dementing disorder, such as short-term memory dysfunction. They are usually easy to distinguish, for example, from victims of Alzheimer's disease, multi-infarct dementia, and the dementias associated with Parkinson's disease, Huntington's chorea, or multiple sclerosis.

Fourth, instead of deteriorating, the schizophrenic's intellectual functions become misdirected or psychologically deranged. Schizophrenics often speak in unusual and complex metaphors dealing with psychological and spiritual conflicts over the meaning of love, life, or God. Often they display enormous passion around the concept of their own presumed evil or exalted nature. Quite frequently only one or two specific false ideas (delusions) will appear in an otherwise normal mental life. These delusions will be defended with intellectual vigor and a high degree of mental acuity indicating that overall brain function itself is normal and often above average.

In summary, there is almost no reason to believe that findings of brain atrophy and dementia are caused by schizophrenia, while there is overwhelming evidence to indict neuroleptic therapy.

Psychiatric Denial of Neuroleptic-Induced Dementia

It took psychiatry 20 years to recognize tardive dyskinesia as an iatrogenic illness, although it afflicted a large portion of hospitalized patients (Gelman, 1984). As noted in chapter 4, resistance to dealing adequately with tardive dyskinesia continues (Breggin, 1983a; Brown & Funk, 1986; Cohen & McCubbin, 1990; Wolf & Brown, 1987). An even greater reluctance to recognize tardive dementia and brain atrophy is likely, since the damage is still more catastrophic. Furthermore, it is easier to overlook cognitive defects and dementia than to ignore dyskinesias, and easier as well to mistakenly attribute the deficits to the patient's psychiatric disorder.

The "Newer" Atypical Neuroleptics

Because the atypical neuroleptics have received so much publicity, and because information about them is not so readily available to many readers, I will single them out for a somewhat more detailed discussion.

The last several years have seen the introduction of several new neuroleptics in the United States. The most publicity has been given to clozapine (Clozaril), a drug that has been covered in the news media as if it were a newly discovered miracle. While not introduced into this country until 1990, clozapine is in fact an old drug. It was synthesized in 1960 and caused so many deaths in Europe by the mid-1970s that it was banned in some European countries and its development was curtailed in this country. Its tendency to suppress white cell production in the bone marrow (agranulocytosis) can result in lethal infections and requires close supervision and regular blood counts. That the FDA approved clozapine indicates its growing leniency toward drug companies (see chapter 11).

Clozapine causes a particularly high rate of grand mal seizures, estimated at 4%–5% in the first year. This is a very serious hazard. The drug frequently produces severe low blood pressure and increased heart rate, potentially resulting in collapse. It can also cause hypertension. It can cause fever and a flu-like syndrome. Respiratory arrest has been reported (Westlin, 1991). It can be particularly hazardous for the elderly who may risk falls, cardiovascular problems, or delirium (Pitner et al., 1995).

Clozapine, like more typical neuroleptics, blocks dopaminergic neurotransmission. It seems to be more potent in this regard in the limbic (emotion-regulating) system than in the striatal region (which controls both emotion and voluntary movement) (Chiodo & Bunney, 1983). Because of the drug's greater impact on the frontal lobes and limbic system, it was thought that it would produce more therapeutic effect with fewer extrapyramidal side effects. The drug probably does produce a more profound deactivation or lobotomy-like syndrome in some patients, accounting for its reputation for sometimes working better than other neuroleptics. As a result, it probably has a greater risk of producing permanent frontal lobe damage and tardive dementia or tardive psychosis.

Concern about clozapine's especially damaging effect on higher brain functions was voiced as early as 1977 by Ungerstedt and Ljungberg, based on the European experience. Chouinard and Jones (1982) pointed to observations on reactive psychoses following withdrawal from clozapine and commented, "This convincing evidence of clozapine's ability to induce supersensitivity psychosis might be related to both the short half-life of the drug and its greater affinity for mesolimbic dopamine receptors." More recent observations have also pointed to the possible existence of clozapine withdrawal psychoses (see Adams & Essali, 1991). There is a report of a clozapine withdrawal syndrome that includes new symptoms of agitation, restlessness, shakiness, dyskinesia, confusion, sweating, aggression, and suicidal behavior ("Clozapine withdrawal syndrome," 1994; Richardson & Partridge, 1993).

Clozapine's anticholinergic effects can cause confusion and delirium, as well as sedation and lethargy. It can aggravate or cause hypersalivation, glaucoma, constipation and ileus, and urinary retention (Baldessarini & Frankenburg, 1991). Weight gain is a serious problem.

While it may in some studies cause fewer extrapyramidal reactions, clozapine can produce every one of the neurological reactions associated with neuroleptic use, including neuroleptic malignant syndrome (Anderson & Powers, 1991; DasGupta & Young, 1991) and tardive dyskinesia (Weller & Kornhuber, 1993).

Overall, caution is necessary concerning claims that atypical neuroleptics do not cause as much extrapyramidal side effects as other neuroleptics. This book has already documented how easy it has been for psychiatry to overlook or minimize severe drug-induced neurological reactions. Furthermore, the relative absence of obvious neurological syndromes may lull psychiatrists into overlooking the more devastating damage these drugs may end up inflicting on the frontal lobes and limbic system, and hence on the mental life of patients.

Clozapine's efficacy has been highly touted to the public but in reality is questionable even by conventional standards (see comments of psychiatrist Herbert Meltzer in Winslow, 1990). Furthermore, in the arena of neuroleptics, a better or stronger drug is in reality a more suppressive and potentially more destructive drug.

Risperidone (Risperdal) is a more recently marketed (1994) atypical neuroleptic and its newness limits the availability of information on harmful effects. The clinical trials, most of which lasted a few weeks, were too short to determine the rate of tardive dyskinesia and many other adverse effects. Indeed, the brief controlled clinical trials used for the approval of both clozapine and risperidone do not provide sufficient information to determine either efficacy or safety, since the drugs will be used for months and years in individual patients rather than weeks (see chapter 11). Patients taking the medications over the coming years will provide the experimental data. Meanwhile, the FDA has required the same tardive dyskinesia and neuroleptic malignant syndrome warnings on the labels of clozapine and risperidone as on the labels of the older neuroleptics.

Risperidone has a particular tendency to produce adverse stimulant effects, including insomnia, agitation, and anxiety. Probably because of these stimulant effects, it may have an increased risk of causing mania (Dwight, Keck, Stanton, Strakowski, & McElroy, 1994). Stimulation may also account for risperidone-induced rage attacks and the urge to resume substance abuse, although the author of the report believes these reactions are due to despair from increased psychological insight (Post, 1994). In addition to stimulation, the drug frequently causes fatigue, sleepiness, or insomnia.

Risperidone causes all the extrapyramidal reactions found with other neuroleptics, including tardive dyskinesia (Addington, Toews, & Addington, 1995) and neuroleptic malignant syndrome (Mahendra, 1995; Singer, Colette, & Boland, 1995; chapter 4 of this book). It is too early to tell if the rate of tardive dyskinesia will differ from that of other neuroleptics.

A recent report found that even small doses of risperidone (average dose of 1.7 mg/day) produced or worsened acute extrapyramidal reactions in one-third of an elderly population suffering from dementia (Baker, 1996). Among 41 patients, 6 developed new parkinsonism, 5 had a worsening of previous parkinsonism, one developed cervical dystonia, and one developed neuroleptic malignant syndrome while also taking Tegretol and Mellaril.

Like most neuroleptics, risperidone can cause mammary cancer in rats and mice but this finding has not been taken seriously enough by the FDA, the profession, or the drug companies (reviewed in Breggin, 1991a).

Because of the interest in these newer agents, I have described their broad array of adverse effects in more detail than with the older neuroleptics. The most important point, however, is their brain-disabling effect. Neuroleptics have their effect by producing deactivation and a lobotomy syndrome. If more potent ones can be developed, they will be worse, rather than better, for the patients.

Drugs to Treat Acute Extrapyramidal Side Effects

A variety of drugs are used to control neuroleptic-induced acute extrapyramidal effects, such as tremors, rigidity, akathisia, and dystonia. Most of these agents suppress the cholinergic nervous system. They include benztropine (Cogentin), biperiden (Akineton), procyclidine (Kemadrin), and trihexyphenidyl (Artane). These agents produce multiple anticholinergic side effects, including glaucoma, severe constipation, ileus, and the inability to empty the bladder. Since many of the neuroleptics also produce anticholinergic effects, the likelihood of these adverse reactions is increased when they are combined.

From the brain-disabling viewpoint, anticholinergic drugs can cause confusion, organic brain syndromes, and psychoses. Far too little attention has been paid to their adverse effects on memory and learning that could interfere with everyday living, rehabilitation, or school (Marcus, Plasky, & Salzman, 1988; McEvoy, 1987).

There is widespread concern that these drugs may contribute to or worsen tardive dyskinesia. They can cause withdrawal symptoms in the form of rebound hyperactivity of the cholinergic system, including a flu-like syndrome and emotional discomfort.

CONCLUSION

There is convincing evidence that long-term treatment with neuroleptic medication frequently produces persistent cognitive deficits, dementia, and atrophy of the highest centers of the brain. Much of the evidence is accumulated from brain imaging, human postmortems, animal autopsies, clinical evaluations, and neuropsychological testing. The association of tardive dyskinesia with irreversible cognitive dysfunction and dementia in itself demonstrates that the neuroleptics frequently cause permanent mental dysfunction. The lessons of functional neuroanatomy made that association inevitable. In addition, there is evidence that neuroleptics also produce tardive psychosis. By contrast, there is little or no reason to believe that schizophrenia causes dementia and brain atrophy.

The most consistent information on prevalence has been generated by brain scans which measure brain atrophy. We can estimate a prevalence of 10%–40% among neuroleptic-treated patients. It probably exceeds 50% in older patients and in more intense, long-term treatment. Not surprisingly, these figures are somewhat parallel to those for tardive dyskinesia, which strikes the same anatomical region.

Even if the rate turns out to be in the lower range, we are confronted with an epidemic of iatrogenic brain damage of large proportions with serious consequences. Millions of patients, some with tardive dyskinesia and some without, have developed drug-induced damage to the higher brain and mental processes.

CHAPTER 6

Antidepressants, Including Prozac-Induced Violence and Suicide*

The antidepressants include tricyclics, the monoamine oxidase inhibitors (MAOIs), the "second generation" antidepressants (Appleton, 1982; Kielholz, 1980), and the recent selective serotonin reuptake inhibitors (SSRIs). The SSRIs will receive special attention in this chapter.

It remains important to remember that children and the elderly are especially susceptible to toxic effects. Older populations are very prone to the brain-disabling impact of antidepressant drugs (Leipzig & Saltz, 1992).

THE SSRIs

The SSRIs include the antidepressants fluoxetine (Prozac), sertraline (Zoloft), and paroxetine (Paxil), as well as fluvoxamine (Luvox) for the treatment of obsessive-compulsive disorder. To a great extent, they can be treated as one group of similar agents. These drugs have their greatest

---

*A small portion of the material on Prozac is adapted from *Talking Back to Prozac* (Breggin & Breggin, 1994a). I wish to thank St. Martin's Press for permission to use this material, some of which is presented in much greater detail in the 1994 book.

impact on the brain by preventing the removal (reuptake) of serotonin from the synaptic cleft, in effect flooding the space between the neurons with serotonin. This can increase the activity of postsynaptic neurons, making them fire more frequently. However, the brain resists the toxic intrusion by activating mechanisms that compensate for or stop this process, producing an unpredictable imbalance (Breggin & Breggin, 1994a).

Theoretical attempts have been made to explain why hyperactivity of this system should relieve depression, but they are at present speculative. They also raise the specter that when the brain produces compensatory "sluggishness" in the system, it could lead to opposite and untoward effects, such as depression and suicide or violence (see below and Breggin & Breggin, 1994a).

Venlafaxine (Effexor), another recently approved antidepressant, inhibits the reuptake of serotonin but not selectively and it is therefore not considered an SSRI. It also inhibits the reuptake of norepinephrine and to a lesser extent dopamine. However, as its FDA-approved label documents, it shares nearly all the adverse effects of SSRIs, such as Prozac, that will be discussed in this chapter. It is known to cause the basic stimulant profile of agitation, anxiety, nervousness, insomnia, anorexia and weight loss, and mania. Consistent with this, severe abnormal behaviors and emotional reactions have been reported in association with its use, including paranoid reaction, hostility, psychotic depression, delusions, and psychosis. Again, like the SSRIs, it can produce various abnormal movements, including painful torticollis (spasm of the neck muscles) and hyperactivity. Like the SSRIs, it can cause impairments of sexual function.

Drugs with stimulant profiles, including Effexor and Prozac, can have a variety of effects, including paradoxical sedation and fatigue. Frequently their dominant impact is to produce a flattening or blunting of all feeling.

Background Information on Prozac

In *Talking Back to Prozac,* Breggin and Breggin (1994a) offered a detailed analysis of the clinical and scientific data pertaining to Prozac safety and efficacy, including an examination of the FDA approval process (see chapter 11). Before presenting new material on Prozac, the following sections will highlight some of the earlier information from the 1994 book.

Prozac Acts Like a Stimulant

After all the data had been collected during Prozac's NDA[1] approval process, FDA psychiatrist Richard Kapit (March 28, 1986) wrote the official "Safety Review" of adverse reactions or side effects. Kapit summarized: "Most frequently this new drug caused nausea, insomnia, and nervousness, which resembles the profile of a stimulant rather than a sedative drug." He thought this stimulant profile would "give rise to the greatest clinical liabilities in the use of this medication," including "insomnia, nervousness, anorexia, and weight loss." Later in his report, Kapit repeated his observations, stating that Prozac's "profile of adverse effects more closely resembles that of a stimulant drug than one that causes sedation and gain of weight." Kapit concluded:

> It is possible that these adverse effects of fluoxetine treatment may negatively affect patients with depression. Since depressed patients frequently suffer from insomnia, nervousness, anorexia, and weight loss, it is possible that fluoxetine treatment might, at least temporarily, make their illness worse.

He repeated this concern in his summary, stating "It is possible, therefore, that fluoxetine may exacerbate certain depressive symptoms and signs." He recommended that the label warn physicians about these dangers.

Later, in his "Safety Update" of the NDA on October 17, 1986, Kapit spoke of several cases of a "syndrome of fluoxetine-induced hyper-arousal and excessive stimulation . . . [which] resemble episodes of stimulant drug intoxication." It was especially likely to occur at higher doses; but it could occur at the standard 20 mgs. The state of overstimulation included "anxiety, agitation, insomnia, headache, confusion, dizziness, obnubilation [mental clouding], memory dysfunction, tremor, impaired motor coordination. Hyperactivity, hypomania, and mania may sometimes occur." In overdose, the drug produces an even more flagrant stimulant syndrome culminating in seizures. Thus there is a continuum of stimulation effects.

Showing concern for possible abuse potential that might show up in the future, Kapit warned about "the fact that fluoxetine causes a set of adverse effects which resemble those caused by amphetamine" (p. 23).

---

[1]NDA stands for new drug application, the manufacturer's basic documentation for the FDA in support of marketing the drug (see chapter 11).

Despite Kapit's function as the chief safety investigator for Prozac, the Division of Psychopharmacological Drug Products, under psychiatrist Paul Leber, allowed none of Kapit's concerns to appear on the drug's label. The label does not indicate that Prozac is a potentially stimulant drug or that it can cause or worsen depression.

In a December 10, 1987, "Review and Evaluation," Kapit recommended that the company conduct postmarketing tests to study Prozac's potential to worsen the condition of patients already suffering from "weight loss, anorexia, and agitation." Neither the FDA nor the manufacturer followed up on this.

The actual data contained in the label confirms a stimulant profile, but the conclusion must be dug out from all the "noise" (see Breggin & Breggin, 1994a). A table of Prozac's stimulant symptoms, drawn from various parts of the label and including the percentage of patients afflicted, would look like this:

The Prozac Stimulant Profile

I. Psychiatric and Neurological
headache (20.3%)
nervousness (14.9%)
insomnia (13.8%)
anxiety (9.4%)
tremor (7.9%)
hypomania and mania (1%)
agitation (frequent)
abnormal dreams (frequent)
seizures (0.2%)

II. Digestive System
significant weight loss (13%)
nausea (21.1%)
diarrhea (12.3%)
mouth dryness (9.5%)
anorexia (8.7%)
dyspepsia (6.4%)
abdominal pain (3.4%)
vomiting (2.4%)

III. Skin
excessive sweating (8.4%)

As I will document, the stimulant profile should also have included another category:

IV. Behavioral
paranoia
violence
depression ("crashing")
suicide
withdrawal and drug abuse

Prozac, Suicide, and Violence

Shortly after Prozac was approved, a flood of media reports connected Prozac to suicide and violence (summarized in Breggin & Breggin, 1994a). Very quickly, more than 100 lawsuits were brought against Eli Lilly, most of them concerning violence against self or others.

Teicher, Glod, and Cole from Yale (1990) published a summary of clinical reports on increased suicidality on Prozac and concluded that the drug was causal. They followed this with a review of the overall problem, and proposed a series of potential clinical and neurological mechanisms (Teicher et al., 1993). More reports appeared in the literature (Breggin & Breggin, 1994a).

In clinical trials, King and Yale colleagues (King et al., 1991) confirmed "Emergence of Self-Destructive Phenomena in Children and Adolescents During Fluoxetine Treatment." One statistical analysis of anecdotal reports, published as a confirmation that Prozac was harmless (Fava & Rosenbaum, 1991), actually tended to incriminate it in causing suicidality. Another report describing violent reactions in youngsters was suppressed. A medical examiner's report found a disproportionately large number of successful suicides among patients taking Prozac (Bost & Kemp, 1992; these reports are discussed in Breggin & Breggin, 1994a).

A unique study of self-reports from a large cohort of patients obtaining antidepressant medication from pharmacies was conducted in Texas by Fisher, Bryant, and Kent (1993). They found that Prozac causes "a higher incidence of various ACEs [adverse clinical events] including delusions and hallucinations, aggression, and suicidal ideation." They concluded that all physicians should be alerted to the danger.

The prestigious British journal *Lancet* ("5-HT Blockers," 1990), warned in an editorial that SSRIs were associated with "the promotion of suicidal thoughts and behavior."

Fogel and Stone (1992) have observed:

Antidepressants, given to improve impulsive behavior by correcting depressed mood and perhaps indirectly by improving frontal lobe function . . . may at times induce a hyperarousal state with an increase in impulsive behavior. This issue has recently been raised in connection with suicidal or violent behavior in patients initiating therapy with fluoxetine, but hyperarousal can be seen with any of the antidepressants (Teicher et al. 1990). It is perhaps less common with the more sedating agents, such as trazodone and amitriptyline.

Mechanisms of SSRI-Induced Violence and Suicide

There are a number of potential mechanisms for SSRI-induced violence and suicide. One is the clinical association between agitated depression and both violence and suicide. The SSRIs, through their stimulant effects, can produce agitated depression in previously depressed patients and commonly in patients who were not previously depressed (see below).

On a biochemical level, "sluggish serotonin"—that is, an underactive serotonergic system in the brain—has been postulated as the cause of depression, as well as of impulsive, violent behavior. In theory, the SSRIs are supposed to correct this imbalance. But the brain attempts to compensate for this stimulation through a temporary compensatory shutdown of the production and release of serotonin and then through a persistent reduction in the number of serotonin receptors. These mechanisms, aimed at reducing overstimulation of the serotonergic system, could themselves lead to sluggish serotonin, for example, when serum levels drop several hours after each dose or after termination of treatment.

Clinicians Discover the Stimulating Effects of Prozac

Prozac was so stimulating that during the approval process Lilly principal investigators, breaking the rules of their own protocols, frequently gave sedative drugs and minor tranquilizers to their Prozac patients (Breggin & Breggin, 1994a). In one large set of trials, Prozac was no better than placebo unless it was combined with sedating drugs.

The FDA approved Prozac as if the drug, by itself, had passed muster in the trials. In reality, the trials featured Prozac often in combination with sedatives and tranquilizers to treat the agitation and anxiety caused by Prozac. The addition of sedatives and tranquilizers exposed patients to increased risks of cognitive dysfunction, addiction, withdrawal reactions, and other adverse effects. The failure to inform the profession and the public about the frequent need to combine Prozac with sedatives and tranquilizers was also potentially disastrous. It left doctors and patients unprepared to recognize or to treat Prozac-induced agitation and related adverse reactions, such as violence toward self and others.

More Recent Disclosures Concerning Prozac

Since the publication of *Talking Back to Prozac*, there have been a number of new developments surrounding the issue of whether or not Prozac can induce or aggravate violence and suicide. Much of this information is reviewed or published here for the first time.

Recent Cases of Severe Stimulation

Severe stimulation reactions were recently reported in 4 of 6 fluoxetine-treated patients with posttraumatic stress disorder, requiring 3 of them to withdraw from the study: "Two experienced agitation and worsening of hyperarousal symptoms; one patient's panic symptoms markedly worsened. A fourth patient also suffered severe agitation and greater anxiety . . . " (Marshall, Printz, Cardenas, & Liebowitz, 1995, p. 1238).

Research Confirmation of Prozac-Induced Suicide

A recent British epidemiological study has reconfirmed the danger of Prozac-induced suicide. To estimate the rate and means of suicide among people taking 10 different antidepressants, Jick, Dean, and Jick (1995) reviewed computer data from general practices in the United Kingdom involving 172,598 patients. They found, "Rates of suicide were higher in patients who received fluoxetine, but this may be explained by selection biases which were present for those drug users."

Jick, Dean, and Jick stretched beyond reason to take their position that Prozac might not be the cause of the suicides.[2] They found that "when the analysis was restricted to those without a history of having felt suicidal or who had taken only one antidepressant, the increased risk for those

---

[2]A footnote explains that the "drug surveillance programme" is supported in part by ten different drug companies, at least one of which makes an SSRI. However, Eli Lilly was not among them.

who took fluoxetine was reduced.'' Thus, the increased risk was reduced by these manipulations, but not eliminated. Data in a table show that after taking into account a past history of suicidal behavior and/or antidepressant use, Prozac remained *twice* as likely to be associated with suicide as any other antidepressant. In fact, Prozac became the *only* antidepressant that was associated with *increased* risk of suicide.

In comparison to three of the more sedating antidepressants—doxepin, imipramine, and amitriptyline—Prozac remains more than *4* times more likely to be associated with suicide. Since the danger of Prozac lies in its stimulating effect, it makes medical sense that the risk of Prozac was especially increased in comparison to the older, sedating drugs. Probably Prozac was causing more suicide than even these data indicate. Because of the much greater lethality of tricyclic antidepressants, overdosing with them would have been much more likely to have been noticed and interpreted as a suicide attempt.

What Really Happened
in the Wesbecker Prozac Murder/Suicide Trial

At present, there are approximately 160 product liability cases against Eli Lilly pertaining to Prozac, most claiming that the drug has caused murder or suicide. Most of the new revelations in this chapter concerning Prozac were generated through my work as a medical expert in the first product liability case to go to trial against Eli Lilly concerning Prozac (Fentress, 1994; see Breggin, 1994 for my testimony). In that case, Joseph Wesbecker entered his former place of employment in 1989, shot 20 people, killing 8 of them, and then committed suicide. He had been taking Prozac, as well as other medications. The plaintiffs argued that Eli Lilly had failed to adequately study and then to warn physicians about the potential for Prozac-induced violence toward self and others.

Although the Wesbecker case was seemingly won by Eli Lilly by a divided 9–3 jury vote,[3] the presiding judge, John W. Potter, later concluded that Lilly settled secretly with the plaintiffs before the case went to the jury (Castellano, 1995; Gibeaut, 1996; Potter, 1995; Scanlon, 1995; and most extensively, Varchaver, 1995). The judge had not been informed of

---

[3]One more vote against Lilly and it would have been a hung jury.

the settlement during the trial. To the contrary, both sides denied its existence to the judge (Varchaver, 1995).

As a part of the settlement, in addition to receiving money and agreeing not to appeal the case, the plaintiffs agreed to withhold from the jury certain damaging evidence against Eli Lilly (Gibeaut, 1996; Potter, 1995; and others in previous paragraph). Meanwhile, the trial went on as if no special arrangements had been made. This created a mock or fake trial.

Judge Potter tried to amend the official outcome of the case from "dismissed by the jury without prejudice" to "settled with prejudice." The judge's attorney stated, "There was a payment of money to withhold evidence" (Wolfe, 1995). Initially, an appeals court overruled Judge Potter on the grounds that too much time had elapsed before his attempt to change the verdict (Varchaver, 1995; Wolfe, 1995) but the judge won his appeal to the Supreme Court of Kentucky (Gibeaut, 1996).

On May 23, 1996, the Supreme Court of Kentucky unanimously agreed in Potter v. Eli Lilly & Co. that Judge Potter could proceed to hold a hearing on the secret settlement under an inherent-powers doctrine allowing courts to protect the integrity of their procedures (Gibeaut, 1996). The Supreme Court justices wrote, "In this case, there was a serious lack of candor with the trial court and there may have been deception, bad faith conduct, abuse of judicial process or perhaps even fraud" ("Trial Court's Authority . . . ," 1996, p. 35; Gibeaut, 1996, p. 18).

Estimates of the secret settlement made by Eli Lilly & Co. in the Wesbecker case have come through unrelated divorce suits. One plaintiff's attorney, presumably privy to the Lilly settlement amount involved in his client's divorce suit, stated, "The amount boggles the mind" (Gibeaut, 1996, p. 18).

Not only was the Wesbecker case settled secretly during the trial, but the plaintiff's lead attorney, Paul Smith, settled all of his several other cases against Lilly at that time. Eli Lilly can no longer claim it has never settled a Prozac case. It has settled several of them involving different attorneys. It also seems that the drug company cannot claim to have won a legitimate trial.

Lilly Acknowledges to the FDA
That Prozac Frequently Causes Depression

In preparing my testimony in the Wesbecker case, I went through an additional mass of FDA documents obtained under the Freedom of Information Act (FOIA). I discovered a section of Lilly's final draft of its

Prozac label that was submitted to the FDA. The section, in conformity with the standard label, was entitled, "Other Events Observed During the Premarketing Evaluation of Prozac" (Eli Lilly, 1987). It drew on the total database of 5,600 patients given Prozac. The label notes that "It is important to emphasize that, although the events reported did occur during treatment with Prozac, they were not necessarily caused by it."

In this final version of their label, under "Nervous System," the company listed "depression" as a *frequent* adverse effect of the drug. Frequent is equivalent to common and means occurring at least once in a hundred cases. But the FDA, in a last-ditch editing attempt to shorten what it called Lilly's "laundry list" concept, scratched a line through "depression" (Temple, 1987). The approved and current label lists only "abnormal dreams" and "agitation" as frequent or common. Depression went from being listed as a frequent adverse effect in the proposed label to being wholly unmentioned in the final approved label. This transformation took place at the very last minute before the FDA's final approval of the drug for marketing.

The admission that the drug was frequently reported to cause both agitation and depression is of great importance. Through research, clinical experience, and consulting as a medical expert, I have learned that many of the murders and suicides reported to have occurred during Prozac treatment seem driven by a combination of agitation and depression, specifically, Prozac-induced agitated depression (Breggin & Breggin, 1994a).

As a result of the current label, physicians have no awareness that Prozac is a possible cause of depression. Therefore, when a patient on Prozac becomes more depressed, rather than less, the physician is likely to increase the dose, rather than to stop or taper the drug.

Prozac-Induced Mania

Even in the short clinical trials for the NDA, Prozac caused mania in slightly more than 1% of patients (Kapit, October 17, 1986). But material that I recently found in the NDA indicates that Prozac poses a considerably greater danger of causing mania than the tricyclic antidepressants (Kapit, October 17, 1986, p. 18). In the studies for the FDA, only 0.3% of patients on tricyclics became manic—a rate one-third that of Prozac's. In addition, all the patients who became manic on tricyclics turned out to have a prior history of mania. Among the 33 reported cases of mania on Prozac, 23 occurred in patients who had never been manic before.

Mania frequently results in very destructive behavior toward oneself or others, including outright violence. The manic person can experience intense paranoid feelings and often feels enormous hostility, especially if thwarted in his or her own ambitions of the moment. The increased rates on Prozac once again confirm its stimulant quality.

An example of Prozac-induced mania with potential violence was presented by Jerome (1991), who described a 10-year-old boy who became depressed when his family moved to a new neighborhood and he was placed on 20 mg of Prozac by his family physician. The youngster immediately became "hyperactive, agitated . . . [and] irritable," and his speech was pressured. He gained energy, required less sleep, and developed a "somewhat grandiose assessment of his own abilities." Then he began to make a number of anonymous phone calls, threatening to kill a stranger in the neighborhood. When the telephone calls were traced back to him, the Prozac was discontinued and all of the hypomanic symptoms resolved within 2 weeks. Mania and hostility frequently go together and suggest one of the mechanisms for Prozac-induced violence. "Crashing" after mania could cause depression and suicide as well.

Jafri and Greenberg (1991) described the case of a 15-year-old boy who became psychotic "directly related to his receiving fluoxetine." After his medication was stopped, he improved over about one week's time. Hersh, Sokol, and Pfeffer (1991), physicians from Cornell University Medical College, described an 11-year-old girl who developed a delusional system on Prozac. There are many other reports of varying degrees of psychosis caused by Prozac (Chouinard & Steiner, 1986; Lebegue, 1987; Settle & Settle, 1984; Turner, Jacob, Beidel, & Griffin, 1985) and also by Zoloft (Laporta, Chouinard, Goldbloom, & Beauclair, 1987).

Recently, *Clinical Psychiatry News* (Sherman, 1995) headlined "Prozac for Kids: 'Landmark' Study Affirms Drug's Use." It described a placebo-controlled clinical trial involving Graham Emslie from the University of Texas Southwestern Medical School in Dallas. When I evaluated the data from the newspaper report, the rate of drug-induced mania turned out to be an extraordinary 6% (Breggin, 1995). In addition, during the question period after the paper was presented, Emslie admitted to an increase in aggressivity as well (Sherman, 1995).

Lilly Researcher Secretly Defined and Documented the Prozac Stimulant Syndrome

Lilly asked Charles Beasley, from their Division of Clinical Neurosciences, to count the cases of agitation in their clinical trials (Breggin,

1994). He produced a secret in-house report entitled "Activation and Sedation in Fluoxetine Clinical Studies" (Fentress Trial Exhibit 70), dated November 8, 1988. The report found that 333 Prozac patients became agitated in the trials but only 16 placebo patients. Beasley called it an "activation" effect, including "nervousness, anxiety, agitation, insomnia." He found that 38% of patients developed this effect on Prozac and 19% on placebo.

The totals for Prozac stimulation should have been even higher, however, because Beasley didn't count several stimulant categories, including euphoria, mania, nightmares or bad dreams, and hyperactivity. The rates of agitation would also have been higher if a large percentage of the Prozac patients hadn't been prescribed concomitant benzodiazepines and other sedatives.

Meanwhile, there were publicity concerns inside Lilly caused by doctors who felt that Prozac was so stimulating it might worsen agitated depressions. In fact, doctors put pressure on Lilly, which it resisted for some time, to make a smaller (10 mg) pill to facilitate prescribing less stimulating doses.

In going through mountains of documents, I found no evidence that the FDA ever saw the crucial Beasley study that confirmed FDA investigator Kapit's frequently expressed concerns about the drug's similarity to stimulants, including amphetamine (e.g., Kapit, October 17, 1986).

Spontaneous Reports of Aggressive or Violent Behavior on Prozac

As I described in *Talking Back to Prozac* (Breggin & Breggin, 1994a, p. 164), the FDA made a presentation at its 1991 hearings on antidepressants and abnormal behavior that showed a disproportionately high frequency of reports of "hostility" and "intentional injury" on Prozac (Food and Drug Administration, 1991). The reports were sent to the FDA through its postmarketing spontaneous reporting system. The FDA representative projected the data onto a screen but the data was not included in the transcript of the meeting. Although this issue was of overriding, central importance to its deliberations, the FDA advisory panel paid absolutely no attention to it. It was as if the data, so critical to their conclusions, had been presented to an empty room.

In response to a Freedom of Information Act (FOIA) request from me, the FDA claimed that the data could no longer be found. However, Eli Lilly was compelled to produce the data under court order in the Wesbecker case (Trial Exhibit 120) and I used it in my court testimony (Breggin, 1994, October 18).

The FDA study compared Prozac and the antidepressant trazodone. After taking into account the greater number of patients taking Prozac (based on numbers of prescriptions), Prozac reports of hostility and intentional injury remained 8 times more frequent. This avalanche of reports began prior to the adverse publicity surrounding Prozac. It was therefore truly spontaneous and not generated by increased publicity.

Some drug companies have tried to defend themselves by suggesting that controlled clinical trials are the best or only reliable source of data to demonstrate the existence of adverse drug reactions; but in fact the relatively short and small trials often turn out to be a very poor source of data on adverse reactions (see chapter 11). Postmarketing data, such as those pertaining to Prozac, are a frequent source of major conclusions concerning adverse drug reactions, commonly leading to label changes or withdrawal from the market (chapter 11).

Suicide Attempts on Prozac
in Lilly's Own Controlled Clinical Trials

In materials gained through discovery in the Wesbecker case, I found in-house documents from Eli Lilly clearly demonstrating an increased rate of suicide attempts in Prozac patients compared to placebo and to tricyclic antidepressants (Breggin, 1994[4]). This was a shocking discovery, as Eli Lilly claimed and continues to claim that no such data exist.

In the summer of 1985, Eli Lilly set out to respond to accusations, including those from the German regulatory agency, that Prozac could cause or contribute to suicidality. The company evaluated data from their basic 4- to 6-week controlled clinical trials. Twelve reported suicide attempts were found among the Prozac patients but only one each in the placebo group and the comparison drug group (tricyclic antidepressant). This 6:1 ratio could not be explained by differences in size between the Prozac group and the placebo/tricyclic group. When the total patient days of exposure were taken into account, the ratio remained a significant 3:1 for increased suicide attempts in the Prozac group.

Consultants hired by Eli Lilly pruned down the original reports, excluding 6 of the suicide attempts on Prozac and 1 on either the comparison drug or placebo. The ratio remained 6:1, and the consultants continued

---

[4]The judge did not allow the material to be entered as a court exhibit and so I have cited my testimony (p. 3126).

to find a borderline statistically significant ($p=.051$) increased rate for suicide attempts among the Prozac patients.

Furthermore, the removal of several of the Prozac suicide attempt reports was wholly unjustified. For example, one discarded case involved a patient who took 10 fluoxetine capsules spaced at 2-hour intervals over 5 hours while drinking a bottle of rum. Taking the pills slowly in this manner, along with alcohol, is done during genuine suicide attempts to avoid vomiting the medication. The complete data on another exclusion was as follows: "The patient had suicidal ideation at the beginning of the study and made a self-inflicted laceration of the skin with a razor blade" (Breggin, 1994, p. 3129).

In throwing out these cases, the Lilly consultants second-guessed their own clinical investigators, who had categorized these reactions as drug-related suicide attempts. The consultants made their decisions on the basis of a mere few lines of clinical description. According to one of the company's executives, they did not contact the authors of the reports—their own clinical investigators—for more information (Beasley, 1994a, p. 245). Yet these clinical investigators, based on firsthand knowledge, had cited the cases as suicide attempts.

Eli Lilly's own consultant, biopsychiatrist David Winokur, offered an explanation for how Prozac could increase the suicide attempt rate: "A possibility which comes to mind is that Prozac might be somewhat more stimulating as a drug and that individuals may be slightly more impulsive although their thinking had not changed" (Breggin, 1994, pp. 3129–3130). Independently, in my writing and testimony, I had also developed the concept of Prozac as a stimulating drug causing impulsive behavior and suicide.

As far as I can ascertain, these extremely important facts and analyses about Prozac-induced suicidality were never submitted to the FDA or in any way made available to the government, the profession, or the public. To the contrary, Lilly has maintained—and continues to maintain—that there is no evidence whatsoever for increased suicidality on Prozac. As an example, Eli Lilly did not make known their analysis of increased suicidality on Prozac at the 1991 FDA conference (Food & Drug Administration, 1991). Nor did they present the Beasley data on increased activation.

There is a high probability that there were even more Prozac-induced suicide attempts in the premarketing controlled trials that went unreported by the principal investigators. As I stated in my testimony, the principal investigators in charge of testing Prozac on patients had been notified by Eli Lilly not to report depression as a drug effect. Thus, Lilly and its investigators may have excluded suicide attempts from the list of adverse drug reactions by calling them "depression" or even "failure to improve" (Breggin & Breggin, 1994a, pp. 162–163). Furthermore, Lilly instructed its principal investigators not to report possible adverse drug events if they could be attributed to the patient's mental disorder (Beasley, 1994b, p. 155), encouraging them not to report suicide attempts in their depressed patients.

Adverse Reactions to Prozac in Lilly's Earliest Research

In the March 1986 Safety Review of the NDA (Kapit, 1986), the FDA psychiatrist summarized five "serious clinical events" in the first 77 patients given Prozac, including one paranoid psychosis and one manic psychosis. There was also evidence in Lilly's files—presented in my testimony—that some of the first human subjects responded very adversely to Prozac. In his deposition, Lilly's top scientist, Ray Fuller (1994), confirmed an early in-house memo (Exhibit 11) in which he wrote:

> Some patients have converted from severe depression to agitation within a few days. In one case the agitation was marked and the patient had to be taken off the drug. In future studies, the use of benzodiazepines to control agitation will be permitted.

This is a "smoking gun" indicating that Lilly knew from the beginning that Prozac would make many patients so agitated that they would need others drugs to control it. Fuller admitted in deposition that the decision was made to add benzodiazepines to the NDA clinical studies because patients reportedly were becoming agitated on Prozac. As noted, the use of concomitant sedatives and minor tranquilizers became a common practice in the protocols preceding drug approval.

It should be emphasized, however, that giving tranquilizers or sedatives along with Prozac by no means guarantees that the patient will escape undergoing drug-induced agitation, depression, suicide, or violence. The benzodiazepines can have paradoxical effects, including agitation. They, too, can cause or aggravate depression, violence, and suicide (chapter 10). In general, the greater number of psychoactive drugs a patient takes, the greater the risk of an adverse drug reaction.

Prozac-Induced Aggression in Lilly's Earliest Animal Studies

In preparing for the Wesbecker trial, I found more evidence than I origi-nally suspected concerning Prozac-induced agitation and even violence in animals. I testified at trial concerning a Lilly animal study, documented by Brophy, a Lilly project leader. He reported, ''A total of six dogs, two males and four females, from the high-dose group were removed from treatment for periods of 1 to 17 days due to severe occurrences of either aggressive behavior, ataxia, or anorexia.'' In his deposition (p. 368), Ray Fuller, Lilly's highest ranking scientist, stated that 6 of 20 dogs in the high-dose study group became unexpectedly aggressive. A number of mice were getting hyperactive, but not aggressive, on Prozac.

Slater, Jones, and Moore, from the Lilly Research Labs, published a paper in 1978 concerning the inhibition of REM sleep in cats. Disruption of REM sleep can cause emotional disturbances. The Lilly researchers report: ''The present authors are at a loss to explain why cats receiving fluoxetine for several days began to hiss and growl or why this behavior decreased with continued treatment.''

In defense of their company and their drug, these authors then explained, ''The subjects who received fluoxetine in Phase I clinical trial (Lemberger, unpublished data) have not described any change in mood nor have observ-ers noted any change in affect.'' This claim is not supported by the facts as disclosed in the NDA or in Lilly's own documents. As the previous section documented, some of the first subjects given Prozac showed drastic, even deteriorating,[5] changes.

I can find no evidence that follow-up studies were done to further evaluate Prozac-induced agitation or aggression in animals. No primates were tested for behavioral effects.

British and German Regulatory Authorities Inquire About Prozac-Induced Stimulation, Agitation, and Depression

The FDA was not the only regulatory agency to show concern about Prozac-induced agitation, stimulation, and depression. In my Wesbecker testimony, I described how the British Committee on Safety of Medicines (CSM), prior to approval of Prozac, raised the same issue:

> It is possible that these adverse effects of fluoxetine treatment may nega-tively affect patients with depression. Since depressed patients frequently

---

[5]We must also doubt Lilly's methods of selecting Phase 1 subjects (see ahead, this chapter).

suffer from insomnia, nervousness, anorexia and weight loss [Prozac effects], it is possible that fluoxetine might at least temporarily make their illness worse. (quoted in Breggin, 1994, p. 3094)

For a time, the CSM seemed determined to make Prozac contraindicated in underweight, anorexic, or agitated patients; but apparently nothing came of it.

During the mid-1980s, the BGA, the German equivalent of the FDA, also raised doubts about approving Prozac. The BGA found that doctors in clinical studies were more positive about the drug than the actual patients. The agency worried about a possible increase in the suicide rate. They shared Kapit's concern about stimulating effects.

In 1984 Lilly employees in Germany named Schenk and Weber wrote in a company memo, "The BGA suspects fluoxetine to be a stimulating/ activating drug (side-effect profile, suicides, suicide attempts)" (quoted in Breggin, 1994, p. 3151). Remarking on suicide associated with Prozac, they declared "This is a very serious issue in the opinion of the BGA." According to the memo, the BGA had stated: "Considering the benefit and the risk we think this preparation totally unsuitable for the treatment of depression." The BGA was especially concerned about Prozac's potential to cause agitation before its antidepressant effect took place. The BGA, unknowingly echoing Kapit, but more strongly, warned: "During treatment with the drug, some symptoms of the underlying disease (anxiety, insomnia, agitation) increase, which as adverse effects exceed those which are considered acceptable by medical standards."

The conflict between the BGA and Eli Lilly went on for many years. On February 6, 1991, Hans Weber, representing Lilly in Germany, wrote to Ray Fuller at Eli Lilly. He described a meeting held between Lilly representatives and the BGA. Weber stated, "The question was raised whether fluoxetine could be an amphetamine-like drug, which may explain its stimulating and anorectic effects" (quoted in Breggin, 1994, p. 3154).

Eventually the BGA did approve Prozac. Unlike the FDA, however, they required a label warning under the heading of "risk of suicide." It states that the patient may need an additional sedative along with Prozac until the antidepressant effect takes over. It notes that this would also apply to patients with extreme sleep disturbances or excitability.

Lilly's undisclosed in-house studies of increased activation and suicidality on Prozac were probably done in the hope of allaying fears expressed in Germany and elsewhere. When the studies instead confirmed the worst fears about stimulation and suicidality, they were apparently never made known to the relevant agencies in England, Germany, or the United States.

Stimulant and Behavioral Abnormalities Associated with Other SSRIs

Zoloft (sertraline), Paxil (paroxetine), Luvox (fluvoxamine), and all SSRIs, have stimulant effects similar to those of Prozac. The main difference between Zoloft and Prozac is Zoloft's greater tendency to produce somnolence and sexual dysfunction, especially in males. Both insomnia and somnolence may be increased with Luvox.

In Zoloft's label, in the section entitled "Other Events Observed During the Premarketing Evaluation," under "Psychiatric Disorders," the following reactions are among those listed as *infrequent* (between 1/100 and 1/1,000): Suicide ideation and attempt, depression, aggravated depression, aggressive reaction, paranoid reaction, abnormal thinking, abnormal dreams, emotional lability, euphoria, hallucination, and delusion. Confusion was found to be *frequent*; but it was placed under "Central and Peripheral Nervous System Disorders" rather than under "Psychiatric Disorders," so it is likely to be missed in a quick reading.

These reactions were gathered from the overall database of 2,700 patients receiving the drug. The label points out that these reports do not necessarily establish a causal relationship.

Through FOIA, I have had the opportunity to review the Zoloft Summary Basis of Approval (1988). Many of the problems that plagued the NDA of Prozac were also rampant in the NDA for Zoloft, including numerous violations of protocol, the use of concomitant long-acting benzodiazepines, high dropout rates, many negative studies, and no evidence of efficacy in hospitalized patients. As in the Prozac studies, "agitation" and "insomnia" were among the reasons for the dropouts. In fact, the efficacy of Zoloft was considered questionable until the last minute before its final approval (discussed in chapter 11).

As documented in its official label, Paxil displays a similar pattern of stimulant effects: insomnia, tremor, nervousness, and anxiety. Like Zoloft, it produces more somnolence and more sexual dysfunction than Prozac. In fact, somnolence (23.3%) is almost twice as frequent as insomnia (13.3%).

For Paxil, the list of psychiatric disorders reported in association with drug treatment is categorized under "nervous system." Again, the company makes the point that these reactions were reported but not necessarily causally related. The database included 4,126 patients. The list of *frequently* reported reactions includes, among others, CNS stimulation, depression, and emotional lability. The Paxil list of infrequent CNS reactions is lengthy, including psychotic depression, antisocial reaction, and hostility.

Prozac Interaction with Monoamine Oxidase Inhibitors and Tryptophan

When combined with other drugs that stimulate the serotonergic system, such as monoamine oxidase inhibitors (MAOIs) antidepressants and tryptophan,[6] Prozac can produce a well-documented, severe stimulant condition called the serotonin syndrome (Sternbach, 1991). This disorder looks somewhat like the serotonin stimulant syndrome and shares with it the symptoms of euphoria and hypomania, agitation, confusion, and gastrointestinal upset, including diarrhea. The serotonin syndrome additionally involves overstimulation of the brain stem and spinal cord, producing symptoms not typically seen with the stimulant syndrome, such as fever and chills, severe incoordination, muscle spasms, and hyperactive reflexes.

Prozac in Combination with Tricyclic Antidepressants

Psychiatrists and other physicians too frequently combine Prozac with other antidepressants, including the tricyclics, such as Tofranil (imipramine) and Elavil (amitriptyline). The combination is extremely dangerous. In a 1992 study conducted in Lilly's own research laboratory by the team of Bergstrom, Peyton, and Lemberger, Prozac was found to increase the blood concentrations of tricyclics by as much as *10 times*.

The tricyclics become toxic at blood levels not much higher than their therapeutic ones. A tenfold or more increase in concentration of a tricyclic could produce, among other things, a fatal heart arrhythmia, a severe drop in blood pressure, central nervous system depression, or a grand mal

---

[6]The brain synthesizes serotonin from tryptophan, an essential amino acid found in a variety of foods. The ingestion of large amounts of tryptophan increases the production of serotonin.

seizure. It could also cause abnormal mental reactions, such as confusion, panic, mania, or even depression.

Lilly's label does not do justice to the dangerousness of Prozac's interaction with tricyclics. Describing Prozac interactions with other antidepressants, it states ''There have been greater than 2-fold increases'' in blood concentrations with the combination of Prozac. The tricyclic antidepressants are not mentioned by name, vastly reducing the physician's capacity to respond to the warning. Furthermore, the difference between ''greater than 2-fold'' and the actual figure of *tenfold or greater* is enormous. It is a potentially lethal difference.

One rat brain study shows that Prozac and tricyclics given together accelerate their joint impact on the brain (Baron et al., 1988). Down-regulation of adrenergic receptors (discussed in a later section) was greatly increased in rapidity and intensity by the combination.

Akathisia, Dystonia, and the Risk of Permanent Neurological Disorders from Prozac

As early as 1979, H. Y. Meltzer and a team at the University of Chicago recognized that Prozac suppresses dopaminergic neurotransmission. Concerned about reports of neurological side effects that might stem from this dopamine suppression, Ross Baldessarini and Elda Marsh from McLean Hospital and Harvard demonstrated the effect in Prozac-treated animal brains in 1990.

Drug-induced disruption of dopamine neurotransmission is known to produce a variety of neurological side effects (see chapters 3 and 5). The neuroleptics suppress dopamine neurotransmission, causing a reactive hyperactivity of the system that produces a high rate of irreversible dyskinesias, cognitive dysfunction, and dementia.

Prozac can cause most of the acute, *reversible* neurological disorders that are also produced by the neuroleptic drugs. Prozac's pharmacological mechanism for suppressing dopamine is more indirect than that of the neuroleptics. However, the clinical result can be very similar. Prozac can cause akathisia (agitation with hyperactivity), parkinsonism (''Fluoxetine,'' 1990), and dystonia (muscle spasms) (Meltzer et al., 1979; Recoppa, Welch, & Ware, 1990).

Drug-induced akathisia, dystonia, and parkinsonism can produce extreme discomfort. They can be disabling and feel like torture (chapter 3 for details). In brief, akathisia can become an inner torment and anguish that drives the individual into hyperactivity. Akathisia can contribute to the development of psychosis, as well as violence against self or others (chapter 3). Dystonia often produces agonizing muscle spasms in the region of the eyes, head, and neck, but can also cause spasms that disable the whole body. Parkinsonism produces emotional dulling and immobilizes the body.

Under "Adverse Reactions of the Nervous System," the Prozac label mentions akathisia as "infrequent." By contrast, the June 1990 *Health Letter* (Public Citizen Health Research Group, 1990) estimates that akathisia affects a whopping 15%–25% of Prozac patients.

In the September, 1989, issue of the *Journal of Clinical Psychiatry*, Joseph Lipinski and his colleagues from McLean Hospital and Harvard Medical School described five cases of Prozac-induced akathisia, which they believe occurs "fairly frequently." They estimate the rate of akathisia in Prozac patients at between 9.7% and 25%. They state that their cases were indistinguishable from neuroleptic-induced akathisia.

Five days after starting Prozac, one woman "reported severe anxiety and restlessness. She paced the floor throughout the day, found sleep at night difficult because of the restlessness, and constantly shifted her legs when seated" (Lipinski, Mallaya, Zimmerman, & Pope, 1989). Another woman kept her roommate awake as she moved her legs so vigorously in bed it was like riding a bicycle.

How could such a frequent, distressing side effect go almost wholly unrecognized among the thousands of patients tested by Eli Lilly during the FDA drug approval process? Typically, psychiatrists have tended to blame akathisia on the patient's emotional state.

The FDA's Kapit warned, "it is possible that a tardive syndrome related to fluoxetine may exist. It will be necessary to be on the lookout for such events" (October 19, 1986, p. 32). By January 1993, more than two dozen reports of Prozac-induced TD had reached the FDA (Food and Drug Administration, 1993) but the profession has not taken notice.

Meanwhile, as demanded by the FDA, in March, 1990, Lilly added "dyskinesia" to the list of side effects. This in no way alerts the physician to the frequency, severity, or nature of the multiple neurological disorders now associated with the drug, including agonizing akathisia and dystonia, and probably tardive dyskinesia.

Psychiatrists too often keep patients on Prozac even after they have developed distressing neurological symptoms. Lipinsky's group at Harvard, for example, continued their patients on Prozac while giving them a drug that somewhat relieved their akathisia. Despite the tragic lessons learned from the neuroleptics, they showed no concern in their report about the risk of producing permanent disorders, such as TD, through continued exposure to the offending toxic agents.

Down-Regulation of Serotonergic Receptors

While Prozac in theory is supposed to energize the serotonin system by making more serotonin available in the synapses, in reality the brain reacts to Prozac as a toxic intrusion and tries to overcome its effects. One compensatory mechanism, called down-regulation, quickly begins reducing the number of receptors in the brain for serotonin (Wamsley et al., 1987; Wong & Bymaster, 1981; Wong, Reid, Bymaster, & Threlkeld, 1985). After being exposed to serotonin for periods of time, the receptors actually die off or disappear. The end result of down-regulation is called subsensitivity. At lower doses, there were both increases and decreases in receptor density in various areas of the brain, according to Wamsley, indicating the complexity of the brain's response (also see Fuller, Perry, & Molloy, 1974).

Down-regulation begins to occur in rats after 2 days of treatment with Prozac and the reductions continue over several weeks of testing. Up to 60% of some classes of serotonin receptors can disappear. The down-regulation is widespread, involving the frontal lobes and cortex, which regulate the emotional and intellectual life of the individual. Down-regulation of serotonin will reduce the capacity of the serotonin system for activation. Especially between drug doses or during drug withdrawal, this could theoretically produce sluggish serotonin, associated with increased impulsivity, depression, suicide, and murder.

Do the lost or down-regulated serotonergic receptors come back to life or replace themselves once Prozac is stopped? No studies have been done to show whether or not the brain recovers from Prozac-induced receptor loss. The FDA does not require these studies, and Lilly has seemingly not carried them out. Yet they would be very easy and relatively inexpensive to incorporate into existing animal studies.

Ray Fuller, Lilly's top researcher, explained in deposition testimony that he did not recall any experiments on the possible recovery of down-regulated serotonin receptors. When asked if he thought these experiments might be important, Fuller declared "I don't see that that would be of any value to know that" (Fuller, 1994, p. 266).

Meanwhile, seemingly oblivious to the possible danger of irreversible brain dysfunction from down-regulation following the prolonged use of Prozac, many psychiatrists urge their patients to stay on Prozac for years or even for a lifetime. As far as I know, Lilly has issued no warnings or "Dear Doctor" letters showing concern about this trend toward long-term therapy.

Can Prozac Impair Mental Process?

Before a psychiatric drug is marketed, the FDA does not require extensive neuropsychological testing of its effects on mental processes such as memory, learning, abstract reasoning, reaction time, short- and long-term memory, and so on. The drug companies themselves do not routinely conduct this critical research. In the case of Prozac, even postmarketing cognitive testing is sparse and inconclusive. As of 1993, two studies were available. One found no impairment (Fudge, Perry, Garvey, & Kelly, 1990) and the other found some memory impairment (Murray & Hooberman, 1993).

Prozac and the Brain-Disabling Principle

Prozac once again illustrates the principle that the differences between therapeutic effects and adverse effects are merely steps along a continuum from mild to extreme toxicity. Drug-induced feelings of well-being can be understood as an early stage along the continuum from mild euphoria to mania, sometimes combined with a generalized dulling or flattening of emotional responsiveness and social sensitivity.

Many patients who feel better on Prozac are probably experiencing the initial stages of euphoria or mania. That is, the early signs of stimulant toxicity will be subjectively experienced as beneficial—a sense of increased alertness and energy, and a narrowing of focus and loss of emotional responsiveness. But even among patients who feel benefited, a large percentage will also suffer from nervousness or jitters, anxiety, insomnia, disturbing dreams, or loss of appetite, sometimes requiring the addition of a minor tranquilizer and sometimes leading to discontinuation of the drug. As the dose is increased, it becomes even more likely that these effects will become very uncomfortable, and at very high doses, mania and other psychoses are more likely to develop.

Harmonizing Neurotransmitters or Disabling the Brain?

Patients are frequently told that Prozac and the other SSRIs benefit the brain by correcting imbalances or harmonizing neurotransmitters. Prozac is said to enhance serotonergic neurotransmission, but in fact it grossly impairs the process of neurotransmission. Some of these impairments can be measured, such as the blockage of the normal reuptake process of serotonin, as well as the brain's attempts to compensate by shutting down the system or by reducing the number of receptors. In contrast to these proven drug-induced abnormalities, we can only speculate about the alleged improvement—that somehow improved mental functioning will result from disrupting the brain's normal processes. If Prozac sometimes improves a biochemical imbalance in the brain, it is surely a stroke of luck. Nearly always, if not always, it will disrupt the brain's normal activities.

Taking Prozac introduces a toxic interference into the brain. Due to drug-induced emotional blunting or euphoria, or the placebo effect, the patient may feel benefited, but the apparent benefit comes at the cost of diminished mental function.

Withdrawal Symptoms and Addiction

Patients can "crash" coming off SSRIs and undergo severe depression, and suicidal ideation (Breggin, 1992c; Breggin & Breggin, 1994a). They can also undergo behavioral abnormalities. There are also suggestions that Prozac has addictive potential and is, on occasion at least, being abused (Breggin & Breggin, 1994a).

Einbinder (1995) describes a patient who felt fatigue and dizziness with falling on withdrawing from Prozac. Interestingly, Einbinder states "The manufacturer was unaware of any reports of withdrawal symptoms on cessation of fluoxetine."

It is most remarkable if Eli Lilly did indeed tell Einbinder that it was unaware of any reports of withdrawal symptoms associated with the use of Prozac. By January 24, 1993 the spontaneous reporting system of the FDA had received 94 reports of "withdrawal syndrome" from Prozac, as well as 26 reports of drug dependency and 4 of drug addiction (Food & Drug Administration, 1993).

I myself made a report in the literature on Prozac dependency, addiction, and withdrawal (Breggin, 1992c) and I sent it directly to the company as well. The company acknowledged receipt of the document (Marvel, 1993) and filed it with the FDA using several event terms, including "withdrawal syndrome."

There is seemingly no way that Eli Lilly & Co. could have been unaware of reports of withdrawal reactions from Prozac.

There are reports of physical withdrawal from Paxil and Zoloft. Debattista and Schatzberg (1995) report on physical symptoms associated with a case of paroxetine withdrawal with vomiting, headache, and tremulousness, which they compared to a similar report concerning sertraline withdrawal (Louie, Lannon, & Ajari, 1994).

TRICYCLIC ANTIDEPRESSANTS

The tricyclics as a group have been used for several decades. I have previously described their CNS toxic effects in some detail (Breggin, 1983a; also see Breggin, 1991a). This section will therefore be abbreviated.

The tricyclic antidepressants include the following drugs (trade names in parentheses): imipramine (Tofranil, Imavate, Presamine, SK-Pramine, Janimine), desipramine (Pertofrane, Norpramin), amitriptyline (Elavil), nortriptyline (Aventyl, Pamelor), protriptyline (Vivactil), doxepin (Sinequan, Adapin), trimipramine (Surmontil), and amoxapine (Asendin). Maprotiline (Ludiomil) is often placed in this class of antidepressant.

They are called tricyclic because their chemical nucleus has the basic tricyclic structure of the original phenothiazine neuroleptic, chlorpromazine or Thorazine (Bassuk & Schoonover, 1977; Pauker, 1981). Of extreme importance, the antidepressant amoxapine (Asendin) is turned into a neuroleptic in the body, producing the same problems as any other neuroleptic, including tardive dyskinesia (chapters 3 and 4).

Bassuk and Schoonover (1977) note that tricyclic antidepressants can cause a toxic syndrome similar to the neuroleptics:

Tricyclics may also cause psychomotor slowing and difficulties in concentration and planning. Although more attenuated than with the phenothiazines, some of these properties are similar to the neuroleptic syndrome.

These effects should be explained to the patient if he is in a setting where active physical or mental performance is required. Weakness and fatigue, nervousness, headaches, agitation, vertigo, palsies, tremors, ataxia, paresthesia, dysarthria, nystagmus, and twitching are central symptoms that occasionally occur. Tricyclics also lower the seizure threshold in a manner similar to the phenothiazines.

In discussing animal behavior Jarvik (1970) notes, ''Despite its clinical antidepressant effects, imipramine produces a depression of spontaneous motor activity in laboratory animals.'' He notes that it produces ''difficulty in concentrating and thinking comparable to that experienced during the course of similar treatment with chlorpromazine.'' He states: ''Its effect has been described as a dullness of depressive ideation . . . '' Byck (1975) takes the same position in a later edition of the same book, including the observation that ''Imipramine seems to produce greater impairment of cognitive and affective processes and less reduction in physical movement than does chlorpromazine.'' Other studies of tricyclics indicate that they produce ''measurable cognitive impairment in normal subjects following acute or chronic administration'' (Judd, Squire, Butters, Salmon, & Paller, 1987).

Withdrawal from Tricyclics

Tricyclic antidepressants commonly produce withdrawal, frequently in the form of cholinergic rebound, with flulike symptoms such as nausea and vomiting, diarrhea, myalgia, headache, fatigue, and anxiety (Breggin, 1991a). McMahon (1986) summarized:

> Autonomic symptoms are most common and include gastrointestinal disturbance (nausea, diarrhea), general somatic distress (myalgias, malaise, headache, rhinorrhea), sleep disturbances (insomnia, nightmares), and cardiovascular symptoms (arrhythmias, ventricular ectopy). Psychotic decompensation, withdrawal mania, and general anxietylike symptoms have been attributed to abrupt withdrawal of cyclic antidepressants.

More recently, Maxmen and Ward (1995) have provided an extensive list of tricyclic antidepressant withdrawal symptoms. One group of withdrawal symptoms includes a flulike syndrome without fever: anorexia, nausea, vomiting, diarrhea, queasy stomach, and cramps. A second group involves sleep disturbances: insomnia, hypersomnia, excessive dreaming, and nightmares. A third group includes mania and hypomania.

Maxmen and Ward point out that these symptoms can also be experienced between doses as the blood level drops.

Withdrawal symptoms can begin soon after stopping the medication and build up over a period of days or a couple of weeks. I have seen patients suffer from withdrawal symptoms for months and, in some cases, permanently. Withdrawal symptoms often compel patients to continue taking these drugs.

The Tragedy of Drug-Induced Mania

The hazards surrounding drug-induced mania during treatment or during withdrawal have not received enough attention. In the short trials used for obtaining approval, most antidepressants produce mania in about 1% of patients. If hypomania, excitement, and agitation are included, the overall rate is much higher even during these controlled trials.

In actual clinical practice, the risk to many patients is much higher due to the predisposition of some patients toward mania and due to other factors such as larger tricyclic doses, concomitant stimulating medications, and lack of adequate clinical supervision.

Mania, it should be emphasized, is a psychosis characterized by behavior that is often dangerous to oneself and others. An otherwise ordinary citizen can, during a drug-induced mania attack, end up spending a family fortune in a matter of days. With no previous history of aggressive behavior, he or she can become violent, injure someone, and land in jail with serious criminal charges—all in less than 24 hours.

Many millions of people around the world take these drugs every year. Hundreds of thousands develop drug-induced symptoms along a continuum from agitation to mania. The toll in terms of human suffering and wasted resources is enormous and yet largely ignored by the medical profession.

Tricyclic Antidepressants and the Brain-Disabling Principle

The therapeutic effect of tricyclics can result from any number of effects that vary from individual to individual, including emotional blunting, sedation, and stimulation. They frequently cause organic brain syndromes, which—as in the case of electroshock treatment—tend to relieve depression by causing emotional apathy or an artificial high. A study from the Yale University Department of Psychiatry by Davies, Tucker, Harrow, and Detre (1971) indicates that acute organic brain syndromes are very common during routine tricyclic antidepressant therapy (reviewed in detail in Breggin, 1983a). Symptoms included "forgetfulness, agitation, illogical thoughts, disorientation, increased insomnia, and, at times, delusional states" (Davies et al., 1971).

My own experience and clinical reports confirm that many clinicians purposefully administer tricyclics until they produce toxic reactions. Goodwin and Ebert (1977) advise giving the tricyclics in doses that produce "confusion" and other signs of toxicity. Amphetamine-like toxic effects are considered a good sign. Wells and Mendelson (1978) observe, "In our practice, an adequate trial often constitutes the highest dose that the patient can tolerate."

As described in chapter 1, the patient who experiences drug-induced brain dysfunction and the psychiatrist who induces it collaborate in a mutual denial of what is going on. Both end up denying the patient's drug-induced brain dysfunction and the patient's real-life personal problems. When euphoria is present, it becomes especially easy for the patient and the psychiatrist to deny the reality of what is happening. A drug with sufficient neurotoxicity to produce a mild to severe organic brain syndrome is especially suited to creating the illusion of improvement in depressed patients.

Tricyclics: More Cause than Cure for Suicidality?

There is no substantial published evidence that any antidepressants, new or old, ameliorate suicidal tendencies. Instead, there is clinical evidence that the tricyclic antidepressants, like the SSRIs, can cause suicide. Baldessarini (1978) warns, "The risk of suicide may even increase with initial improvement, since activity usually increases before mood elevation." This is similar to the explanation offered by Eli Lilly's consultant psychiatrist to explain the increased rate of suicide attempts on Prozac.

Damluji and Ferguson (1988) reviewed "Paradoxical worsening of depressive symptomatology caused by antidepressants" and reported four cases of their own caused by amoxapine, desipramine, nortriptyline, and trazodone. The American Psychiatric Association Task Force report on benzodiazepines (1990) also cites the problem of depression and suicide from tricyclic antidepressants.

Tragically, while these drugs cannot prevent suicide, in relative small amounts they can become lethal instruments in the hands of suicidal patients. As little as one week's supply of most tricyclics can cause death, often due to cardiac dysfunction. In combination with other drugs, their lethality increases. Thus, millions of depressed, suicidal patients are given the tool with which to kill themselves. By 1981 ("Tricyclics") the tricyclics were overtaking the barbiturates as the medications most frequently involved in serious overdose. The tricyclics remain a major public health problem as agents of suicide (Henry, Alexander, & Sener, 1995).

Chapter 9 will discuss the use of antidepressants in children.

Other Antidepressants

Several other "atypical" antidepressants are currently on the market in the United States. This brief review is not intended to be comprehensive in regard to their adverse effects.

Venlafaxine (Effexor), approved by the FDA in December 1993, was described in more detail early in this chapter. It is a nonselective serotonin reuptake inhibitor that also strongly inhibits the reuptake of epinephrine. Its profile is very similar to SSRIs in producing stimulation, including anxiety, nervousness, insomnia, anorexia, and weight loss. It causes the various emotional and behavioral abnormalities that go along with stimulation, such as agitation and mania, and has been associated with hostility, paranoid reaction, psychotic depression, and psychosis. It can cause hypertension.

Nefazodone (Serzone) was approved by the FDA in December 1994. It inhibits the reuptake of serotonin and norepinephrine, but also blocks some of the receptor groups for those neurotransmitters. It is more likely to produce somnolence than stimulation. It can produce lightheadedness, confusion, and memory impairment, as well as hypotension. A range of abnormal behaviors have been reported in association with its use, including hostility, paranoid reaction, suicide attempts or ideation, derealization and depersonalization, and hallucinations.

Trazodone (Desyrel) and Buproprion (Wellbutrin) are somewhat older "atypical" antidepressants that do not fit the pattern of other groups of agents. Buproprion has an unusually high rate of seizures associated with its use. It can be very stimulating and agitating. Trazodone tends to cause sedation and can also cause dizziness and fainting. It can cause cardiac difficulties for recovering heart patients. It also produces the potentially disastrous side effect of priapism—uncontrolled, irreversible penile erection, sometimes requiring surgical intervention.

In my experience, any of the antidepressants can produce a variety of unexpected and sometimes severe emotional reactions including apathy, lethargy, and depression, or euphoria, paranoia, and mania. Frequently these adverse effects are mentioned as possibilities in the FDA-approved label.

Keep in mind that as a group antidepressants affect diverse neurotransmitter systems in a complex, little-understood manner. Even the supposedly selective SSRIs end up producing generalized dysfunction in the brain and hence the mind.

Recent research challenges the concept of antidepressants in general, suggesting that they have no therapeutic effect beyond placebo (see ahead).

PSYCHOSTIMULANTS IN ADULTS

Many antidepressants, including SSRIs and tricyclics, have stimulant effects. The classic psychostimulants include dextroamphetamine (Dexedrine), methylphenidate (Ritalin), and pemoline (Cylert). When I wrote *Psychiatric Drugs: Hazards to the Brain* (1983a), these agents had gone out of fashion for the treatment of depression. The FDA, in fact, has removed depression from the list of approved uses for these drugs. But the prescription of psychiatric drugs is not driven by empirical data, and stimulants are once again coming back into fashion as a treatment for depression. Too often they are given to add ''punch'' to antidepressants, creating potentially dangerous adverse reactions, including insomnia, agitation, mania, and organic brain syndromes.

As the use of these stimulants increases, Baldessarini's (1978) original observations remain valid:

Thus current indications for the use of amphetamines in medical practice are very limited. Moreover, there is a considerable risk of abuse of this class of agents. Although the risk of true physiological addiction is often exaggerated, some dysphoria and depression of mood ("crashing") commonly follow the abrupt discontinuation of high doses of amphetamines. In very high and prolonged doses, stimulants can induce a paranoid psychosis, responsive to antipsychotic drugs, and in lower doses they can induce psychotic exacerbations in schizophrenic patients. Since they are ineffective antidepressants and poor anorexic agents, it is remarkable that their production and prescription continue at high rates.

In comparing Prozac to the stimulants in *Talking Back to Prozac* (Breggin & Breggin, 1994a), the brain-disabling impact of amphetamine and related drugs was documented in detail. Chapter 9 will examine the use of psychostimulants in children.

MAOIs: "ENERGIZING" TUBERCULOSIS PATIENTS

In the late 1940s certain analogs of nicotinic acid used in the treatment of tuberculosis were found to have an energizing effect on patients. From this observation developed the use of iproniazid (Marsilid) as one of the first allegedly specific antidepressants. These drugs were labeled monoamine oxidase inhibitors (MAOI) because of their action on this biochemical system in the brain, and on the basis of the unconfirmed belief that the clinical effect is directly related to this action.

Iproniazid, after initial rave reviews, became a subject of great controversy and was eventually taken off the market in the United States because of its high toxicity (Kalinowsky & Hippius, 1969). In *The Therapeutic Nightmare*, Morton Mintz describes how its successor, Parnate (tranylcypromine), caused so many fatalities, mostly from hypertension and stroke, that it was almost removed from the market. Its efficacy was also in doubt. Last-minute lobbying by the combined forces of industry (Smith-Kline & French) and the American Psychiatric Association kept it on the market (Mintz, 1965).

Currently available MAOIs include Parnate, Marplan (isocarboxazid), and Nardil (phenelzine). Marplan and Nardil are related to iproniazid. Parnate is chemically similar to amphetamine. Eldepryl (selegiline) was approved for the treatment of Parkinson's disease, but some psychiatrists prescribe it for depression.[7]

---

[7]Eldepryl was approved as an orphan drug for limited purposes; physicians should be wary of extending its use to depression.

The history of initial enthusiasm for the MAOIs is of great illustrative importance. In one of the few early critiques of the antidepressants in the psychiatric literature, Robert Liberman (1961) cast doubts on the already burgeoning enthusiasm for these drugs:

> When isoniazid was first tried in tuberculosis, the patients were photographed dancing in the hospital corridors. . . . Patients, however, are no longer dancing and it is now clear that isoniazid does not induce euphoria. The early patients who received the drug were euphoric without a doubt, but the euphoria was not a result of the pharmacologic properties of the drug. It was due to the fact that the doctors in the sanitariums had just been suddenly converted from jailers to therapists, and it was their renewed hope and pleasure from this event that affected their patients.

I have observed (1983a) that the MAOIs "in their clinically effective range are so toxic that they have been largely discarded in recent years. They represent one more class of miracle cures whose miracle has somehow evaporated." Yet as a part of the resurgence of biological psychiatry, they are back in vogue.

Consistent with the brain-disabling hypothesis, MAOIs can produce severe brain dysfunction, including a lowered seizure threshold, memory deficits, and frequent euphoric psychoses resembling mania (Kalinowsky & Hippius, 1969). Indeed, the original observations assigning an antidepressant effect to isoniazid probably derived from its capacity to produce toxic psychoses (e.g., see Noyes & Kolb, 1958, p. 187).

Patients often report to me that the MAOIs can have very numbing effects on the brain and mind. Sometimes they compare the impact to that of the neuroleptics.

The MAOIs are very toxic to the nervous system. They can cause a variety of CNS disorders that can be missed by the clinician, including myoclonic jerks, peripheral neuropathy, and paresthesia (see Schatzberg & Nemeroff, 1995). They can cause insomnia, agitation and anxiety or, more rarely, sedation. Like most antidepressants, they can cause organic brain syndromes and manic psychoses. Patients often have to be given concomitant sedatives, exposing them to additional adverse effects.

If combined with any one of a variety of medications or foods, MAOIs can cause disastrous stimulant hypertensive crises leading to fatal strokes or heart attacks, as well as more generalized CNS dysfunction. These toxic reactions can occur when MAOIs are mistakenly combined with psychostimulants such as amphetamine, dopamine, ephedrine, isoprotere-

nol, metaraminol, epinephrine, phenylepherine, methylphenidate, phenyl-
propanolamine, and pseudoephedrine. Many of these agents are found in
cold and asthma medications. Severe CNS toxic reactions can also occur
when MAOIs are combined with other antidepressants, such as tricyclics
and SSRIs, as well as buproprion and tryptophan. Central nervous system
toxic reactions can also occur when MAOIs are combined with Demerol
(meperidine) or L-Dopa. Hypertensive crisis can develop when MAOIs
are combined with foods that contain tyramine, including beef and chicken
liver, fermented sausages, caviar, fava beans, yeast, some alcoholic beverages, and a variety of others. A list of hazardous foods can be found in
most handbooks of pharmacology (e.g., Hyman, Arana, & Rosenbaum,
1995; Schatzberg & Cole, 1991).

SCIENTIFIC EVIDENCE
FOR ANTIDEPRESSANT EFFICACY

At the height of enthusiasm for tricyclic antidepressants, Baldessarini
(1978) found little scientific confirmation. Spontaneous remission and
placebo effect, he concluded, might account for why it usually takes several
weeks to obtain a positive response. Even in more severe depressions, he
noted, the spontaneous remission rate can exceed 50% in a few months.
Similarly, Klerman and Cole (1965), strong drug advocates, recognized
that "depressions, on the whole, are among the psychiatric conditions
with the best prognosis for symptomatic recovery, with or without treatment." They cite data predating the drug era that show improvement rates
of "44% of all patients within the first year and 56% recovery eventually
over a longer time period." Like Baldessarini, they observe that the time
lapse before the antidepressants are alleged to work may coincide with
the period of spontaneous recovery.

More recently, Fisher and Greenberg (1989, 1995) approached the
subject of antidepressant efficacy with a systematic analysis of the existing
controlled studies. They cast considerable doubt on the efficacy data (see
chapter 9 in regard to children). They do not believe that antidepressants
can be proven superior to placebos that produce sufficient side effects to
convince patients that they have been administered a potent drug.

Antonuccio, Danton, and DeNelsky (1994, 1995) have reviewed the
literature and concluded that psychotherapy is as good as, or better than,
antidepressants. It is certainly safer.

In conclusion, there is growing evidence that antidepressants are not the best treatment for depression. At the same time, there is by now a great deal of evidence that they frequently disable the brain and mind, sometimes producing severe and dangerous behavioral abnormalities, including violence against self and others.

CHAPTER **7**

Lithium and Other Drugs for Bipolar Disorder

Lithium for the treatment of manic episodes or manic-depressive (bipolar) disorder was originally promoted to the public and to the mental health profession as the ultimate example of a specific biochemical treatment for a specific psychiatric disorder. To bolster this claim, it was said that lithium lacks any brain-disabling effects on either patients or normal volunteers. This view of lithium directly challenges the brain-disabling principle of psychiatric treatment.

CLAIMS OF LITHIUM SPECIFICITY

In 1970 a booklet published by the National Institute of Mental Health (NIMH) and intended for public consumption claimed that lithium produces "no unwanted effects on mood and behavior" and "only the symptoms are leached out while the rest of the personality remains unaffected." The NIMH report concludes, "The drug is unique among psychopharmaceuticals in that it rarely produces any undesirable effects on emotional and intellectual functioning." It calls the substance "the first specific chemical treatment for a mental disease."

Five years later the APA (1975) published "The Current Status of Lithium Therapy: Report of the APA Task Force." Without citing evidence, the authors state, "The task force has concluded that lithium is a

111

more specific anti-manic agent than neuroleptics and that its therapeutic results are achieved in a unique pharmacologic effect rather than non-specific calming action.''

Ronald Fieve is one of the leading advocates of lithium. In his book, *Moodswing* (1989), he stated ''I have not found another treatment in psychiatry that works so quickly, so specifically, and so permanently as lithium for recurrent manic and depressive mood states'' (p. 4). He describes this extraordinary therapeutic effect as occurring with no discernible adverse effects (p. 3). We shall find instead that lithium is neither quick nor specific nor permanent in its impact. Nor is lithium relatively free of adverse effects.

SUBDUING EFFECTS OF LITHIUM

Subduing Effects on Animals

Cade (1949) discovered the potential therapeutic value of lithium accidentally while experimenting with guinea pigs, and immediately decided to try administering it to human beings. Here in his own words is the deductive leap he made:

> A noteworthy result was that after a latent period of about two hours the animals, although fully conscious, became extremely lethargic and unresponsive to stimuli for one to two hours before once again becoming normally active and timid.
>
> It may seem a long distance from lethargy in guinea pigs to the excitement of psychotics, but as these investigations had commenced in an attempt to demonstrate some possibly excreted toxin in the urine of manic patients, the association of ideas is explicable.

Thus Cade leaped from producing a toxic lethargy in animals to experimenting on human beings. As reviews by Schou (1957, 1968, 1976) indicate, no large studies on primate behavior were conducted before the widespread use of lithium in humans. One reason for this may be indicated in Schou's summaries of the rat and mouse literature. In a 1957 review he noted, ''A certain apathy and slowness of reaction have been frequent symptoms in the experimental animals . . . '' Or, as he remarked in a later review (1976), there is ''decreased spontaneous and exploratory activity.''

Lithium is toxic in rats at the same serum concentrations as in humans (Schou, 1976). In a rat study by Smith and Smith (1973) lithium was administered in the low therapeutic range for a period of only one week. The authors summarized, "The most consistent effect of lithium was to decrease the voluntary activity of the rats."

The consistent finding of generalized behavioral suppression in animals would seem to undermine the claim that lithium is a specific "magic bullet" for mania. Suppression of voluntary or spontaneous activity is one of the hallmarks of brain-disabling therapies.

Subduing Effects on Normal Infants

If a drug subdues the human fetus or infant, it is likely that its effect is not specific for a particular psychiatric disorder. Lithium freely crosses the placental barrier in utero, and can be passed through breast milk (Ananth, 1978). The effects of lithium in producing lethargy and hypotonia (loss of muscle function) in babies at relatively low serum levels has been thoroughly documented (Rane, Tomson, & Bjarke, 1978; Strothers, Wilson, & Royston, 1973). Hollister (1976) notes that lithium causes "lethargy, cyanosis, poor suck and Moro reflexes." As in animal studies, clinical reports concerning newborn and nursing babies demonstrate that lithium suppresses and even disables the central nervous system.

DISABLING EFFECTS OF LITHIUM

Disabling Effects on Normal Volunteers

Because they considered lithium to be disease-specific for mania, advocates of the drug initially claimed that it had little or no effect on normal individuals (Dempsey & Herbert, 1977; Hollister, 1976). Even van Putten (1975a), usually a keen observer of drug effects, stated that "lithium prophylaxis does not affect normal mental functioning or deprive a patient of normal human sorrow or elation. . . . "

Claims that lithium has no effect on normal volunteers are often based on a study by Schou and his colleagues (1968) who state: "The most striking observation seems to be how little lithium affects normal mental

functions: in prophylactic dosage not at all and in higher therapeutic
dosage only moderately'' (Schou et al., 1968).

However, their data does not support this view. It is true that they
found no impact in six volunteers when the drug was given at low doses for
only 1 week. However, the authors also administered lithium to themselves
within the therapeutic range (1.0 mEq/l) for 1 to 3 weeks. The authors
experienced the common initial somatic side effects, including "transient
nausea, diarrhea, slight tremor of the hands, etc." In addition they suffered
from a straitjacketing effect: "A feeling of muscular weakness or heaviness
was prominent in all the subjects. They had to overcome a certain resistance
against rising and moving and also had a feeling that mental effort was
needed to undertake any physical task."

The most remarkable effects were subjective. Keep in mind that the
authors are trying to substantiate how *little* effect lithium has on normal
mental function:

> Psychological effects were, on the whole, subtle and ill defined. There was
> no consistent change of the mood level, but irritability or emotional lability
> could at times be noted. There might be hypersensitivity to everyday sights
> and sounds. On other occasions responsiveness to environmental stimuli
> was diminished; this was in one of the cases welcomed by the family
> ("Dad is much easier and nicer than usual"), while the families of the
> two other subjects complained about their being so dull. The subjective
> experience was primarily one of indifference and slight general malaise.
> This led to a certain passivity. The subjects often had a feeling of being
> at a distance from their environment, as if separated from it by a glass
> wall. The subjective feeling of having been altered by the treatment was
> disproportionately strong in relation to objective behavioral changes. The
> subjects could engage in discussions and social activities but found it
> difficult to comprehend and integrate more than a few elements of a situa-
> tion. One of the subjects noted, for example, that whereas he had unaltered
> ability in a game such as chess with only two participants, he was less
> good at bridge with its four players. Intellectual initiative was diminished,
> and there was a feeling of lowered ability to concentrate and memorize;
> but thought processes were unaffected, and the subjects could think logically
> and produce ideas. The assessment of time was often impaired; it was
> difficult to decide whether an event had taken place recently or some time
> ago. (Schou et al., 1968)

In their summary, the authors confirm the overall brain-disabling effects. Echoing neuroleptic deactivation and surgical lobotomy (chapter

2), they speak of "indifference and a feeling of being at a certain distance from the environment" and note that "intellectual initiative is diminished."

Small, Milstein, Perez, Small, and Moore (1972) examined the mental effects of lithium on 11 normal volunteers in a more systematic fashion. Three had such serious reactions that there were "objective indications of impairment in work and school performance." A fourth developed a "severe, precipitous toxic delirium on the tenth day of taking lithium." A fifth volunteer dropped out of the study in the first week with "severe muscle weakness, confusion, and depression," which the authors argue, without evidence, was "more likely" related to psychological factors than to the drug.

Linnoila, Saario, and Maki (1974) focused on behavioral reactions in simulated automobile driving and found impairment in response and reaction times, and in judgment.

Judd and colleagues also studied the reactions of normal volunteers to lithium (mean, 0.9 mEq/l) over a 2-week period. In one study (Judd, Hubbard, Janowski, Huey, & Attewell, 1977; see also Judd, Hubbard, Janowski, Huey, & Takahashi, 1977) they report the effects on mood and personality on 23 subjects. They express surprise at their findings, which included a decreased "sense of well-being" (Judd, Hubbard, Janowski, Huey, & Attewell, 1977) among their volunteers and a "large number of spontaneous complaints." The authors describe their results in no uncertain terms:

> These subjective changes are not mood elevating, but rather mood lowering. In general, these feeling-tone alterations are dysphoric and characterized by lassitude, lethargy, and feelings of negativism and depression. In addition, feelings of agitation, anxiety, tension, and restlessness are related to lithium carbonate maintenance. There is also some evidence that subjects indicated they did not want to have to deal with the demands of interacting with their human environments. Finally, there are consistent self-reports of inability to concentrate, mental confusion, feeling muddleheaded, and a loss of clear-headedness.

In 1979 Judd summarized the results of studies with 42 healthy young men. He concluded that lithium produces a "general dulling and blunting of various personality functions" and a "generalized subjective dysphoria." He attributes the therapeutic effect to a general slowing of cognitive processes.

An especially interesting aspect of Judd's research confirms that trained independent observers are not likely to report adverse drug effects even when they are apparent to those who administered the drug and to those personally associated with the persons receiving the drug (Judd, Hubbard, Janowski, Huey, & Attewell, 1977):

> It was of interest to find that the effects of lithium carbonate in normal subjects were not perceptible to trained independent observers in the experimental situation. We initially speculated that these changes, although profound to the individual experiencing them, were not such that they were easily discernible, even to trained observers. In contrast to this was the fact that the "significant other," an individual who had a much more extensive interpersonal experience with the subject, was able to identify alterations in behavior and mood during the time the subjects were being maintained on lithium carbonate. Further, their observations were completely consistent with qualitative changes obtained from the self-rating data from the subjects themselves. Thus, these changes due to lithium carbonate are not just subjectively experienced, but are apparent to independent observers who are well acquainted with the normal range of behavior of each of the subjects.

The adverse effects most frequently noted by personal associates of the subjects included "increased levels of drowsiness and lowered ability to work hard and to think clearly" (Judd, 1979). The group who reported these changes in the subjects consisted of "friends, roommates, girlfriends, etc." The background of the "trained independent observers" is not described, but presumably they are mental health professionals.

It is striking that the trained observers were "unable to detect any behavioral changes in the subjects induced by lithium" when they were apparent to personal associates and could be measured on testing. Judd seems to attribute their failure to a lack of familiarity with the subjects in their normal surroundings. But various findings in this book confirm that this failure to observe adverse drug effects is characteristic of the vast majority of research reports and review articles in the drug literature. It is the doctor's part in iatrogenic denial—the tendency to deny the brain-disabling effects of psychiatric treatments (chapter 1).

More recent studies have continued to demonstrate adverse effects of lithium on normal subjects (Glue, Nutt, Cowen, & Broadbent, 1987; Kroph & Müller-Oerlinghausen, 1979; Müller-Oerlinghausen, Bauer, Girke, Kanowski, & Goncalves, 1977; Weingartner, Rudorfer, & Linnoila,

1985). Schatzberg and Cole (1991) appropriately warn that the patient's subjective experience of mental dysfunction should be taken seriously:

> Some patients on lithium complain of slowed mentation and forgetfulness and, on testing, a memory deficit has been found. Although such patients are often suspected or accused of "using" such symptoms to avoid necessary lithium therapy, our impression is that these complaints are often real and constitute a basis for lowering the dosage or trying another therapy. (p. 159)

Jefferson (1995) recently summed up:

> Neurologic adverse effects of lithium include reduced reactivity, lack of spontaneity, intellectual insufficiency, memory problems, difficulty in concentration, dysphoria. Some of these effects may be related to the therapeutic action of lithium in reducing hypomania. However, hypothyroidism, weakness and fatigue due to hypercalcemia, and breakthrough depression must be considered in the presence of these symptoms.

The production of thyroid disorders by lithium is common and requires constant concern throughout the treatment. Lithium-induced hypothyroidism can produce depression and other mental dysfunction, greatly confusing and complicating the patient's clinical picture.

In a review of the literature concerning the impact of psychiatric drugs on cognition in normal subjects, Judd et al. (1987) found:

> In summary, lithium often induces subjective feelings of cognitive slowing together with decreased ability to learn, concentrate and memorize. In addition, controlled studies have consistently described small but consistent performance decrements on various cognitive tests, including memory tests. The available data suggest that the slowing of performance is likely to be secondary to a slowing in the rate of central information processing. (p. 1468)

Studies of normal volunteers should lay to rest the claim that lithium only affects a disease process. It should also put an end to the claim that lithium has a specific antimanic effect rather than a generalized brain-disabling effect.

Turning Down the "Dial of Life"

Confirming the brain-disabling principle, lithium has the same subduing effects on psychiatric patients as on normal volunteers. Speaking of successful treatment cases with lithium, Dyson and Mendelson (1968) observed:

> It is as if their "intensity of living" dial had been turned down a few notches. Things do not seem so very important or imperative; there is greater acceptance of everyday life as it is rather than as one might want it to be; and their spouses report a much more peaceful existence.

The comparison to neuroleptic deactivation and to lobotomy again seems apparent.

According to Dyson and Mendelson (1968), even on effective maintenance therapy, the dial of life remains turned down. They quoted some of their patients:

> "I just don't get irritated and upset at things as I used to." "Things that used to bother me don't seem so important anymore." "I don't have any energy, can't accomplish what I used to be able to."

Schlagenhauf, Tupin, and White (1966) found, "When improvement was first noted the patients complained of feeling internally 'curbed,' a subjective experience that all of them had considerable difficulty in describing very precisely." The patients felt "unable to talk, think or move as fast as they would like."

Demers and Davis (1971) examined the attitudes of spouses toward patients treated with lithium. Without intending to emphasize the point, the study makes clear that there is an overall reduction in all forms of lively expression or vitality:

> An apparent unfavorable result of lithium treatment was a reduction in enthusiastic behavior, as well as sexual responsiveness in the manic-depressive. Hypomanic joviality, enthusiasm, and spontaneity are often regarded as social pluses; and manic-depressives and their spouses complain about the loss of these valued attributes. When pressed to discuss the sexual compatibility of the marriage, frequently they will say it is worse since lithium treatment started, as the lithium-treated spouse has less libidinal strivings.

OTHER LITHIUM EFFECTS

Lithium Effects on Creativity

Ronald Fieve of the New York State Psychiatric Institute achieved national attention ("New Old Treatment," 1973) in newspapers and magazines when he presented theatrical producer-director Joshua Logan at the annual meeting of the American Medical Association, where Logan gave a testimonial for lithium.

The entire question of testimonials for various treatments is a difficult and complex one. Quack cures, for example, often have avid supporters. Logan (1976), in his autobiography, describes his many contacts with psychiatric treatment over the years, including earlier public testimonials for psychiatry. He expresses surprise that people are critical of electroshock treatment, which he found to be very "benign."

Logan's own psychiatrist, Fieve, co-authored an article (Polatin & Fieve, 1971) describing three individuals (rare cases, in the authors' opinion) who rejected maintenance lithium, two of whom did so specifically on the grounds that it interfered with their creativity as writers of "bestsellers": "These patients report that lithium carbonate inhibits creativity so that the individual is unable to express himself, drive is diminished, and there is no incentive."

Despite their claim that lithium does not interfere with creativity, Schou and Baastrup (1973) describe its inhibiting, flattening effect:

> It is not always the elation that is missed. An undertaker's customers, mistaking depressive sadness for compassion, complained about his appearance of indifference when he was in lithium treatment. Another patient regretted that in discussions he was unable to attain the level of excitement he considered necessary: "Doctor, I am a communist and I must get excited when I discuss." There are also patients who feel that lithium treatment makes life "flat" and less colorful, "curbs" their activity, and prevents them from going as fast as they would like. In most cases these complaints disappear when the patients become used to the stable life course.

Whether these complaints do in fact disappear in most cases has never been carefully investigated. Even if the complaints become less frequent, there may be many unfortunate reasons for this, including iatrogenic denial.

More recently, Jefferson (1993) and Goodwin and Jamison (1990) have confirmed that loss of creativity is experienced by some patients.

Cognitive Dysfunction, Including Memory Deficits, in Patients Taking Lithium

It is now generally accepted that lithium can impair intellectual function. For example, Shaw, Stokes, Mann, and Manevitz (1987) found impairments of memory and hand motor speed on lithium.

In *Manic-Depressive Illness*, a book written wholly from a biopsychiatric perspective, Frederick Goodwin and Kay Jamison (1990) nonetheless conclude that lithium does cause serious cognitive impairments. They summarize much of the literature and declare:

> Since the drug's primary action is mediated through the central nervous system, it is not surprising that lithium can cause cognitive impairments of varying types and degrees of severity. Indeed, memory problems are among the side effects of lithium treatment that patients report most frequently. Although affective illness itself contributes both to cognitive deficits and complaints about such deficits, it is important to bear in mind that impairment of intellectual functioning caused by lithium is not uncommon and, in many patients, leads to noncompliance. Creativity can also be affected. [citations and chapter references omitted] (p. 706)

Acute Organic Brain Syndromes

Considering how vigorously lithium is promoted as relatively free of overpowering mental effects, it is surprising how frequently the literature has cited cases of toxic delirium during routine lithium therapy (Johnson, Gershon, & Hekimian, 1968; Mayfield & Brown, 1966; Prien et al., 1972; Shopsin, Kim, & Gershon, 1971; Strayhorn & Nash, 1977). Prien et al. (1972) found that almost one-third of the patients in their "highly active" category suffered "severe" reactions, including several with toxic confusion described as "disorientation, confusion, lack of continuity of thought, and reduced comprehension."

Neurotoxic Effects in Low-Dosage Maintenance Therapy

Branchey, Charles, and Simpson (1976) published a follow-up of patients on long-term lithium maintenance (6 months to 7 years). Only 10 of 36 are "free of neurologic symptoms," even with the low maintenance doses employed. Four of 36 patients have parkinson-like symptoms at a "low level of severity."

The existence of extrapyramidal side effects on maintenance lithium is controversial, but has been found in numerous studies (e.g., Kane, Rifkin, Quitkin, & Klein, 1978; Shopsin & Gershon, 1975). Shopsin and Gershon's patients, like those of Branchey et al., did not complain about their neurologic symptoms, suggesting further mental impairment.

Abnormal Brain Waves Produced by Routine Lithium Therapy

The EEG demonstrates significant pathologic response to lithium therapy, confirming the intoxicating effect of the drug (Baldessarini, 1977; Corcoran, Taylor, & Page, 1949; Mayfield & Brown, 1966; Peach, 1975; Schou, 1957; Small et al., 1972). Consistent with the brain-disabling principle, Mayfield and Brown correlated EEG abnormalities with the therapeutic response to treatment. Müller-Oerlinghausen et al. (1977) reported grossly abnormal brain-wave patterns in patients and normal volunteers. These persisted in the volunteers at the final testing seven days after the withdrawal of lithium therapy.

Two review articles confirm reports of persistent brain-wave changes in patients treated with lithium (Friedman, Culver, & Ferrell, 1977; Reisberg & Gershon, 1979). Reisberg and Gershon declare, wholly without proof, that "the evidence is that these effects are benign."

Lithium Disruption of the Compromised Brain

In combination with neuroleptics, especially haloperidol, there is an increased likelihood of severe encephalopathic syndromes that are sometimes irreversible (Baldessarini, 1978; Cohen & Cohen, 1974). There is a case report of a similar reaction from combining lithium with the newer neuroleptic, risperidone (Swanson, Price, & McEvoy, 1995).

Lithium administered in combination with electroshock produces more severe acute organic brain syndromes (Weiner, Whanger, Erwin, & William, 1980). Remick (1978) and Hoenig and Chaulk (1977) report single cases of an acute, severe delirium resulting from this combination. Mandel, Madsen, Miller, and Baldessarini (1980) reported on two more cases of this nature. In 1980 Small, Kellams, Milstein, and Small reviewed 25 patients given electroshock while being treated with lithium and found that the patients had more severe memory loss, more severe confusion, and occasional neurologic dysfunctions. The authors recommend against the use of electroconvulsive therapy (ECT) in patients receiving lithium therapy.

The literature concerning lithium administration to individuals with preexisting brain disease is sparse, but indicates the expected increase in brain disability, including in the elderly (Baldessarini, 1978).

Beitman (1978) has described a case of reactivation of tardive dyskinesia following lithium therapy; the tardive dyskinesia had been quiescent for many years. Crews and Carpenter (1977) describe a case in which lithium aggravated a preexisting tardive dyskinesia.

ASSESSING LITHIUM THERAPY

Cade Supports the Brain-Disabling Hypothesis

There is a particular irony in the date of the first publication on the use of lithium in mental patients; Cade's paper appeared in 1949, the same year that Corcoran et al. published "Lithium Poisoning from the Use of Salt Substitutes" in the *Journal of the American Medical Association.*

In regard to neuroleptics, we found that pioneers in their use were most straightforward about its brain-disabling effects. Cade indicated that lithium when used for other medicinal purposes produced "actual mental depression" in a variety of patients, not just those suffering from mania or manic depression. It forced a "quieting effect" on persons he considered schizophrenic (dementia praecox, in his nosology):

> An important feature was that, although there was no fundamental improvement in any of them, three who were usually restless, noisy and shouting nonsensical abuse . . . lost their excitement and restlessness and became quiet and amenable for the first time in years.

Cade preferred lithium to lobotomy on "restless and psychopathic mental defectives" in order "to control their restless impulses and ungovernable tempers."

The Mechanism of Lithium Effect

Writing from the viewpoint of the pharmacologist rather than the psychiatrist, Peach (1975) observed:

> The accumulation of lithium in the intracellular environment could be envisioned to perturb any event that is modulated by monovalent cations, e.g., sodium or potassium. These possible interactions signify the enormous magnitude of the task of determining precise mechanisms of action of the lithium ion.

Lithium disrupts almost every measurable cellular activity pertaining to nerve transmission, as well as many other vital functions. In addition, its distribution is fairly uniform throughout the central nervous system, with no known areas of specific concentration. It produces what Wilson, Schild, and Modell (1975) call a "non-selective diminution in neuronal activity." The neurophysiology of lithium, even without supporting clinical data, renders absurd the notion of a specific biochemical treatment for a specific disease.

Iatrogenic Helplessness and Denial

The research by Judd, discussed earlier in this chapter, demonstrates how professionals utterly fail to see lithium-induced disabilities that are obvious to friends and detectable on psychological testing. Patients themselves have difficulty evaluating their mental status on lithium. Toxicity often creeps up slowly over many days or weeks so that their judgment is impaired in an almost imperceptibly gradual manner. In fact, patients cannot be relied on to notice when they are becoming severely toxic, even though the toxicity heavily affects mental function. Instead, blood levels must be carefully monitored and the patients carefully watched.

Normal volunteers on small doses suffer impairments of their reflexes, but do not realize or acknowledge the impairment (Linnoila et al., 1974). Lithium patients who report no side effects often have tremors. The failure of patients on maintenance therapy with lithium to notice their own neurologic defects clearly demonstrates that maintenance lithium does have a brain-disabling effect, albeit a milder one than that achieved with the initially larger therapeutic doses.

The Relative Ineffectiveness of Lithium in Acute Mania

The myth of lithium specificity is shattered in exactly that arena in which one would expect to find the most support—clinical use as described by its advocates. Early on, it became generally accepted that the neuroleptics, not lithium, are most effective in stopping acute mania (Baldessarini, 1978; Juhl, Tsuang, & Perry, 1977). Even with the development of combined neuroleptic-lithium therapy, some authorities advocate ECT as well for the control of especially severe cases (Hollister, 1976).

The clinical preference for the neuroleptics as the treatment for acute mania has been confirmed by the single most comprehensive, controlled study, which was conducted by Prien and his colleagues (1972). They specifically contradicted the thesis that lithium has any specificity for mania, or the "underlying manic process." They cautioned that "Unfortunately, these observations have been all but lost in the vast number of unqualified endorsements of lithium carbonate therapy that have deluged the literature." Alexander, Van Kammen, and Bunney (1979) and Growe, Crayton, Klass, Evans, and Strizich (1979) also opined that lithium is not disease-specific for mania.

In the past a great deal was written about the use of lithium for the control of violence (Fieve, 1989; Marini & Sheard, 1977; Micer & Lynch, 1974; Morrison, Erwin, Gionturco, & Gerber, 1973; Sheard, Marini, Bridges, & Wagner, 1966; reviewed in Breggin, 1983a). While these claims have not been confirmed, they focus once again on the tendency to use or to advocate lithium for a variety of purposes.

How Effective Is Lithium
in Preventing the Recurrence of Manic Episodes?

Lithium has been promoted so strongly within psychiatry and to the public as a method of preventing recurrences of mania that few practitioners or consumers doubt its efficacy. In reality, lithium's effectiveness in this regard remains questionable. At the height of lithium's popularity, Prien, Caffey, and Klett (1974) reviewed the literature and found that studies showed a relapse rate as high as 50% over 2 years during lithium prophylactic treatment. Lithium did reduce the number of manic episodes in patients who had a history of infrequent attacks. But in patients with a high rate of past manic episodes, lithium did no better than placebo and all patients in this group eventually relapsed. If lithium were a disease-specific treatment, it surely would have performed better than this.

More recent research has been even more discouraging. Gitlin, Swendsen, Heller, and Hammen (1995) conducted a prospective study of patients treated with lithium for bipolar disorder. The patients were carefully monitored for effective drug treatment. Despite this, 73% of the patients relapsed into mania or depression within 5 years. Of those who relapsed, two-thirds had multiple episodes. Even among those patients who did not completely relapse, many suffered serious emotional difficulties. The authors conclude that "even aggressive pharmacological maintenance treatment does not prevent relatively poor outcome in a significant number of bipolar patients" (p. 1635).

Can Withdrawal from Lithium Cause Mania?

The situation may be even worse than suggested by these studies of treatment failure. There is evidence that stopping lithium in itself can stimulate a new manic episode. Suppes, Baldessarini, Faedda, and Tohen (1991) analyzed 14 studies and found that the rate of relapse into mania increased following the discontinuation of lithium. The patients, who tended to cycle into mania about once a year (mean 11.6 months), developed a new episode less than 2 months (mean 1.7 months) after stopping their medication. In other words, discontinuation of treatment with lithium produced a much more rapid onset of mania than the untreated patients would have endured.

The research by Suppes and her team provided a good argument for not starting lithium treatment. Unfortunately, patients who relapse soon after taking lithium are rarely, if ever, told that their relapse was probably caused by lithium withdrawal.

Many psychiatrists advise patients who are diagnosed bipolar or manic that they must take lithium for many years or even for the rest of their lives. They are told that it is irresponsible for them not to do so. Families and psychotherapists are pressured to urge or to coerce patients to take their lithium. The data do not confirm this strong advocacy for the drug.

Other Adverse Reactions to Lithium Withdrawal

Nearly all psychiatric drugs can cause adverse reactions when abruptly withdrawn, including neuroleptics, antidepressants, and minor tranquilizers. Less has been written about withdrawal from lithium, although some patients have told me about emotional suffering during acute withdrawal of the drug.

Swartz and Jones (1994) have reviewed the literature and presented three cases concerning severe and often persistent adverse reactions to the abrupt withdrawal of lithium in patients suffering from hyperlithemia during routine treatment. One of their own cases became severely demented. In their review of 50 cases obtained from the Lithium Information Center of the University of Wisconsin, they found that many patients became demented or otherwise deteriorated severely when abruptly withdrawn from lithium. Patients subjected to kidney dialysis for lithium toxicity often deteriorated badly with a rapid drop in lithium levels.

Neurologic sequelae persisted in 30% of the 50 patients. The authors found "substantial neurotoxic risks" in rapidly withdrawing patients from high lithium levels.

If rapid withdrawal from high lithium levels can produce mania and disabling neurologic reactions, then it is probable that rapid withdrawal from lower levels may produce more subtle adverse reactions.

LITHIUM IN YOUR DRINKING WATER
AND OTHER POLITICAL IMPLICATIONS

In 1970 Dawson, Moore, and McGanity tried to support a fantastic thesis: Increased rainfall dilutes certain minerals in reservoirs, including lithium, producing a correlation between areas of lesser rainfall, higher lithium levels in drinking water, and a lower incidence of mental illness as measured by hospital admissions. In *Psychiatric Drugs* (1983a) I examined and debunked the study and its various supporters (see Fieve, 1989; "In Texas," 1971). Here I want to emphasize that it demonstrates one of the political hazards of arguing that a psychiatric treatment corrects biochemical imbalances without adversely affecting the brain.

LITHIUM SUBSTITUTES
AND OTHER "MOOD STABILIZERS"

A variety of other drugs are used to control acute mania and to reduce the likelihood of a recurrence of the disorder. None of them are considered specific for the disorder and all of them have some brain-disabling, often sedative, effects. In reality, almost all sedative drugs have been used to subdue or control mania with varying degrees of success. I will review the lithium alternatives briefly.

When lithium fails to control recurrences, neuroleptics such as Haldol or Prolixin are frequently added to the regimen. This exposes the patient to all their brain-disabling effects, including the potentially lethal neuroleptic malignant syndrome and the various irreversible tardive disorders (chapters 3–5).

Several drugs commonly used in neurological medicine for the control of epilepsy—valproic acid, carbamazepine, and clonazepam—are also used extensively in psychiatry. The brain-disabling effects of these agents are more likely to appear in psychiatric practice than in the treatment of epilepsy by neurologists because the drugs are often prescribed in excessive doses by psychiatrists in order to control or subdue behavior. Therefore, the following discussion should not discourage the use of these agents when appropriate for the control of seizures.

Valproic acid (Depakene), sodium valproate (Depakene syrup), and divalproex sodium (Depakote, enteric-coated combination of the other two) are forms of an anti-epileptic agent that has been recently approved by the FDA for the treatment of manic-depressive disorder. The drug can be hepatotoxic, especially in children. From the brain-disabling perspective, it can cause sedation, tremor, and ataxia. More rarely, it can cause adverse changes in mood and behavior, including behavioral automatisms and confusion. Somnolence or delirium can develop, especially when combined with other sedatives (Silver, Yudofsky, & Hurowitz, 1994). There may be "mild impairment of cognitive function with chronic use" (Hyman et al., 1995, p. 127).

Carbamazepine (Tegretol) is closely related to the tricyclic antidepressants. In neurological medicine, its principal uses are as an anticonvulsant for partial complex seizures and in the management of tic douloureux, a facial pain syndrome. It causes similar brain-disabling effects, including sedation, tremor, confusion, depression, psychosis, and memory disturbances (chapter 6). Cognitive disturbances are more common with concomitant use of neuroleptics, with preexisting brain damage and with aging (Hyman et al., 1995). In addition, it poses the threat of potentially lethal agranulocytosis or aplastic anemia. Carbamazepine can cause hyponatremia (low serum sodium), leading to a syndrome that includes lethargy, confusion or hostility, and stupor.

Clonazepam (Klonopin), a benzodiazepine minor tranquilizer, has been used to treat both acute mania and as prophylaxis. It has all the many, sometimes severe, problems associated with the other benzodiazepines, including sedation, rebound and withdrawal syndromes, addiction, and behavioral abnormalities (chapter 11).

Verapamil (Calan and others) is a calcium channel blocker used for the treatment of cardiac disorders. It can produce a variety of cardiovascular side effects.

Clonidine, an antihypertensive drug, also has been used in the treatment of mania. Sudden withdrawal can produce a rebound hypertensive crisis. It can produce many psychiatric symptoms, including sedation, vivid dreams or nightmares, insomnia, restlessness, anxiety, and depression. More rarely, it can cause hallucinations.

Some clinicians will add a variety of antidepressants, including SSRIs like Prozac, to the treatment of patients with manic-depressive disorder. Nearly all antidepressants can cause or worsen mania (chapter 6; also see Goodwin & Jamison, 1990).

The lengthy list of attempts to substitute for lithium suggests, once again, that it is hardly a specific "magic bullet" for mania or manic-depressive disorder.

CONCLUSION

Lithium is a highly neurotoxic substance with a generally suppressive effect on neuronal function and mental function in the commonly pre-scribed therapeutic range. This brain-disabling effect is not specific for manic or manic-depressive (bipolar) patients. Lithium will subdue or suppress the functioning of a variety of patients and inmates with other diagnoses. It has devastating effects on the function of normal volunteers. It will also suppress the newborn infants and nursing infants of mothers who take lithium. Lithium-treated animals also show similar taming effects. The various alternatives to lithium have their own brain-disabling effects, and none of the drugs is specific for mania.

Although lithium possesses these suppressive properties, it is not as effective in controlling mania as the neuroleptics, especially in acute mania or in severe, recurrent mania. This is partly because of lithium's extreme toxicity in doses sufficient to subdue severely disturbed or rebellious individuals.

The claim that lithium is a disease-specific therapy for mania or manic-depressive (bipolar) disorder has no basis in fact; it is a brain-disabling agent. Its efficacy has been exaggerated and its adverse effects on the mind have been too frequently minimized.

CHAPTER 8

Electroshock for Depression*

Sarah Williams was fifty-five years old when her husband died of a sudden heart attack in the early spring. She managed to teach music in high school for the remainder of the year but by the summer her "blues" worsened. She lost weight, had difficulty staying asleep at night, and even lost her zest for visiting with her grown children. Her oldest daughter, Jeannette, became concerned and in June took her to a psychiatrist. On the first visit, he put her on a tricyclic antidepressant, doxepin, that made her feel too groggy so she stopped taking it. Then he put her on Prozac which made her feel agitated. She was now both depressed and agitated, and her psychiatrist admitted her to a hospital for electroconvulsive therapy (ECT).

Jeannette was very reluctant to submit her mother to ECT but she was convinced by the doctor and a video film that shock was the most effective modality for depression. Jeannette and her mother were told that the electrical current and the grand mal convulsion that it produced were virtually harmless. The electrodes would be placed on only one side of the head (unilateral ECT) with the latest modifications to prevent injury.

Mrs. Williams herself protested about having electricity passed through her brain, and she wondered why no one seemed to want to talk with her about her feelings. Didn't psychiatrists do talking therapy anymore? But she was willing to accept anything that promised an end to the hopelessness

---

*This chapter has been greatly modified and expanded from "The Return of ECT" published in *Readings*, March 1992. I wish to thank *Readings* for the use of this material.

that pervaded her life. Especially, she wanted to stop being a burden to her daughter, Jeannette.

After the first shock treatment Mrs. Williams developed a headache and stiff neck. She was somewhat nauseated. By the third treatment, given every other day, she was confused and couldn't recall her daughter's previous visit. Her daughter was reassured by the doctor that this was "normal" for ECT, that all the effects were temporary, and that it would be best if she didn't see her mother until the series of ten ECTs was completed.

The nurses' notes from the hospitalization show increasing "complaints" of memory difficulties by Mrs. Williams as the treatments progressed in number. However, after the eighth ECT she stopped communicating about anything. The doctor's progress note at this point stated "Improved. No longer complaining of feelings of depression." The nurse's progress note indicated "No complaints. Sits quietly."

By the tenth treatment, Mrs. Williams couldn't find her way around the ward. The head of occupational therapy noted that the patient was too "disoriented and confused" to participate in the music and art activities.

When Jeannette visited her mother again at the conclusion of the treatments, she hardly recognized her. The expression on her mother's face was bland and indifferent rather than pained. Sometimes her mother got a silly, almost goofy, look that especially upset Jeannette. Her mother had always been so serious and dignified. To her daughter's dismay, her mother could not remember any of the events of the previous summer, including the visits to the psychiatrist. She couldn't remember who had come to her husband's funeral the previous April. She couldn't remember much about teaching for two semesters during the school year.

Mrs. Williams stayed in the hospital for one week after the completion of the ECT. At that time, her insurance ran out and she was discharged home. Her discharged diagnosis was "Major Depression in remission."

Jeannette could see that her mom looked confused as she drove her home. She didn't seem to recognize the neighborhood where she had lived for thirty years and raised her children. At home, her mother couldn't find the coffee or the sugar. She didn't recognize the blender that Jeannette had bought her the previous Christmas.

A week later, Jeannette went to see the psychiatrist with her mother. The psychiatrist reassured her that he had never seen a case of permanent memory loss following electroshock except for memory blanks for the period immediately around the shock treatment.

In September, two months after the ECT, Mrs. Williams tried to return to teaching but quit after two weeks. She couldn't remember the books or teaching materials she'd been using for several years. The principal, who had started at the school a year earlier, was a stranger. She had trouble recognizing most of her previous students, including some who had been in music class with her for several years.

For the first time in her life, Mrs. Williams found she was having difficulty hearing music in her head. She was slow reading music and was distraught that she couldn't learn new pieces by heart anymore. She felt like a beginner in music, except she couldn't learn as well as a beginner. She became suicidally depressed for the first time in her life.

Jeannette took her mother back to the psychiatrist, who insisted that none of these problems could be from the shocks. He said that Mrs. Williams was depressed and needed more ECT. Instead, Jeannette took her mother home to live with her.

It was now January and her mother wasn't getting any better. Mom seemed like a changed person. Her personality was gone. So was her vitality. She couldn't remember the simplest things, such as a phone call message or a list of three items to get at the grocery store.

Jeannette took her mom to the university medical center for evaluation. Lengthy neuropsychological testing over a two-day period indicated that her mother had major impairments in anterograde memory (learning and recalling new material) and in retrograde memory (remembering past events). Some of her memory losses extended back several years. She had difficulty concentrating and there were impairments of abstract reasoning. Formerly very quick mathematically, she was now poor at calculating. Her overall IQ had dropped twenty points. She became very fatigued and frustrated from the effort of trying so hard on the tests.

The neuropsychologist described the pattern as typical of traumatic brain injury but after a consultation with Mrs. Williams' former psychiatrist, he avoided any suggestion that the deficits could have been caused by a series of electroshocks to the brain. Brain wave studies showed that Mrs. Williams had abnormal slow waves on her EEG consistent with brain injury to the right frontal lobe and the anterior portion of the right temporal lobe (the site of the electrode placement). A brain scan (MRI) showed possible atrophy in the same region.

To this day, Mrs. Williams' psychiatrist states that he has never seen a case of permanent memory loss, or any other permanent neuropsychological deficits, following ECT. He did not report the case in the literature, to the FDA, or to the manufacturer of the shock machine.

Mrs. Williams remains chronically depressed and refuses to go to any doctors for anything. She lives with her daughter, who supports her financially.

Cases like Mrs. Williams's have become increasingly common as psychiatry relies more and more exclusively on drugs and ECT. The last decade has seen a resurgence in the promotion and use of ECT, also called electroshock or simply shock treatment. Recently the press has taken note of the escalating controversy surrounding its use (Boodman, 1996). A critical article by Cauchon (1995) in *USA Today* was followed up by a remarkable editorial ("Patient, public need . . . ," 1996) that declared "the long-term effects can be devastating. They include confusion, memory loss, heart failure, and, in some patients, death."

Electroconvulsive therapy is a treatment that originated in Italy in 1938 for producing convulsions in psychiatric patients. At the time it was thought that convulsions induced by a variety of methods, including insulin coma and stimulant medication, were useful in treating psychiatric disorders, especially schizophrenia.

Nowadays ECT is recommended for major depression, usually when other approaches have failed. However, some doctors quickly resort to it. Probably more than 100,000 patients a year in the United States are shocked. The majority are women and many are elderly. In California, for example, two thirds of shock patients are reported to be women, more than half of whom are 65 or older (State of California, 1989). Recent data (1989–1993) from Vermont concerning ECT show that 77% of shock patients were female (Sullivan, 1996). For all sexes, 58% were at least 65 years old and 20% were at least 80 years old. During this time, one Vermont hospital, Hitchcock Psychiatric, shocked 35 women and one man who were 80 and older. Overall, the hospital shocked 112 women and 26 men during those 5 years.

The use of ECT tends to vary from institution to institution. At Johns Hopkins, for example, a biologically oriented center, 20% of the inpatients may be on a regimen of ECT at any one time (Wirth, 1991, p. 9). Many other hospitals do not even offer ECT.

The Food and Drug Administration and ECT

In 1979, the FDA classified shock devices as demonstrating "an unreasonable risk of illness or injury" (see Food and Drug Administration, 1990).

This would have required animal testing for safety. However, under pressure from the APA, the FDA gave notice of its intent to reconsider its original decision and to reclassify ECT machines as safe. The APA's most recent Task Force report was timed to come out in the midst of the FDA's political squirming over ECT.

The FDA's final report (Food and Drug Administration, 1990) reads remarkably like the APA's 1990 report. Although no large animal studies have been done with shock devices since the 1950s, and although those earlier studies consistently demonstrated brain damage (see ahead), the FDA panel has now recommended defining ECT devices as safe for depressed patients. It did so ambivalently, recommending that the approval be delayed until the establishment of engineering safety standards for the machines. The approval process continues to be delayed by the lack of approved standards and ECT exists in a kind of FDA limbo which has not discouraged psychiatrists from using it.

I have reviewed what the FDA has made available as its complete file on ECT. There are dozens of recommendations from state-funded and private patient rights and advocacy groups to ban ECT, and hundreds more from patients who feel they have been permanently damaged by the treatment. It is astonishing that the FDA has ignored or rejected such an avalanche of official recommendations and personal reports and protests.

In approving the ECT machines as potentially safe, the FDA ignored a most remarkable situation. Before being put on the market, the ECT machines, such as the commonly used MECTA, were not tested for safety on animals or humans. There were no systematic or controlled studies to evaluate their impact on the living brain. The FDA has simply taken the word of organized psychiatry that ECT is safe and effective.

The Politics of the 1990 APA Report

The political nature of the APA task force report (1990b) is reflected in the membership of the panel that wrote it. The chairperson, Richard Weiner, was APA's official representative in defense of ECT at the FDA hearings, and has for some time been APA's chief spokesperson on the subject. Two of the other six members are psychiatrist Max Fink and psychologist Harold Sackeim, among the nation's most zealous promoters of the treatment. Fink (1994, 1995) is currently pressing to increase the use of shock treatment for children and adolescents. Sackeim and his colleagues (1993) have written an article calling for a return to much higher electrical doses, given the "old-fashioned way" with bilateral electrode placement (see below) to increase the intensity of the shocks.

By contrast, the task force sought no input from the several patient organizations that oppose the treatment, and none from psychologists, psychiatrists, neurologists, and other professionals who are critical of it.

The APA task force report in its acknowledgments thanks the manufacturers of electroshock machines for their contributions; company advertising handouts are listed as useful sources of public information; and the names, addresses, and phone numbers of these companies are provided in the report. The task force is particularly positive toward Somatics, Inc., whose sole function is to manufacture the electroshock machine, Thymatron. Somatics, Inc. is acknowledged for providing "input into the guidelines." Under "Materials for Patients and Their Families" the task force cites a pamphlet by Richard Abrams and Conrad Swartz and a videotape by Max Fink, both of which are advertising materials for Thymatron and can only be obtained by writing to the manufacturer.

The report nowhere mentions any link between this company and Richard Abrams, who would appear to be the task force's most valued expert. One of Abrams's articles is recommended under "Materials for Patients and Their Families" and another under "Materials for Professionals." Nine of his publications are cited in the report's general bibliography, making him by far the most heavily represented author. Abrams is also listed among those individuals who "provided comment on the draft of the ECT Task Force Report." However, his most interesting affiliation is absent: Abrams *owns* Somatics, Inc.! In a deposition in which he was a medical expert (DeToma v. Brohamer, 1991), Abrams acknowledged under questioning that Somatics, Inc., is the source of 50% of his income.

LACK OF EFFICACY

Rifkin (1988) noted that the claim is frequently made that ECT is more effective and works more rapidly than drugs in the treatment of depression. He found nine controlled studies comparing the two treatments, but they were badly flawed. He could find no conclusive evidence that ECT was better than antidepressant treatment.

Crow and Johnstone (1986), in a review of controlled studies of ECT efficacy, found that both ECT and sham ECT were associated with "substantial improvements" and that there was little or no difference between the two. Crow and Johnstone concluded, "Whether electrically induced convulsions exert therapeutic effects in certain types of depression that cannot be achieved by other means has yet to be clearly established" (p. 27).

Crow and Johnstone's critical review, which was presented at the largest conference of shock advocates in recent years, is not cited in either the APA or FDA reports on ECT. Instead, the APA task force's proposal for a "Sample Patient Information Sheet" declares that "ECT is an extremely effective form of treatment" (APA Task Force, 1990, p. 160).

At the June, 1985, Consensus Conference on ECT, critics and advocates of ECT debated the issue of efficacy. The advocates were unable to come forth with a single study showing that ECT had a positive effect beyond 4 weeks. Many studies showed no effect and in the positive studies, the improvements were not dramatic. That the treatment had no positive effect after 4 weeks confirmed the brain-disabling principle, since 4 weeks is the approximate time for recovery from the most mind-numbing effects of acute organic brain syndrome.

The Consensus Conference panel stated in its report that ECT had no documented positive effect beyond 4 weeks. This is critical in terms of the concept of maximum therapeutic trade-off. Acute brain damage and dysfunction, with a high probability of permanent adverse effects, are exchanged for a brief period of traumatically induced emotional blunting or euphoria.

ECT and Suicide

ECT is frequently justified as treatment of last resort in cases at high risk for suicide. But research uniformly shows that ECT has no beneficial effect on the suicide rate. In a blatantly misleading fashion, the negative studies are cited by the task force report, the FDA report, and others as showing a positive effect. For example, a retrospective study by Avery and Winokur (1976) found no improvement in the suicide rate compared to matched controls who had no shock treatment: "In the present study, treatment was not shown to affect the suicide rate" (p. 1033). Yet it is presented in the 1990 task force report as supporting the position that

ECT results in "a lower incidence of suicide" (p. 53). The task force also mentions three other studies as supporting a beneficial effect on suicide, yet two of them (Avery & Winokur, 1977; Milstein, Small, Small, & Green, 1986) specifically find *no* such beneficial effect and the third (McCabe, 1977) doesn't even deal with suicide. In two other retrospective studies of relatively large populations of ECT patients and matched controls, ECT had no effect on the suicide rate (Babigian & Guttmacher, 1984; Black, Winokur, Mohandoss, Woolson, & Nasrallah, 1989).

Overall, there is little or nothing in the literature to suggest that ECT ameliorates suicide whereas a significant body of literature confirms that it does not. Once again, treatment opinions are not driven by empirical data. Instead empirical data is ignored, distorted, or misrepresented to confirm treatment opinions.

My own clinical impression is that ECT in reality increases the suicide risk for many patients. It is well known, for example, that Ernest Hemingway attributed his suicide to despair over ECT ruining his memory and rendering him unable to write (Hotchner, 1966, p. 308).

As they attempt to recover from the treatment, electroconvulsive therapy patients frequently find that their prior emotional problems have now been complicated by brain damage and dysfunction that won't go away. If their doctors tell them that ECT never causes any permanent difficulties, they become further confused and isolated, creating conditions for suicide.

Many shock survivors have told me that reading my papers and books about ECT was a life-affirming experience for them. Instead of reacting with more despair to the confirmation of their ECT-induced brain damage and disability, they have felt understood and empowered for the first time. Mental health professionals should be advised that it is both ethical and beneficial to acknowledge to patients in a supportive, empathic manner that they have been injured by the treatment.

ECT, Women, and Memory Loss

Women have always been the main victims of the most destructive psychiatric treatments, including lobotomy. More recently, older women have become the major population for ECT, despite the absence of controlled studies on safety or efficacy in the elderly.

One of the most remarkable reports in the ECT literature was published by Carol Warren (1988) who studied 10 women post-ECT, including their family relationships. Many of the women thought that the purpose of the treatment was to erase their memory. While some felt it was helpful to forget painful memories, they "uniformly disliked the loss of everyday memory, as well as associated effects such as losing one's train of thought, incoherent speech, or slowness of affect. What specifically was forgotten varied from matters of everyday routine to the existence of one or more of one's children . . . " Without reporting on the clinical significance of the women's experience, Warren is describing mild to moderate dementia following closed-head injury.

Family members sometimes approved of the memory loss. One husband said, "They did a good job there," referring to his wife's loss of memory concerning their past marital conflicts. A patient who had been molested by her mother's brother believed that her mother wanted her to have "the full treatment" to "make me forget all those things that happened."

Three of the ten women lived in dread of ECT for years afterward, but were afraid to express their angry feelings for fear of being sent back to the hospital for involuntary shock treatment. In my clinical experience, this is a realistic fear. Doctors frequently respond to complaints about the treatment by deciding that the patient is in need of more treatment. The treatment can almost always be relied on to eventually put an end to all protests.

Shock treatment has been used even more blatantly to erase the memories and even the personalities of patients, usually women. H. C. Tien, in the early 1970s, described the use of unmodified ECT to erase the personalities of women, then to "reprogram" them as more suitable wives—with their husband's help ("Electroshock: Key Element . . . ," 1972; "From Couch to Coffee Shop . . . ," 1972). World-renowned psychiatrist D. Ewen Cameron at McGill University, in part utilizing secret funds from the CIA, used multiple ECTs to obliterate the minds of his patients and then to reprogram them (Cameron, Lohrenz, & Handcock, 1962; for more details on the Tien and Cameron controversies, see also Breggin, 1979 & 1991a).

ECT and the Elderly

As already noted, elderly women have become the most frequent target of ECT. The elderly, of course, have more fragile brains, and are especially sensitive to biopsychiatric interventions, even relatively mild doses of drugs. In addition, many elderly already suffer from memory dysfunction due to a variety of causes, making them especially vulnerable to the worst effects of ECT.

Against all common sense, the task force advises that ECT can be used "regardless of age" (p. 15) and cites the successful treatment of a patient aged 102 (pp. 71–72). It does warn, however, that "some elderly patients may have an increased likelihood of appreciable memory deficits and confusion during the course of treatment" (p. 72).

The aged are, in fact, gravely at risk when exposed to any form of head trauma, including electrically induced, closed-head injury from ECT. There are a growing number of reports of special dangers to the elderly that are not mentioned in the APA or the FDA reviews (Figiel, Coffey, Djang, Hoffman, & Doraiswamy, 1990; Pettinati & Bonner, 1984). In a curious twist, an article by Burke, Rubin, Zorumski, and Wetzel (1987) is listed in the bibliography of the APA report but not cited in the actual discussions of the elderly. Burke and his colleagues found a high rate (35%) of complications among the elderly. They noted, "Common complications in the elderly include severe confusion, falls, and cardiorespiratory problems" (p. 516).

In a study involving three times as many women as men, Kroessler and Fogel (1993) produced data indicating that ECT can cause a devastating decline in longevity:

> This is a longitudinal study of 65 patients who were 80 years old or older at the time they were hospitalized for depression. Thirty-seven were treated with ECT and 28 with medication. Survival after 1, 2, and 3 years in the ECT group was 73.0%, 54.1%, and 51.4% respectively. Survival after 1, 2, and 3 years in the non-ECT group was 96.4%, 90.5%, and 75.0% respectively. (p. 30)

These are extraordinary findings, indicating a very high increase in mortality in the elderly who receive ECT. The authors, however, argue that the patients receiving ECT were more physically ill and hence at greater risk of dying. They provided no data to explain such a vast difference in mortality.

The lethality of ECT was made even more tragically wasteful by its comparative lack of efficacy. ECT patients were much more frequently rehospitalized for depression than non-ECT patients (41% versus 15%). The recurrence rate of depression was more than twice as high among the ECT patients compared to the non-ECT patients (54.1% versus 25%). Lasting recovery from depression was much lower in ECT patients (22% versus 71%).

Elderly women have many reasons—psychosocial and economic, some of them rooted in the ageist and sexist attitudes of our society—for feeling depressed. Often, these women need improved medical care, social services, family involvement, and loving care from friends and volunteers. All of their basic needs may require attention. Meanwhile, they typically do not have the strength to resist a doctor's proposal that they undergo electroshock. There may be no family members available or willing to protect them. One thing the elderly do not need is more brain cell death, mental dysfunction, and memory deficits.

I have been a consultant or a medical expert in several suits in which psychiatrists have tried to administer electroshock against the will of elderly women who had no family to defend them. Each time, the doctors have backed down or, as in the case of Lucille Austwick, they have lost in court (Boodman, 1996, p. 19). However, many other elderly women are probably getting shocked involuntarily without their situation gaining public attention. In addition, in my experience, many seemingly voluntary patients are badgered or misled into taking the treatment.

Electroshock advocates argue that more women than men become depressed and so more women need the treatment. But why do more women become depressed? Multiple research studies have now connected depression in women to patriarchal oppression, including outright sex abuse (American Psychological Association, 1990). Warren's study confirmed that ECT can, in fact, be used to cover up the sexual abuse of women and girls.

INJURY BY ELECTROSHOCK

The Production of Delirium (Acute Organic Brain Syndrome)

After one or more shock treatments, ECT routinely produces delirium or an acute organic brain syndrome. Abrams (1988), although an advocate of the treatment, has himself observed that:

> . . . a patient recovering consciousness from ECT understandably exhibits multiform abnormalities of all aspects of thinking, feeling, and behaving,

including disturbed memory, impaired comprehension, automatic movements, a dazed facial expression, and motor restlessness. (pp. 130–131)

At times, patients are so organically impaired following ECT that they will sit around apathetically on the ward, unable to engage in any activities. On occasion, the patients' neurological dilapidation from routine ECT will reduce them to lying in a fetal position for many hours. In malpractice suits in which I have been a medical expert for plaintiffs, psychiatrists for the defense have claimed that this kind of neurological collapse is normal and harmless following ECT.

Given that ECT routinely produces acute, marked brain dysfunction, there can be no real disagreement about its damaging effects. The only legitimate question is: "How complete is recovery?" Basic neurology warns that it will frequently be incomplete.

ECT As Closed-Head Electrical Injury

Neurology recognizes that relatively minor head trauma—even without the delirium, loss of consciousness, and seizures associated with ECT—frequently produces chronic mental dysfunction and personality deterioration (Bernat & Vincent, 1987). If a woman came to an emergency room in a confusional state from an accidental electrical shock to the head, perhaps from a short circuit in her kitchen, she would be treated as an acute medical emergency. If the electrical trauma had caused a convulsion, she might be placed on anticonvulsants to prevent a recurrence of seizures. If she developed a headache, stiff neck, and nausea—a triad of symptoms typical of post-ECT patients—she would probably be admitted for observation to the intensive care unit. Yet ECT delivers the same electrical closed-head injury, repeated several times a week, as a means of improving mental function. ECT is electrically induced closed-head injury.

The symptoms of mild to severe closed-head injury are listed in detail by J. M. Fisher (1985). They include impairment of every area of mental, emotional, and behavioral function, confirming the multiple adverse effects of ECT on the mind and brain. McClelland, Fenton, and Rutherford (1994) describe the postconcussive syndrome in terms of

the emergence and variable persistence of a cluster of symptoms following mild head injury. Common to most descriptions are somatic symptoms (headache, dizziness, fatiguability) accompanied by psychological symptoms (memory and concentration difficulties, irritability, emotional lability, depression and anxiety).

Between one third and one half experience this symptom cluster over the first few weeks and a "substantial minority" continue to experience it for months or a year or more.

Head-injury victims, including post-ECT patients, frequently develop an organic personality syndrome with shallow affect, poor judgment, irritability, and impulsivity. They seem "changed" or "different" to people around them, much as lobotomy patients often seem to their families. Sometimes they become slightly clumsy, moving awkwardly or dropping things. Often they have "lapses" where they cannot think or cannot voice their thoughts. Sometimes their handwriting deteriorates. Headaches frequently begin with the traumatic treatment and may recur indefinitely.

Many post-ECT patients suffer from irreversible generalized mental dysfunction with apathy, deterioration of social skills, trouble focusing attention, and difficulties in remembering new things. I have worked with a number of them who suffer from dementia, confirmed by neuropsychological testing. Several have developed partial complex seizures or psychomotor epilepsy, permanently abnormal EEGs, and atrophy on brain scans. Many have been deprived of the experience of years of their lives, their professional careers, and their mental ability following ECT (Breggin, 1979, 1981a).

Death, Suicide, and Autopsy Findings

Many deaths were reported in association with ECT in the first few decades of use. An extensive autopsy series indicated that many suffered from trauma to the brain resulting in visible pathology (Impastato, 1957). More recently, advocates for ECT have claimed the death rate is very small or nearly nonexistent; but I have suspected that deaths are simply no longer reported. For example, I have known of deaths of ECT recipients in the Baltimore–Washington area that went unreported.

Recently, there was confirmation of the probability of a significant death rate. A recent law in Texas requires the reporting of death within two weeks after ECT. From June, 1993, through August, 1994, eight deaths were reported among nearly 1,700 patients subjected to shock treatment. Controversy surrounds causation, and critics of ECT are attempting to obtain more autopsy details (Smith, 1995).

Memory Deficits

Memory deficits, retrograde and anterograde, are among the most common early signs of traumatic brain damage, and are seen in virtually all cases of ECT. The only disagreement surrounds the severity and persistence of these deficits; but as I've tried to emphasize, neurological experience indicates that patients frequently fail to recover from much less intense injury to the brain.

Electroshock specialists almost never seriously consider the memory deficits of their patients. In case after case that I have evaluated for clinical or forensic purposes, I have been the first doctor to take the symptoms seriously, let alone to take a complete inventory of memory losses and ongoing mental difficulties. I have previously outlined a method for evaluating memory deficits from ECT (1979).

The APA task force report, like the FDA report, disregards all of the relevant research on memory loss, except for Freeman and Kendell's 1986 study, which the task force mentions and then grossly misrepresents. That study asked patients to assess their memory function a year or more after electroshock treatment. The authors themselves remark that the study was biased toward a low reporting of memory dysfunction because the patients were interviewed by the same doctor who had treated them. Nonetheless, 74% mentioned "memory impairment" as a continuing problem, and "a striking 30% felt that their memory had been permanently affected" (Freeman & Kendell, 1986). In defiance of the facts, the APA task force cites Freeman and Kendell as indicating "a small minority of patients, however, report persistent deficits" (APA Task Force, 1990).

Squire and Slater's 1983 study, also omitted by the APA task force, found that, 7 months after treatment, patients report an average loss of memory spanning 27 months. Squire, in a personal communication to me at the June 1985 Consensus Conference on ECT, explained that one patient lost the recollection of 10 years of her life. He told me that he felt it was not necessary to report this in his actual publication.

The Consensus Conference on Electroconvulsive Therapy (1985) used Squire and Slater's results to conclude that "on average, patients endure memory loss extending from 6 months prior to the treatment to 3 months afterward." These data, while serious enough in themselves, are misleading. The data reported at 7 months following treatment, cited in the above paragraph, are more likely to be accurate. The brain cannot regenerate lost brain cells or lost memories. With the passage of more time, there's little likelihood of increased improvement, but much likelihood of a growing tendency to deny the losses.

The APA task force also ignored older controlled studies by Janis showing extensive, permanent loss of important personal memories and life history following routine ECT. Janis (1948, 1950; Janis & Astrachan, 1951) interviewed 19 patients before and after routine ECT, and 11 control patients with similar diagnoses in the same hospitals. The results 1 month postshock were striking: Every shock patient had significant memory losses. Many patients were unable to recall 10 to 20 life experiences "which had been available to recall prior to electroshock treatment."

Janis (1950) followed up five of the patients at 2 1/2 to 3 1/2 months later. Most of the lost memories remained lost. Another follow-up 1 year later showed continuing losses (see review in Breggin, 1979).

Janis (1948) confirmed the importance of denial and anosognosia, especially the reality that shock patients tend to minimize or even confabulate to cover up their memory losses. One patient, for example, in his pre-ECT interview reported that he'd been unable to work for several months prior to coming to the hospital. The historical facts were confirmed by the family. But after 12 ECTs, he was unable to recall the period of unemployment. Instead, he claimed that he worked right up to his hospitalization. As Janis confirmed, patients often do not complain spontaneously to doctors about their memory loss; they tend to deny it.

Not only was Janis left out of the 1990 APA report, over the years he has been wholly misrepresented by other shock advocates. Two of the more important reviews commonly read during my psychiatric training actually cited Janis as evidence that ECT did not harm memory (reviewed in Breggin, 1979).

In 1986, Weiner, Rogers, Davidson, and Squire attempted to measure the loss of personal subjective recollections following ECT because these are "most consistent with the nature of memory complaints by ECT patients themselves." The memory inventory in the study spanned several years prior to the shock treatment. The group found "objective personal memory losses" that lasted through the 6-month duration of the study.

In an earlier paper by a team that also included Weiner (Daniel, Crovitz, Weiner, & Rogers, 1982), there was emphasis on the potentially injurious effect on the patient and the patient's family of losing autobiographical memories. The authors observed that "autobiographical memory failures, if added across a course of ECT, may produce *gross* autobiographical memory gaps that may be disconcerting to a patient and a patient's family, because the patient's sense of continuity with his or her own past may be disrupted'' (p. 923). In contrast, the paper in which these ECT-induced memory deficits were demonstrated lacks any such commentary (Weiner et al., 1986).

One of the newer techniques of shock treatment—multiple monitored electroconvulsive therapy (MMECT)—employs four electroshocks in one session while recording EEG, EKG, and vital signs. Barry Maletzky, an advocate of the treatment, is one of the few who have asked patients in detail about their memory function following ECT. After pointing out that some psychological testings have failed to confirm cognitive deterioration, he observes:

> However, if one listens to what patients say who are treated with either conventional ECT or MMECT, subtle cognitive deficits, not easily tested, are discussed. Some patients will mention deficits only if careful inquiry is pursued. Most will not identify these problems even if asked, thus indicating that either they are absent or so subtle as to be imperceivable to the patient. (Maletzky, 1981, p. 180)

Maletzky then goes on to describe a series of 47 MMECT patients who were interviewed 3 to 6 months after ECT treatment. Thirty-six percent identified a cognitive problem, including difficulty finding their way around, recalling past events in sequence, and understanding TV shows. In another follow-up by Maletzky using a questionnaire and interviews, 23% reported "long-term memory deficits." The problems described by Maletzky's patients extend beyond memory dysfunction to substantial cognitive deficits, such as a math student's loss of his ability to do computations in his head.

Devanand, Dwork, Hutchinson, Bolwig, and Sackeim (1994) in their review skate over the surface of the many cognitive studies, dismissing most of them, failing to mention any of the Janis studies, ignoring follow-up studies indicating that patients frequently experience permanent memory loss, and raising no issues about the improbability of full recovery from traumatic acute organic brain syndromes.

Appearing in the *American Journal of Psychiatry* amid growing controversy surrounding ECT, Devanand et al.'s review was seemingly intended as an establishment response to criticism. For this reason, I shall examine its conclusions at relevant points in this chapter.

STUDIES OF BRAIN DAMAGE FROM ECT

There is an extensive literature confirming brain damage from ECT. The damage is demonstrated in many large animal studies, human autopsy studies, brain wave studies, and an occasional CT scan study.

Animal and human autopsy studies show that shock routinely causes widespread pinpoint hemorrhages and scattered cell death. While the damage can be found throughout the brain, it is often worst beneath the electrodes. Since at least one electrode always lies over the frontal lobe, it is no exaggeration to call electroshock an electrical lobotomy.

In 1976, Friedberg published the first review of brain damage from ECT. This was followed by my own detailed critiques (1979, 1981a, 1986). None of these important studies and none of the reviews on brain damage are mentioned in the 1990 APA task force report.

The original animal studies are from the 1940s and 1950s, but they are still valid. Several of them were elegant by any scientific standard. The model for these studies was conducted by Hans Hartelius on cats and published in 1952 in a book-length publication, "Cerebral Changes Following Electrically Induced Convulsions."

In the double-blind microscopic pathology examination, Hartelius was able to discriminate between the eight shocked animals and the eight nonshocked animals with remarkable accuracy. The experimental animals showed vessel wall changes, gliosis, and nerve cell changes:

> The *vessel wall changes* found more frequently and more distinctly in the animals subjected to ECT consist of characteristic sac-like dilatations of the perivascular spaces, which in some cases contain histiocytic elements. The *glial reaction*, of the progressive type, consists of an increase in the number of the small glial elements in the parenchyma and satellitosis beside the nerve cells. The *nerve cell changes* observed are in the form of various stages of chromophobia, frequently with coincident nuclear hyperchromatism. The arrangement of such cells is mainly focal.

The changes were statistically significant. Confirming their basis in sound pathology, the abnormalities were found most heavily in the animals given the greater numbers of ECTs, were most dense in the frontal lobe, and were correlated with increased age of the animal (implying increased vulnerability).

Hartelius was cautious in his determination of irreversibility. He required shadow cells and neuronophagia (the removal of dead or diseased nerve cells by phagocytes). On the basis of these findings, he concluded, "The question whether or not irreversible damage to the nerve cells may occur in association with ECT must therefore be answered in the affirmative."

Hartelius used relatively small doses of ECT. In fact, the amount of electrical energy he used was a fraction of that currently applied to the heads of shock patients.

Hartelius's conclusions supported a number of earlier studies using dogs and monkeys, often employing clinical amounts of electrical energy, often less than currently used (see ahead in this chapter). Neither the Hartelius study, nor any of the studies using large animals, are included in the 1990 American Psychiatric Association task force report on ECT.

The Russians have carried out a variety of neuropathology studies on animals subjected to clinical ECT in order to determine if there is permanent brain damage. Babayan called for a ban on the treatment in 1985, citing work at the USSR Academy of Medical Sciences as, "convincing proof . . . pointing to grave changes in the central nervous system, the nerve cells, the glial-tissue apparatus . . . " (p. 37). At another institute, studies of the brains of animals led to a "drastic reduction in the use of electroshock therapy in clinical practice" (p. 134). Babayan compares the treatment to lobotomy.

There have been no studies of large animals using modified ECT under clinical conditions. Meldrum and Brierley (1973) studied drug-induced (bicuculline) lengthy seizures in baboons and found widespread ischemic (due to lack of blood flow) changes. Meldrum, Vigouroux, and Brierley (1973) repeated their earlier experiment, now employing modified ECT, and found similar but lesser ischemic changes in neurones. They concluded that modifying the ECT gave some incomplete protection. However, the seizures were very long. Meldrum, Horton, and Brierley (1974) once again studied the impact of drug-induced (allylglycine) seizures in baboons under modified conditions. They used 13 animals, and in 8 the seizures were brief, recurring 6–63 times in 2 to 11 hours, followed by recovery. The short-duration seizures produced no detectable pathology.

Templer (1992) reviewed the question of ECT and permanent brain damage. In regard to animal studies, he focused on Hartelius and also pointed out that animals given artificial ventilation (modified ECT) in other studies also had "brain damage of somewhat lesser magnitude."

If ordinary medical ethics were applied to psychiatry, based on nothing more than the original large-animal studies, shock treatment would be prohibited. It would then be up to shock advocates to use similar studies to prove that modern ECT is safer. The possibility that modern ECT is safer is practically nil, however, since the doses of electrical energy are uniformly higher today than they were in the animal experiments. With the trend confirmed by Sackeim et al. (1993), much more excessive doses of electricity are becoming more common.

While few psychiatrists are willing to say in public that ECT causes brain damage, a large survey of the APA membership, conducted with anonymity in the 1970s, showed that 41% of the respondents agreed with the statement that "It is likely that ECT produces slight or subtle brain damage." Only 26% responded that it did not (American Psychiatric Association, 1978, p. 4).

Devanand et al. (1994) reviewed "Does ECT Alter Brain Structure?"[1] They conclude that animals studies do not show brain damage. They do this by dismissing the best studies. Hartelius, for example, is criticized for applying a series of four ECTs with each one spaced at 2 hours. But there is no reason to assume that this method is more damaging than larger numbers of shocks spaced over longer intervals. As currently used, multiple-monitored ECT inflicts four shocks within the space of an hour or so. In addition, it is extremely misleading to focus on that one group of animals. Some of Hartelius's animals, for example, were given one ECT per day for 4 days and others were treated "with clinical frequency" (three per week).

Devanand et al. dismiss Ferraro and Roizen (1949) for using a "large number of ECSs [electroconvulsive shocks] relative to clinical practice," but in fact many patients are given 32 or more treatments, sometimes in one series, sometimes in several. Ferraro, Roizen, and Helfand (1946), utilizing fewer shocks, are dismissed on the speculation that the current went through the brain stem.

Devanand and colleagues do not deal with the fact that almost every study using large animals, by their own table, shows damage. My review indicates that even purportedly negative studies, on actual reading, indicate harmful effects (Breggin, 1979). For example, Devanand et al. describe Lidbeck's (1944) three dogs as developing "minimal perivascular and ischemic changes" (Devanand et al., 1994). They leave out that in two of the four animals "nerve cells were shrunken and there was a decrease

---

[1]Devanand is one of the authors in Sackeim et al. (1993) calling for the use of intensive ECT using 2.5 times the electrical current required to produce a convulsion.

in the number of stainable granules" (Lidbeck, 1944). Nor do they mention that one of the animals developed blood clots in its brain.

One cannot prove the safety of ECT by criticizing a raft of studies that show damage. To be ethical and scientific, shock advocates would have to produce carefully conducted, large-animal studies that show no damage. This has not been done. In fact, the only studies that Devanand et al. find acceptable were performed on rats rather than dogs, cats, and primates whose brains are more akin to humans and more sensitive to damage.

Brain Scans

There has been contradictory evidence of ECT damage in brain-scan studies, most of which have been carried out by staunch advocates of the treatment. Using CT scans, Weinberger et al. (1979) found that chronic schizophrenic patients who had ECT had more enlargement of their ventricles (cerebral atrophy) than those who had no ECT. Stretching to exonerate ECT, they declare, "Either EST further enlarged the ventricles of the patients treated with it, or it was used with greater frequency in patients who tended to have larger ventricles." In another CT study, Calloway, Dolan, Jacoby, and Levy (1981) found a correlation between frontal lobe atrophy and ECT in 41 "elderly depressives."

Coffey et al. (1991), using Magnetic Resonance Imaging (MRI), studied 35 patients before and after ECT. The follow-ups were 2 or 3 days after and 6 months after. In five subjects, they found "an apparent increase in subcortical hyperintensity." Coffey, a strong ECT advocate who has performed shock on many patients, dismissed his own finding as "most likely secondary to progression of ongoing cerebrovascular disease during follow up" (Coffey et al., 1991). I have seen several other patients with very similar post-ECT MRI findings.

Pande, Grunhaus, Aisen, and Haskett (1990) found no MRI pathology in 7 ECT patients. However, the studies were performed 1 week after the last ECT, so that late-maturing pathology would not have been discovered. Bergsholm, Larsen, Rosendahl, and Holsten (1989) found no pathology on MRI in 40 patients, with the exception of a 69-year-old man who suffered a dilatation of the left temporal horn, which the authors dismiss as unrelated to ECT.

Devanand et al. (1994) reviewed the brain scan literature and found the evidence for brain damage unconvincing. They accept Coffey's unsubstantiated claim that the four damaged patients had progressive cerebral vascular disease rather than ECT pathology. They dismiss studies showing damage.

MODIFIED ECT

For the past two to three decades, a modified form of ECT has been standard, involving sedation with a short-acting barbiturate, muscle paralysis with a curare derivative, and artificial respiration with oxygen. The purpose of these modifications was not, as some advocates claim, to reduce memory loss and brain damage. Muscle paralysis was intended to prevent fractures from severe muscle spasms, while the artificial respiration kept the paralyzed patient breathing.

The modifications used in contemporary ECT make clear that ECT-induced convulsions are far more severe than the spontaneous convulsions in grand mal epilepsy. Patients with spontaneous seizures of unknown origin, or with seizures due to brain injury, rarely break their limbs or their vertebrae during the convulsion. The muscle spasms are not intense enough to produce these effects. Yet these fractures were common with unmodified ECT.

Shock advocates claim that recent modifications have made the treatment much safer, and that its negative public image is unfairly based on the older methods. However, the most basic modifications—anesthesia, paralysis, and artificial respiration—are not new at all. I prescribed and administered such modified treatment more than thirty years ago (1963–64) as a resident at Harvard Medical School's main psychiatric teaching facility, the Massachusetts Mental Health Center.

The public's "mistaken" image of ECT is, in reality, based on modern modified ECT, which has been around for a long time. It is actually more dangerous than the older forms. The electrical currents must be more intense in order to overcome the anticonvulsant effects of the sedatives that are given during modified ECT (Breggin, 1979). Too frequently, the patient is routinely given a sleeping medication or tranquilizer the night before, further increasing the brain's resistance to having a seizure. In addition, the patient is exposed to the added risk of anesthesia. Other modifications include changes in the type of electrical energy employed and the use of unilateral shocks applied to the nondominant (nonverbal) side of the brain. However, these modifications remain controversial.

Since the APA task force does not exclusively endorse them, the claim that modern ECT is somehow much safer is again undercut. Besides, as already emphasized, some ECT advocates give excessive doses—beyond the dose required to produce a convulsion.

There is no reason to believe that shocking the nonverbal side of the brain is less harmful. As Blakeslee (1983) has confirmed, damage and dysfunction on the nonverbal side are more difficult for the individual to recognize or to describe (see discussion of anosognosia in chapter 1). But the defects are no less devastating. Injury to the nonverbal side impairs visual memory, spatial relations, musical and artistic abilities, judgment, insight, intuition, and personality. It is ironic that biopsychiatry promotes sacrificing the nonverbal side of the brain, while humanistic psychology is emphasizing its importance to the full development of human potential.

No matter how ECT is modified, one fact is inescapable: Evolution has assured that human beings do not easily fall victim to convulsions. Therefore sufficient damage must be inflicted to overcome the brain's protective systems.

THE BRAIN-DISABLING PRINCIPLE

Beginning with Cerletti and Bini, who introduced electroshock in 1938, many advocates of the treatment have not wanted to make the treatment less harmful to the brain. They considered brain damage necessary for the cure (reviewed in Breggin, 1979).

Fink, himself a member of the 1978 and 1990 APA task forces, for decades argued and demonstrated scientifically that ECT's therapeutic effect is produced by brain dysfunction and damage. He pointed out in his 1979 textbook that "patients become more compliant and acquiescent with treatment" (p. 139). He connected the so-called improvement with "denial," "disorientation," and other signs of traumatic brain injury and an organic brain syndrome (p. 165).

Fink was even more explicit in earlier studies. In 1957, he stated that the basis for improvement from ECT is "craniocerebral trauma." In 1966, Fink cited research indicating that after ECT "the behavioral changes [after ECT] related to the degree of induced trauma . . . " (p. 475). Referring to the multiple abnormalities produced in the brain following ECT, he wrote "In these regards, induced convulsions in man are more similar to cerebral trauma than to spontaneous seizures'' (p. 481). He stated that improvement depends on the development of an abnormal EEG and other changes in the brain and spinal fluid typical of trauma and compared ECT to ''cerebral trauma'' (p. 48). Fink cited Tower and McEachern (1949), correctly stating that they ''concluded that spinal fluid changes in induced convulsions were more like those of craniocerebral trauma than those of spontaneous epilepsy'' (Fink, 1966). He then gave further evidence for this comparison between ECT and traumatic brain injury.

As recently as 1974, Fink continued to propose that ECT has its effect by traumatizing or damaging the brain. He begins his discussion by noting that psychiatric ''treatments have been often drastic'' and then cites, among other examples, heat and burning, bleeding, water immersion, and craniotomy. He then goes on to present several axioms of ECT, including the connection between the supposed therapeutic effect and traumatic changes in the brain. He speaks directly of the producing ''cerebral 'trauma' '' reflected in EEG slow wave activity (p. 9). He compares induced convulsions to ''craniocerebral trauma'' (p. 10). He attributes improvement to the increased use of ''denial'' by the patient and to the development of ''hypomania''—both signs of profound irrationality caused by brain damage and dysfunction (p. 14).

The 1990 task force report, despite Fink's participation, made no such comparisons between head injury and ECT; instead the report dismissed any suggestion that the treatment is severely traumatic. In depositions in defense of doctors who give ECT, Fink now takes the position that ECT causes no brain damage.

The 1990 APA task force report notes that low-dose unilateral ECT is often less effective than forms of ECT that deliver more electrical energy. This observation tends to confirm the brain-disabling principle that efficacy depends on the degree of damage.

More recently Sackeim et al. (1993) have covertly revived the principle that a therapeutic response depends upon the degree of brain damage and dysfunction. The tendency to increase the electrical dose wholly undermines the promotional campaign aimed at convincing the public that modern shock is safer. They have advocated bilateral ECT—the most obviously damaging method—using a dose of electricity 2.5 times that required to produce a convulsion in the patient. I evaluated a case in which a doctor followed Sackeim's published recommendation and gave his patient the increased dosage. The patient suffered severe, irreversible memory loss and chronic mental dysfunction, rendering her permanently unable to work at her previous high intellectual level.

Psychiatric drugs are nowadays frequently justified on the grounds that they correct biochemical imbalances. Like Prozac, shock treatment is said to work by enhancing serotonin (for example, Abrams, 1988, pp. 159–161). Accepting this rationale requires ignoring the more gross damage being done: The shocked brain is so traumatized that the patient is rendered too confused and blunted to feel any subtle emotions. Even psychosurgery is nowadays sometimes justified on the grounds that it corrects biochemical imbalances. One advocate looks forward to delivering serotonin "psychosurgically" to "serotonin-depleted sites" in the brain (Rodgers, 1992, p. 106).

Iatrogenic Helplessness and Denial

ECT provides a prototype for the concept of iatrogenic helplessness and denial (see chapter 1). Controlled studies of ECT show that any therapeutic effect evaporates after 4 weeks—the approximate time it takes to recover from the most severe symptoms of the organic brain syndrome or delirium. Except for psychosurgery, ECT provides the most extreme example in which the psychiatrist denies the damage he is doing to the patient, and then utilizes the effects of that damage to produce a less emotionally aware, less autonomous, and more manageable patient. As Max Fink's work openly describes, through brain damage and the exercise of medical authority, patients are pushed deep into denial about the harm done to them as well as about their still unresolved personal problems.

Consistent with other victims of central nervous system damage, most ECT patients minimize or deny their real losses of mental function. This denial of mental dysfunction in brain-damaged patients is called anosognosia (discussed in chapter 1). While damage to either side of the brain can produce anosognosia, it seems more common following damage to the nondominant side (in right-handed individuals, the right is usually nondominant). In electroshock treatment, at least one electrode lies over the nondominant side. In contemporary ECT, both electrodes are frequently placed over the nondominant side.

Nondominant shock starkly illustrates the principle of iatrogenic helplessness and denial: The doctor damages the brain in such a way as to confound the patient's ability to perceive the resulting dysfunction.

Advocates of ECT are well aware that shock patients suffer from anosognosia and denial, and therefore cannot fully report the extent of their memory losses and mental dysfunction. Yet these same advocates claim that patients exaggerate their post-ECT problems.

Interviews with family and friends of patients often disclose that they are painfully aware of the damage done to their loved ones. Often, the psychiatrist is the only one who consistently and unequivocally denies the patient's damaged state.

THE CONTROVERSY

The 1978 APA task force report labeled electroshock treatment as controversial. The 1985 Consensus Conference report stated, "Electroconvulsive therapy is the most controversial treatment in psychiatry" and referred to forty-five years of dispute surrounding issues such as efficacy and "possible complications" (Consensus Conference, 1985). In the opening sentence of the introduction to Abrams's 1988 book, Fink referred to the "more than 50 years of controversy" (Abrams, 1988) surrounding ECT.

By contrast, the 1990 APA task force report says not a word about controversy. ECT is presented as if no one in the profession has ever criticized it. Since a number of psychiatrists have been sued for failing to inform patients about the controversial nature of the treatment, the APA report was in part intended as a step toward cleansing the treatment of controversy.

Psychosurgery remains the only treatment surrounded by more controversy than ECT; but it is used much less frequently (Breggin & Breggin, 1994b). The two treatments are closely related in many ways. Electroshock can be understood as "closed-head electrical lobotomy."

The most significant challenge to ECT within the medical profession was launched by neurologist John Friedberg (1976), whose book for laypersons was followed by a journal review (Friedberg, 1977). Friedberg's publications were quickly followed by a volume edited by "shock survivor" Leonard Frank (1978), and a book by this writer (1979). Reviews of ECT-induced damage to the brain and mind have continued to be published in professional journals (Cameron, 1994; Frank, 1990; Templer, 1992). Templer and Veleber (1982), for example, summarized their review of the literature:

Some human and animal autopsies reveal permanent brain pathology. Some patients have persisting spontaneous seizures after having received ECT. Patients having received many ECTs score lower than control patients on psychological tests of organicity, even when degree of psychosis is controlled for.

A convergence of evidence indicates the importance of the number of ECTs. . . . [O]ur position remains that ECT has caused and can cause permanent brain pathology.

Boyle (1986) reviewed the literature and stated:

In conclusion, there is considerable empirical evidence that ECT induces significant and to some extent lasting brain impairment. The studies cited above are but a few which suggest that ECT is potentially a harmful procedure, as indeed are most naturally occurring episodes of brain trauma resulting in concussion, unconsciousness and grand mal epileptic seizures. Accordingly, the continued use of ECT in psychiatry must be questioned very seriously. (p. 23)

After hearing evidence presented to the Food and Drug Administration's Respiratory and Nervous System Device Panel, consumer representative Susan Bartlett Foot (1983) reported back to the FDA:

Evidence of the safety and efficacy of ECT devices remains controversial and conflicting. The "new evidence" submitted [by the American Psychiatric Association] petition did not, by any means, eliminate the unanswered or troubling questions surrounding safety and efficacy of the machines. (p. 2)

Survivors of shock treatment have become an increasingly active force. In addition to writing and appearing in the media, many who have undergone ECT continue to protest at national psychiatric conventions and shock symposia, and even chain themselves to the gates and doors of "shock mills." Most recently, a new organization of several hundred shock survivors—the National Association of Electroshock Survivors (NAES)—has been formed in Texas. It is calling for a ban on ECT. This kind and degree of consumer resistance against a commonly used medical treatment seems unprecedented.

More than 30 states have passed legislation to monitor ECT, set limits on the number of treatments or the age at which it can be given, and require second opinions and informed consent. Four states have banned its use on children, most recently Texas, under NAES leadership. While efforts to require informed consent have proved almost impossible to enforce in the face of psychiatric resistance, they have raised further questions about the use of shock treatment.

The most dramatic threat to shock treatment became known as the "Berkeley ban." Ted Chabasinski, who had been subjected to electroshock as a child, organized a grassroots citizens' movement in support of a referendum to ban ECT in Berkeley, California. After the proposition was overwhelmingly approved by the electorate, the psychiatric establishment, led by the APA, intervened and had the ban overturned in court. But the survivors could claim a partial victory—a "power outage" of 41 days at Herrick Hospital, the city's only ECT facility, in the winter of 1982.

Recently, California again became the center of public criticism of electroshock. Inspired by a coalition of former patients and concerned professionals, Angela Alioto, a member of the San Francisco Board of Supervisors, held hearings on ECT. About two dozen "shock survivors" testified about permanent damage to their brains and minds. Although both sides had ample time to organize, no shock patients showed up to offer testimonials in favor of the treatment (Breggin, 1991b, 1991c; Frank, 1991).

The recommendations of Alioto's committee were adopted by the city's governing body and signed by Mayor Art Agnos on February 20, 1990. The resolution declares the Board of Supervisors' opposition to the "use and financing" of ECT in San Francisco (Figueroa, 1991). It also calls for the state legislature to develop more strict requirements for informed consent, including the exposure of potential patients to live or videotaped presentations by critics of the treatment. The resolution, which follows the recommendations made in my testimony at the Alioto hearings, is not legally binding. While the resolution has been an important moral and educational victory for electroshock opponents, its actual impact may be negligible.

THE NEED TO BAN ELECTROCONVULSIVE THERAPY

The 1990 APA task force report represents a disillusioning and disappointing watershed for my own reform activities around ECT. I have long argued that ECT is an ineffective, dangerous, anachronistic treatment that should be abandoned by modern psychiatry. Yet, despite the urging of many victims of ECT, I refused for many years to endorse public or legislative efforts to ban it. It was my position that the practice of medicine and the rights of patients were better served by insisting on informed consent—and by holding liable those psychiatrists who fail to convey to their patients the controversial nature of ECT and its potentially damaging effects. Unfortunately, the 1990 APA report and the APA's political pressuring of the FDA demonstrate that organized psychiatry is determined not to inform professionals or patients about the risk of ECT. Despite the disclaimer tucked away on its copyright page, the APA report provides a shield for those who recommend and administer ECT—an "official" conclusion that there is no serious risk of harm. Doctors who prescribe or recommend ECT can try to hide behind this report when their injured patients protest to them or bring legal actions.

In the environment created by the APA, informed consent for ECT becomes a mirage. Therefore, after much hesitation, I now endorse public efforts to ban ECT. The banning of ECT should be supported by all concerned mental health professionals.

Some patients do feel "helped" by ECT. Often they have been so damaged that they cannot judge their own condition. They suffer from iatrogenic denial and helplessness. But should a treatment be banned when some people believe they are helped by it? In fact, it is commonplace in medicine and psychiatry to withdraw treatments and devices that have caused serious harm to a small percentage of people, even though they may have helped a very large percentage. The risk of serious injury to a few outweighs helping many.

In the case of ECT, a large percentage of people are being harmed, and there's little evidence that many are being helped. There's no evidence that the treatment prevents suicide or rescues desperate cases. At best the treatment offers a very poor trade-off—potentially irreversible brain damage and mental dysfunction in exchange for the docility and temporary emotional blunting or euphoria that result from the damage.

Stimulants and Other Drugs for Children, Including an Analysis of Attention-Deficit Hyperactivity Disorder*

We are in the midst of a massive increase in the prescription of Ritalin (methylphenidate) to children. In 1990–91, the National Institute of Mental Health (NIMH) and other sources estimated that Ritalin was being administered to 1 million children (Breggin, 1991a). Because Ritalin is a schedule II (highly addictive) controlled substance, the federal Drug Enforcement Administration (DEA) allots and monitors its production. According to the DEA (1995b), the total production of methylphenidate went from 1,361 kg in 1985 to 10,410 in 1995, with the largest increase in the last 5 years. The DEA also found a 6-fold increase in methylphenidate production in the United States since 1990. Meanwhile, the total annual prescriptions reportedly tripled during the period 1990–1994 from 3,144,000 to 9,399,000 (Batoosingh, 1995). Based on earlier estimates of 1–2 million children on Ritalin, this indicates that as many as 5 million

*Some of this chapter is rewritten and expanded from *The War Against Children* (Breggin and Breggin, 1994b). I wish to thank St. Martin's Press for permission to use this material. Because of the great interest in this topic, a version of this chapter is being simultaneously published in the *Review of Existential Psychology and Psychiatry* and the *Journal of College Student Psychotherapy*.

or more children are now being prescribed the drug. This is consistent with the widespread increase in Ritalin usage that many observers have witnessed.

According to the DEA (1995b), "data on physician prescribing practices imply that few general practitioners or pediatricians provide treatment other than pharmacotherapy with psychostimulants" (p. 10). Also, "a small percentage of primary care physicians are writing nearly half of all methylphenidate prescriptions for children" (p. 10). This goes on despite the fact that "studies indicate that treatment with psychostimulants alone does not improve the outcomes of most ADHD children" (p. 10).

The increase in Ritalin usage has been largely restricted to the United States, which consumes five times more than the rest of the world combined (Drug Enforcement Administration, 1995b). Meanwhile, the quotas set by the DEA lagged so far behind the rampant growth of Ritalin prescribing that supplies supposedly ran low in 1994 (Karel, 1994).

According to the Drug Enforcement Administration (1995b), the supply problem never became critical but CIBA-Geigy, the manufacturer of Ritalin, turned it into a public relations blitz. Working with CHADD, the parents' group that it funds, the drug company lobbied Congress and contacted the media to pressure the DEA to make more Ritalin available. It became a public relations event in support of Ritalin. The DEA reports that CIBA-Geigy mailed more than 400,000 letters warning about the impending shortage, causing a panic among parents.

In addition, large numbers of children are also being given the stimulants amphetamine (Dexedrine) and pemoline (Cylert). Most of the observations and conclusions about methylphenidate in this chapter also apply to amphetamine, as well as to Cylert. As the DEA observed, "Methylphenidate is a psychomotor stimulant structurally and pharmacologically related to amphetamines" (pp. 15–16).

The focus throughout much of this book has been on the brain-disabling principle with less attention to surrounding issues, such as efficacy or the presumed validity of the psychiatric diagnoses (issues dealt with in Breggin, 1991a and Breggin & Breggin, 1994b). Because psychiatry is casting an increasingly broad pharmacological net over America's children, this chapter will also examine the diagnoses themselves.

Few professionals can recite the APA diagnostic criteria as delineated in the *Diagnostic and Statistical Manual of Mental Disorders, 4th Edition* (*DSM-IV*) (APA, 1994), even for the diagnoses they routinely use. But their existence creates a strong, if misleading, impression of validity for psychiatric diagnosing in general, as well as for the individual diagnostic categories. The prescription of medication to children, for example, is largely justified on the basis of these diagnoses.

The diagnoses also influence how millions of parents and teachers view the children in their care. Most teachers and many parents of young people have heard of "hyperactivity" and, more specifically, attention-deficit hyperactivity disorder (ADHD). Many nonprofessionals believe they can diagnose it.

THE DISRUPTIVE BEHAVIOR DISORDERS

Along with "conduct disorder" and "oppositional defiant disorder," ADHD was originally considered one of the "disruptive behavior disorders" in the *DSM-III-R* (American Psychiatric Association, 1987). In the *DSM-IV*, an attempt is made to separate ADHD from the other two disruptive disorders, at least when ADHD manifests itself primarily as inattention rather than hyperactivity. The DSM committee found that while disruptive behavior and attention problems "often occur together . . . some" (Fasnacht, 1993, p. 8) ADHD children are not hyperactive and disruptive.

Despite any attempt to separate them, the three diagnoses often overlap each other and research projects often refer to them as one group, the DBDs. The *DSM-IV* observed that "A substantial portion of children referred to clinics with Attention-Deficit/Hyperactivity Disorder also have Oppositional Defiant Disorder or Conduct Disorder." An NIMH study similarly concluded that pure conduct disorder or pure oppositional disorder are "relatively rare" (Kruesi et al., 1992) with most cases also qualifying for an attention-deficit disorder diagnosis. All this casts doubt on the meaningful existence of any one of the diagnoses. It adds up to saying, "A kid in trouble is a kid in trouble" regardless of how you count up the problems.

The *DSM-IV* does not discuss the definition of disruptive behavior disorder. The *DSM-III-R* stated that DBD children are "characterized by behavior that is socially disruptive and is often more distressing to others than to the people with the disorders." The "illness" consists of being disruptive to the lives of adults—a definition that seems tailored for social control and for the self-exoneration of adults.

ATTENTION-DEFICIT/HYPERACTIVITY DISORDER

The *DSM-IV* distinguishes between two types of ADHD, one marked by inattention and the other by hyperactivity-impulsivity. The official standard for ADHD requires any six of nine items under each category. For hyperactivity-impulsivity the first four items in descending order include:

(1) often fidgets with hands or feet or squirms in seat
(2) often leaves seat in classroom or in other situations in which remaining seated is expected
(3) often runs about or climbs excessively in situations in which it is inappropriate (in adolescents or adults, may be limited to subjective feelings of restlessness)
(4) often has difficulty playing or engaging in leisure activities quietly. (p. 84)

The first four items in the list for diagnosing the inattention form of the disorder include:

(1) often fails to give close attention to details or makes mistakes in schoolwork, work, or other activities
(2) often has difficulty sustaining attention in tasks or play activities
(3) often does not seem to listen when spoken to directly
(4) often does not follow through on instructions and fails to finish schoolwork, chores, or duties in the workplace (not due to oppositional behavior or failure to understand instructions) (pp. 83–84)

As the list of criteria demonstrates, ADHD is one more DBD—another way a child gets labeled as a source of frustration or disruption. This is true even in regard to some of the criteria for the inattention aspect of the disorder. As Gerald Golden (1991) observes: "The behavior is seen as being disruptive and unacceptable by parents and teachers, and the child is socially handicapped as a result."

Russell Barkley (1991) stated, "Although inattention, overactivity, and poor impulse control are the most common symptoms cited by others as primary in hyperactive children, my own work with these children suggests that noncompliance is also a primary problem" (p. 13). It is not surprising that some children are noncompliant with Barkley. He not only wants to medicate them, he blames the child for conflicts that the child is having with family and school. As he put it, " . . . there is, in fact, something 'wrong' with these children'' (p. 4). He did not make a similar indictment of the authorities in the child's life, such as parents or teachers, although they have far more influence over the child's pain and suffering than does the child himself or herself.

A Disease That Goes Away with Attention

The symptoms or manifestations of ADHD often disappear when the children have something interesting to do or when they receive a little adult attention. This is agreed upon by most or all observers and indirectly finds its way into the *DSM-III-R* and *DSM-IV*. The *DSM-IV* specified that the symptoms may become apparent when the child is in settings "that lack intrinsic appeal or novelty" and may be minimal or absent when "the person is under very strict control, is in a novel setting, is engaged in especially interesting activities, is in a one-to-one situation," including being examined by the doctor. Most advocates of ADHD as a diagnosis also note that it tends to go away during summer vacation.

If the list of criteria for ADHD has any use, it identifies children who are bored, anxious, or angry around some of the adults in their lives or in some adult-run institutions, such as the school and family. These "symptoms" should not red-flag the children as mentally ill. They should signal to adults that renewed efforts are required to attend to the child's basic needs (for a discussion of basic needs, see Breggin, 1992a).

When a small child, perhaps 5 or 6 years old, is persistently disrespectful or angry, there is always a stressor in that child's life—something over which the child has little or no control. Sometimes, the child is not being respected. When treated with respect, children tend to respond respectfully. When loved, they tend to be loving. While the source of the child's upset may ultimately be more complicated—perhaps the parent is too afraid or distracted to apply rational discipline and lets the child run wild, or perhaps the child is being abused outside the home—the source of the child's anguish or failure lies in the larger world. Small children do not, on their own, create severe emotional conflicts within themselves and with the adults around them. When older children end up generating severe conflict, it usually comes from a long history of prior conflicts with adults. Children aren't born bored, inattentive, undisciplined, resentful, or violent; but the stigmatizing psychiatric labels imply that they are.

In my experience, children labeled ADHD are usually more energetic and more spirited, or more in need of an interesting environment, than their parents and teachers can handle. One of the early advocates of hyperactivity as a diagnosis describes them as unusually dynamic bundles of energy (Wender, 1973). Yet they are being diagnosed with a mental illness—a label that can follow them into adulthood to ruin their future lives.

What Kind of Attention?

Many and probably most so-called ADHD children are receiving insufficient attention from their fathers, who may be separated from the family, too preoccupied with work and other things, or otherwise impaired in their ability to parent. In many cases the appropriate diagnosis is "dad attention-deficit disorder" (DADD) (Breggin, 1991a; Breggin & Breggin, 1994b).

The "cure" for these children is more rational and loving attention from their fathers. Young people are nowadays so hungry for the attention of a father that it can come from any male adult. Seemingly impulsive, hostile groups of children will calm down when a caring, relaxed, and firm adult male is around. Arlington High School in Indianapolis was canceling many of its after-school events because of unruliness, when a father happened to attend one of them (Smith, 1993):

> That evening there was an odd quietness on [the father's] side of the auditorium. It turned out that when he would tell his group to settle down, some students would second him. One said: "That's Lena's father. You heard him. Be quiet; act right." (p. 5)

Since then the school has begun to enlist volunteer dads for its after-school events.

At other times, the so-called disorder should be called TADD: "teacher attention-deficit disorder." Due more to problems in our educational system than to the teachers themselves, few students get the individualized educational programs that they need.

Overall in our society, parents and teachers receive too little support for their tasks, which are among the most difficult in society. The average parents receive more training in how to breathe during the delivery of their children than they will receive in how to relate to their offspring over the ensuing 18 years. The average teacher has difficulty keeping herself afloat amid the pressures of teaching poorly disciplined children in overcrowded classes. She has little time to individualize her instruction to particular educational needs and even less to develop relationships with her students. But as burdened as parents and teachers may feel, they should not try to escape their responsibilities by drugging children. Instead, they should find the support they need to continue improving their skills, while also working toward improving their schools and families.

PROFESSIONALLY DISCREDITED

In 1993 neurologist Fred Baughman, Jr., noted that studies have failed to confirm any definite improvement from the drug treatment of ADHD-labeled children. Baughman cites estimates of the frequency of attention-deficit disorder that vary from 1 in 3 to 1 in 1,000. He therefore asks, "Is attention-deficit hyperactivity disorder, after all, in the eye of the beholder?"

The eye of the beholder theme echoes Diane McGuinness, who has systematically debunked ADHD as the "emperor's new clothes." In a chapter in *The Limits of Biological Treatments for Psychological Distress* (1989), she observed,

> The past 25 years has led to a phenomenon almost unique in history. Methodologically rigorous research . . . indicates that ADD [Attention Deficit Disorder] and hyperactivity as "syndromes" simply do not exist. We have invented a disease, given it medical sanction, and now must disown it. The major question is how we go about destroying the monster we have created. It is not easy to do this and still save face. . . . (p. 155)

According to Richard E. Vatz (1993), "Attention-deficit disorder (ADD) is no more a disease than is 'excitability.' It is a psychiatric, pseudomedical term."

Frank Putnam (1990), a director of one of NIMH's research units, recently applauded "the growing number of clinicians and researchers condemning the tyranny of our psychiatric and educational classification systems." Putnam finds that it is "exceedingly difficult to assign valid classifications [to children, and yet] children are by far the most classified and labeled group in our society." He warns against "the institutional prescriptions of a system that seeks to pigeonhole them."

Comorbidity and Misguided Diagnoses

The notion of a specific ADHD syndrome is further undermined by the tendency to give the same child a combination of several diagnoses. This reality appears throughout the literature. Dulcan and Popper (1991) observe that multiple diagnoses for a single child are common and that hospitalized children average four diagnoses at once. Like the proverbial cookie cutter, the diagnoses chop the child into various predesigned shapes which bear little or no resemblance to the child's underlying psychosocial problems, family or school conflicts, and unmet needs.

Without fully exploring the implications, Dulcan and Popper also point out that the diagnosed behaviors may turn out to be assets:

> Certain individuals may even learn to turn childhood deficits such as excessive sensitivity (separation anxiety), unrelenting stubbornness (oppositional defiant disorder), or uncontrolled activity and enthusiasm (attention-deficit hyperactivity disorder) into strengths in adulthood. (p. 2)

Unfortunately, Dulcan and Popper miss the point. The child does not have "deficits" to begin with. These positive qualities frequently run afoul of adults who, due to their own deficits, cannot live with them or direct them into positive forms of expression. Furthermore, once the child is labeled as having a "disorder" or "deficit," neither the child nor the responsible adults are likely to encourage the offending personal characteristics. Worse yet, when the child is drugged, the potentially positive traits are driven underground by a combination of drug toxicity and stigmatization.

The Supposed Physical Basis for ADHD

A study led by NIMH's Alan Zametkin (Zametkin et al., 1990) received a great deal of publicity for finding increased brain metabolism in positron emission tomography (PET scans) of adults with a history of ADHD in childhood. However, when the sexes were compared separately, there was no statistically significant difference between the controls and ADHD adults. To achieve significance, the data were lumped together to include a disproportionate number of women in the controls. In addition, when individual areas of the brain were compared between controls and ADHD adults, no differences were found. It is usually possible to massage data to produce some sort of statistical result and Zametkin's study is a classic illustration.

Since ADHD is not a disorder but, in most cases, a manifestation of conflict between children and adults, we doubt that a biological cause will ever be found. Golden (1991) put it simply:

> Attempts to define a biological basis for ADHD have been consistently unsuccessful. The neuroanatomy of the brain, as demonstrated by neuroimaging studies, is normal. No neuropathologic substrate has been demonstrated. . . . (p. 36)

Meanwhile, the emphasis on possible genetic and biological causes of upset behaviors in children obscures the growing body of research confirming their psychosocial origins (reviewed in Breggin, 1992a; Green, 1989).

A Nonspecific Treatment

Consistent with the brain-disabling principle, experts generally agree that Ritalin affects normal children in the same way it affects diagnosed children. Golden (1991) observes, " . . . the response to the drug cannot be used to validate the diagnosis. Normal boys as well as those with ADHD show similar changes when given a single dose of a psychostimulant" (p. 37).

Within an hour after taking a single dose of a stimulant drug, any child tends to become more obedient, more narrow in focus, more willing to concentrate on humdrum tasks and instructions. Parents in conflict with a little boy can hand him a pill, knowing he'll soon be more docile.

It is commonly held that stimulants have a paradoxical effect on children compared to adults, but these drugs probably affect children and adults in the same way. At the doses usually prescribed by physicians, children and adults alike are "spaced out," rendered less in touch with their real feelings, and hence more willing to concentrate on boring, repetitive schoolroom tasks.

At higher doses, both children and adults become more obviously stimulated into excitability or hyperactivity. There is, however, great variability among individuals and a number of children and adults will become more hyperactive and inattentive at the lower doses as well.

An Ineffective Treatment

It's not surprising that giving "speed" to children doesn't do them much good in the long run. As NIMH succinctly stated, "The long-term effects of stimulants remain in doubt" (Regier & Leshner, 1992). The FDA-approved information put out by the drug company CIBA-Geigy admits that "long-term effects of Ritalin in children have not been well established" (*Physicians' Desk Reference*, 1996). Yet methylphenidate is typically advocated as a long-term treatment.

NIMH further states that studies have demonstrated short-term effects such as reducing "class room disturbance" and improving "compliance and sustained attention" (Regier & Leshner, 1992). But it recognizes that the drugs seem "less reliable in bringing about associated improvements, at least of an enduring nature, in social-emotional and academic problems, such as antisocial behavior, poor peer and teacher relationships, and school failure."

Dulcan (1994) reviewed stimulant treatment for ADHD children. In regard to long-term control, she found "Stimulants have not yet been demonstrated to have long-term therapeutic effects . . . " The "not yet," it should be emphasized, refers to three decades of trying to prove its effectiveness.

In regard to improvement in learning or educational performance, the record is even worse. There's no convincing evidence for either short-term or long-term improvement in cognitive ability or academic performance (reviews by Breggin, 1991a; Coles, 1987; McGuinness, 1989; and Swanson et al., 1992).

Dulcan also makes clear that for the drug to be effective, an array of other interventions are required:

> Specific learning disabilities and gaps in knowledge and skills due to inattention require educational remediation. Social skills deficit and family pathology may need specific treatment. Parent education and training in techniques of behavior management are virtually always indicated. (p. 1214)

A program such as Dulcan suggested would in reality do away with the need for drugging children. As a consultant to state programs and clinics, I have found that such a comprehensive program can help the most disturbed and disabled children, including those with more severe diagnoses than ADHD. Such programs are offered to very few children, and even fewer once the decision to medicate has been made.

RITALIN, AMPHETAMINE, AND COCAINE

An editorial comment in the 1995 *Archives of General Psychiatry* states: "Cocaine, one of the most reinforcing and addictive of abuse drugs, has pharmacological actions very similar to those of MPH [methylphenidate], one of the most commonly prescribed psychotropic medications for children in the United States." Using PET, Volkow et al. (1995) found that the distributions of cocaine and methylphenidate in the brain were identical, but that the latter remained for a longer period of time.

Parents are seldom told that methylphenidate is "speed"—that it is pharmacologically classified with amphetamines and causes the very same effects, side effects, and risks. Yet this is well known in the profession. For example, *Treatments of Psychiatric Disorders* observes that cocaine, amphetamines, and methylphenidate are "neuropharmacologically alike" (APA, 1989, p. 1221). As evidence, the textbook points out that abuse patterns are the same for the three drugs, that people cannot tell their clinical effects apart in laboratory tests, and that they can substitute for each other and cause similar behavior in addicted animals (APA, 1989, p. 1221. Also see Breggin, 1991a; Breggin & Breggin, 1994a, 1994b). The *DSM-IV* confirms these observations by lumping cocaine, amphetamine, and methylphenidate abuse and addiction into one category. The federal government classifies methylphenidate in a high addiction category, schedule II, which also includes amphetamines, morphine, opium, and barbiturates (Goodman, Rall, Nies, & Taylor, 1991).

Before it was replaced by other stimulants in the 1980s, methylphenidate was one of the most commonly used street drugs (Spotts & Spotts, 1980). In my suburban hometown, youngsters nowadays sell their prescribed methylphenidate to classmates who abuse it along with other drugs, often by snorting it. In working with community groups, we often hear anecdotal reports of individuals who have graduated from using medically prescribed methylphenidate to alcohol or street drugs. I have seen cases in my own practice.

Youngsters selling their prescribed Ritalin even made the *Washington Post* (Welsh, 1995) in a discussion of conditions at local private schools:

> Students report that at two prestigious Virginia boarding schools, boys with prescriptions for Ritalin—a drug for attention deficit disorder—have been selling their pills to classmates looking to get high. At one school, a student said, "Ritalin rivals acid and marijuana."

Like any addictive stimulant, methylphenidate can cause withdrawal symptoms, such as "crashing" with depression, exhaustion, withdrawal, irritability, and suicidal feelings. Parents will not recognize a withdrawal reaction when their child gets upset after missing even a single dose. They will mistakenly believe that their child needs to be put back on the medication.

Concern at the DEA

On October 25, 1995, the Drug Enforcement Administration published a press release (1995a) as an introduction to a substantial document (1995b) concerning the extensive use of methylphenidate and the serious hazards associated with it. The press release began with the following series of points:

> Methylphenidate (MPH), most commonly known as Ritalin, ranks in the top 10 most frequently reported controlled pharmaceuticals stolen from licensed handlers.

> Organized drug trafficking groups in a number of states have utilized various schemes to obtain MPH for resale on the illicit market.

> MPH is abused by diverse segments of the population from health care professionals and children to street addicts.

> A significant number of children and adolescents are diverting or abusing MPH medication intended for the treatment of ADHD.

> In 1994, a national high school survey (Monitoring the Future) indicated that more seniors in high school in the U.S. abuse Ritalin than are prescribed Ritalin legitimately.

Students are giving and selling their medication to classmates who are crushing and snorting the powder like cocaine. In March of 1995, two deaths in Mississippi and Virginia were associated with this activity.

The DEA press release concludes its list of concerns with the following statement:

> Every indicator available, including scientific abuse liability studies, actual abuse, paucity of scientific studies on possible adverse effects associated with long-term use of stimulants, divergent prescribing practices of U.S. physicians, and lack of concurrent medical treatment and follow-up, urge greater caution and more restrictive use of MPH.

The Brain-Disabling Effects of Stimulants

The British are much more cautious about using stimulants for children. Grahame-Smith and Aronson (1992), authors of the *Oxford Textbook of Clinical Psychopharmacology and Drug Therapy*, suggest that stimulants may work in children in the same way they work in rats, by "inducing stereotyped behavior in animals, i.e., in reducing the number of behavioural responses . . . "(p. 141). Stereotyped behavior is simple, repetitive, seemingly meaningless activity, often seen in brain-damaged individuals. The textbook states somewhat suggestively, "It is beyond our scope to discuss whether or not such behavioural control is desirable" (p. 141).

The stereotypical behavior mentioned by Graham-Smith and Aronson (1992) has been carefully studied in the laboratory in regard to both amphetamine and methylphenidate, which produce identical results in animals. Randrup and Munkvad (1970) described the stereotypical behavior produced in rats by subcutaneous injections of amphetamine:

> It begins within one hour after the injection and lasts for an hour or two. The behavior consists of continuous sniffing, licking, or biting the cage floor or the animal's own forelegs. The rat sits in a crouched posture and usually presses its body against the cage wall. Normal activities such as grooming, eating, rearing, and forward locomotion are absent; backward locomotion is seen occasionally.

Randrup and Munkvad noted that the stereotypical behavior varies from species to species but always involves the suppression of normal behavior:

The stereotyped activities are always performed continuously in the absence of normal activities, but the form of the stereotypy depends on the species. Rodents gnaw, lick, or sniff; cats move their head from side to side; and dogs run in circles or back and forth along a fixed route. The monkeys perform various repetitive movements with their hands, limbs, body or head, and locomotion along a fixed route has been observed in a few cases. [citations omitted]

The authors considered stereotypical behavior similar to certain obsessive and compulsive behaviors seen in humans taking stimulants. They cite Scher (1966), who observed,

One of the most peculiar phenomena which may occur in the course of the use of amphetamines, especially methamphetamine, is what is called "being hung up."

An individual who is "hung up" will literally get stuck in a repetitious thought or act for hours. He may sit in a tub all day long, clean up the house or a particular item, hold a note or phrase of music, or engage in nonejaculatory intercourse for extended periods. The danger of getting "hung up" in this way seems to be peculiar to amphetamines. . . . (Scher, 1966)

In a discussion of the effect of amphetamines on children, Everett Ellinwood (Kramer, Lipton, Ellinwood, & Sulser, 1970) pointed out that in response to the drugs, some animals and people are stimulated in such a fashion that they are totally driven to distraction.

Others, however, develop stereotypy, which Ellinwood identified as the sought-after effect in children and some adults:

They are no longer hyperresponsive to their environment and, for the first time, they focus on the object or task before them. For the first time in their lives they can accomplish a task like reading, which requires concentration, without responding to someone who's talking in the room. Some adults also take amphetamines before going to a party, because it cuts down on the peripheral distraction and the noisy background din. . . .
Cats who are in this stereotypy mode cannot be distracted by stimuli in their periphery; you can wave your arms, etc., to no avail.

More Extreme Intoxications

One way to understand the routine effect of any psychiatric drug is to look at its more extreme or toxic effects (Breggin, 1991a). The clinical or therapeutic effect is likely to be a less intense expression of the toxic effect. In discussing methylphenidate's "cognitive toxicity," James M. Swanson (1992) and his coauthors summarized the literature:

> In some disruptive children, drug-induced compliant behavior may be accompanied by isolated, withdrawn, and overfocused behavior. Some medicated children may seem "zombie-like" and high doses which make ADHD children more "somber," "quiet," and "still" may produce social isolation by increasing "time spent alone" and decreasing "time spent in positive interaction" on the playground. [citations omitted]

These findings are very similar to even more extreme reactions with larger, chronic doses. Schiorring (1977) studied amphetamine intoxication in monkeys and in humans. In monkeys, mothers on amphetamine lost contact with their infants and became obsessed in a stereotypical fashion:

> In mother-infant dyadic relationships, amphetamine eliminated the eye contact, the specific gaze that is an important cue for contact in these animals. In addition, the parental care behavior pattern was disrupted. The mother lost her interest in the infant. She did not react to the calling signals of the infant, spent most of the time away from the infant and was preoccupied with stereotyped self-grooming behavior. (abstract of Schiorring, 1977, in Spotts & Spotts, 1980)

In amphetamine addicts, similar behaviors were observed, including stereotypical, bizarre movements, repetition of single words or phrases, stereotyped writing or drawing, talking without listening, and social withdrawal and isolation.

In discussing amphetamine abuse, John Kramer (1970) again compares the stereotypical behavior of animals to some of the reactions in human beings:

> Perhaps the most curious effect of amphetamines is their capacity to induce behavior which is persisted in or repeated for prolonged periods. If the issue is not too disorganized the activity may, on the surface at least, be useful. Dwellings may be cleaned, automobiles polished, or items arranged to an inhuman degree of perfection. . . . Analogous to this compulsive behavior in man is what has been termed *stereotypy* in animals. Rats, mice, guinea pigs, cats, and squirrel monkeys, almost without exception, perform repetitive acts. . . . [citation omitted]

Notice the author's remark that the behavior may "on the surface at least, be useful." In treating children with Ritalin and other medications we settle for a surface or cosmetic change in behavior without dealing with the underlying problems in the family, school, and elsewhere. We do so at grave risk to the child's physical and mental integrity.

RITALIN DAMAGE

Brain Damage

There is reason to be concerned about brain tissue shrinkage as a result of long-term Ritalin therapy. Nasrallah et al. (1986) found brain pathology in more than half of 24 young adults. Since all of the patients had been treated with psychostimulants, "cortical atrophy may be a long-term adverse effect of this treatment."

Giedd et al. (1994) published an MRI study of hyperactive boys, mean age 11.9 years, in a day treatment program at NIMH. Anterior portions of the corpus callosum were found to have significantly smaller areas in the ADHD group. The authors attribute the size difference to ADHD.

The study has a most remarkable and wholly excusable flaw: It never discusses whether the children were taking psychiatric drugs, including Ritalin. In reality, given their diagnosis and their place of treatment, they probably had been prescribed a variety of psychiatric drugs, especially stimulants, over several years. There is reason to suspect that this is another incriminating study in regard to brain damage from Ritalin. That the authors don't even mention the drug history of the children—and that the journal editors didn't insist upon the details—is very telling about the willingness of modern psychiatry to deny the potential damage of its treatments.

In the same vein, Hynd et al. (1991) published an MRI study suggesting that ADHD children, in comparison to normal controls, have a smaller corpus callosum. No consideration is given to the possibility of an adverse drug effect. No attempt was made to correlate the brain changes with intensity of exposure to Ritalin or to a combination of drugs the children may have received over the years. Yet we know the children were given Ritalin because the authors state, "Although not a criterion for inclusion in this study, all children with ADHD were judged to be favorable responders to methylphenidate (Ritalin) by both their parents and physicians."

It is now well established that amphetamine derivatives, MDMA and MDA, can cause "long-lasting neurotoxic effects with respect to both the functional and structural integrity of serotonergic neurons in the brain" (Battaglia et al., 1987). We need to show more concern about the impact of the seemingly less toxic amphetamines on the especially vulnerable growing brain of the child.

It is also known that stimulants, including Ritalin, can delay growth in height and weight, while the degree of recovery on termination of treatment remains undetermined. A relatively small head and brain in a normal person does not indicate any limitation on brain function, but a head and brain rendered smaller than its genetic program by toxic medication is certainly something to be concerned about.

The Drug Enforcement Administration (1995b) provides a summary comparing the adverse effects of methylphenidate and amphetamine. For the central nervous system, it found excessive CNS stimulation, psychosis, dizziness, headache, insomnia, irritability, attacks of Gilles de la Tourette or other tic syndromes. It also lists for both drugs a variety of cardiovascular symptoms, including increased blood pressure and heart rate; various gastrointestinal symptoms, including vomiting, stomach pain, and anorexia; and weight loss and growth suppression. For methylphenidate alone, it lists leukopenia (abnormally low white cells in the blood), anemia, hypersensitivity reaction, and blurred vision. For amphetamine it lists skin rash or hives.

The DEA also observes that adverse effects of irritability or sadness have not been well studied but have been reported in up to 22% of children on stimulant medication. Elsewhere in the same document, the DEA notes that with both Ritalin and amphetamine, "Psychotic episodes, violent behavior and bizarre mannerisms have been reported" (p. 16). Emotionally disturbing adverse effects are even more common with the youngest children. Dulcan and Popper (1991) note that in preschool children there is a greater risk of side effects, "especially sadness, irritability, clinging, insomnia, and anorexia" (p. 188).

Moral, Psychological, and Social Harm

Children are given Ritalin during a period of time in which they are developing their psychological and social skills, and their very identity. What does it mean to a child, and later to the grown adult, to be told of "crossed wires" or a "biochemical imbalance"? What are the repercussions of the child hearing that medication is necessary to produce behavior that conforms to the family or school standard?

It is far more demoralizing for a child to be told that his or her brain is defective than to be called "bad." The diagnosed child gets the same message—"You are bad"—plus a message that he or she is a hopeless "freak"—a person with an abnormal brain and mind.

Dulcan (1994; also see Whalen & Henker, 1991) summarizes some of the harmful moral, psychological, and social effects on children who are prescribed Ritalin:

> . . . indirect and inadvertent cognitive and social consequences, such as lower self-esteem and self-efficacy; attribution by child, parents, and teachers of both success and failure to medication, rather than to the child's effort; stigmatization by peers; and dependence by parents and teachers on medication rather than making needed changes in the environment. (p. 1218)

An unpublished report (circa 1989), "Why Johnny Can't Sit Still: Kids' Ideas On Why They Take Stimulants," was based on research conducted by physicians Peter Jensen, Michael Bain, and Allen Josephson. Jensen is an experienced researcher from the Division of Neuropsychiatry at Walter Reed Army Institute of Research. Using interviews, child psychiatric rating scales, and a projective test entitled "Draw a Person Taking the Pill," the authors systematically evaluated 20 children given Ritalin by their primary care physicians.

The researchers concluded that taking the drugs produced (a) "defective superego formation" manifested by "disowning responsibility for their provocative behavior;" (b) "impaired self-esteem development;" (c) "lack of resolution of critical family events which preceded the emergence of the child's hyperactive behavior;" and (d) displacement of "family difficulties onto the child."

Many of the children thought they were "bad" and were taking the pill to control themselves. They often attributed their conduct to outside forces, such as eating sugar or not taking their pill, rather than to themselves. Jensen and his colleagues warn that the use of stimulant medication "has significant effects on the psychological development of the child," and distracts parents, teachers, and doctors from solving important problems in the child's environment.

The authors conclude, "Research investigating children's perceptions of the meanings of stimulant medication, as mediated by the family context, adult and child attributions, and the child's developmental level, are long overdue."

IS ADHD AN AMERICAN DISEASE? A BOY'S DISEASE?

ADHD is rarely diagnosed in countries with more evident concern for children, such as Denmark, Norway, and Sweden, where psychiatric drugs of any kind are much more rarely given to children. A doctor working in England's National Health Service is not allowed to give methylphenidate in routine practice because it is not on the approved drug list. The doctor could prescribe amphetamines, which have a similar effect, but this is discouraged and relatively rarely done. However, media requests for information coming to me personally and to the Center for the Study of Psychiatry and Psychology indicate that there are growing attempts to promote the use of stimulants in Europe and Australia.

Males are far more frequently given DBD diagnoses than females. According to the *DSM-IV*, ADHD occurs in boys up to 4 to 9 times more frequently than in girls and conduct disorder is "much more common in males," in whom the rates vary from 6% to 16%. Aside from feeling bored or in conflict with adults, why would boys ordinarily tend to act resentfully and rebelliously toward the authority of their mothers and female teachers? The simplest answer is that they are trained to be that way toward women in general. In fact, most grown men in the world today resent being told what to do by women.

A multiplicity of factors contribute to the conflicts and confusion in little boys. Respect for authority in general is on the decline in society. Boys are culturally encouraged and even trained to suppress their tender ("feminine") side. Meanwhile, they are taught to be domineering and hostile toward women. These lessons are imprinted through TV and other entertainment media, and reinforced in sports and on the playground, as well as in the family.

In our modern society, in which girls receive increasingly confusing messages about assertiveness, more and more young girls are being diagnosed with one or another DBD. Often they are children with special enterprise and boldness.

CH.A.D.D.

Founded in 1987, Children with Attention Deficit Disorders (CH.A.D.D.) is an organization of parents who have children labeled with attention-deficit disorders. CH.A.D.D.'s official policy views these children as suffering from genetic and biological problems. In the words of CH.A.D.D. president, Sandra F. Thomas (1990), "Our kids have a neurological impairment that is pervasive and affects every area of their life, day and night."

CH.A.D.D. leaders claim that their children's emotional upset and anger is in no way caused by family conflicts, poor parenting, inadequate schools, or broad social stressors. In a recent CH.A.D.D. brochure entitled *Hyperactive? Inattentive? Impulsive?*, a headline announces: "Dealing with parental guilt. No, it's not all your fault" (CH.A.D.D., undated). After stating that ADHD is a neurological disorder, the brochure goes on to explain:

> Frustrated, upset, and anxious parents do not cause their children to have ADD. On the contrary, ADD children usually cause their parents to be frustrated, upset, and anxious. (p. 1)

There could be no better example of child-blaming and parental exoneration.

CH.A.D.D. has followed the model of its adult counterpart, the National Alliance for the Mentally Ill (NAMI) (Breggin, 1991a). Parents who belong to NAMI usually have grown offspring who are severely emotionally disabled, and they promote biochemical and genetic explanations, drugs, electroshock, psychosurgery, and involuntary treatment. The organization also tries to suppress dissenting views by harassing professionals who disagree with them (Breggin, 1991a). Now NAMI has developed an affiliate, NAMI-CAN—the National Alliance for the Mentally Ill, Child and Adolescent Network (Armstrong, 1993). Both NAMI-CAN and CH.A.D.D. believe in what they call BBBD—biologically based brain diseases.

The Power Base of the Parent Groups

Parent members of CH.A.D.D. and NAMI have developed enormous influence by joining forces with biologically oriented professionals, national mental health organizations, and the drug industry. But where is the money coming from to support high-pressure lobbying, media campaigns, and upscale national conventions at hotels like the Chicago Hyatt Regency? *Pathways to Progress*, CH.A.D.D.'s convention program, states (CH.A.D.D., 1992):

> CH.A.D.D. appreciates the generous contribution of an educational grant in support of our projects by CIBA-Geigy Corporation.

CIBA-Geigy manufactures Ritalin, the stimulant with the lion's share of the ADHD market.

I have been able to obtain a complete list of contributions to CH.A.D.D. by CIBA-Geigy. The escalating totals are as follows:

1989 to year ending June 30, 1992 ....$170,000

year ending June 30, 1993 .... $ 50,000

year ending June 30, 1994 ....$200,000

year ending June 30, 1995 ....$398,000

In 1995, they also had smaller grants from Abbott Laboratories ($37,000) and Burroughs Wellcome ($18,000). Abbott is the manufacturer of the stimulant Cylert (pemoline), used to treat ADHD. Burroughs Wellcome makes several medications used in pediatric medicine, including well-known antibiotics and cold medications. They also make the highly stimulating antidepressant Wellbutrin.

The adult counterpart of CH.A.D.D., NAMI, has had equal success in its political efforts. It too is closely aligned with biological psychiatry and accepts money from the drug companies.

On-the-Spot Diagnosis

A recent CH.A.D.D. *Educators Manual* was written with the collaboration of professionals, including Russell Barkley (Fowler, 1992). It makes clear the intention to diagnose (and subsequently drug) children who fail to conform to strict discipline:

> Attention Deficit Disorder is a hidden disability. No physical marker exists to identify its presence, yet ADD is not very hard to spot. Just look with

your eyes and listen with your ears when you walk through places where children are—particularly those places where children are expected to behave in a quiet, orderly, and productive fashion. In such places, children with ADD will identify themselves quite readily. They will be doing or not doing something which frequently results in their receiving a barrage of comments and criticisms such as "Why don't you ever listen?" "Think before you act." "Pay attention."

TREATING CHILDHOOD BEHAVIOR PROBLEMS WITH NEUROLEPTICS

Neuroleptics such as Mellaril are too frequently given to children with behavioral problems. The risks are enormous. As already documented, tardive dyskinesia is common in children, often in a particularly disabling form (chapter 4). The neuroleptics frequently cause irreversible intellectual, emotional, and behavioral deterioration in children (chapter 5).

Dulcan (1994) warns about the array of EPS:

Acute extrapyramidal side effects, including dystonic reactions, parkinsonian tremor, rigidity and drooling, and akathisia, occur as in adults. Laryngeal dystonia is potentially fatal. . . . Adolescent boys seem to be more vulnerable to acute dystonic reactions than are adult patients. . . . (p. 1225)

TREATING CHILDHOOD TOURETTE'S WITH NEUROLEPTICS

One of the most tragic situations in the treatment of children today involves the use of neuroleptics for the control of Tourette's Disorder. Tourette's involves a combination of tics and spontaneous, inappropriate vocalizations, such as curse words. While claims have been made for a biological origin, none has been demonstrated. On the other hand, it is extremely well documented that neuroleptics frequently produce tardive dyskinesia in children with far more disabling tics, spasms, and other abnormal movements.

The devastating effects of neuroleptics in children diagnosed with Tourette's often go unrecognized. Dulcan (1994) reports that the symptoms of Tourette's can be exacerbated for several months following withdrawal from neuroleptics. Bruun (1988) reviewed 208 cases. She found that 34 suffered from drug-induced dysphoria that appeared in the form of an "organic affective syndrome," 9 from a drug-induced worsening of their Tourette's, 5 from aggression and hostility, 3 from "fog states," and 2 from "frank psychomotor seizures." A number of the children endured drug-induced akathisia, which worsened their emotional and neurological condition. The author also noted the appearance of withdrawal dyskinesias. Three of the children developed symptoms of tardive dyskinesia which, the author reports, resolved over a period of weeks or months.

Neurologist Fred Baughman (1996) observes that "Most of the single tics of childhood such as blinking, shoulder hiking, and throat clearing are wholly benign and disappear or nearly so with time and patience." He warns against treating these children with drugs like Haldol that cause permanent tics.

The use of neuroleptics for the treatment of Tourette's does not meet a reasonable medical standard in terms of its risk/benefit ratio.

TREATING CHILDREN WITH ANTIDEPRESSANTS

It is increasingly common to treat depression in children with antidepressants, although they have not been approved for this by the FDA and although there is no evidence that they are effective. Sometimes they are used, equally without scientific justification, for the treatment of behavioral problems. At the very moment that their use is on the increase, the scientific literature confirms that they have no proven clinical efficacy. As a headline in *Clinical Psychiatry News* indicates, "Though Data Lacking, Antidepressants Used Widely in Children" (Baker, 1995).

Sommers-Flanagan and Sommers-Flanagan (1996) reviewed all double-blind, placebo-controlled efficacy trials for tricyclic antidepressants (TCAs) with depressed young people published in 1985–1994. They also looked at all group studies of Prozac. They summarized: "Results indicate that neither TCAs or SSRIs have demonstrated greater efficacy than placebo in alleviating depressive symptoms in children and adolescents, despite the use of research strategies designed to give antidepressants an advantage over placebo" (p. 145). They conclude, "There has never been a double-blind, placebo controlled study published indicating that antidepressant medications are more effective than placebo in treating child or adolescent depression'' (p. 151).

Fisher and Fisher (1996) explore the ethical issues surrounding the use of antidepressants in children. They point out how published recommendations for the use of antidepressants fly in the face of data within the same publications. They observe, ''The prescribing of antidepressants for children clearly illustrates how a significant group of practitioners (child psychiatrists and pediatricians) can persist in using a procedure that is actually contradicted by research data and at the same time muster justifications for doing so'' (p. 101).

While antidepressants lack efficacy in the treatment of children, they do not lack severe adverse effects. We have already noted that Prozac can cause or exacerbate behavioral problems in children (chapter 6). In discussing the use of tricyclic antidepressants in children, Dulcan (1994) observed:

> Behavioral toxicity may be manifested by irritability, worsening of psychosis, mania, agitation, anger, aggression, forgetfulness, or confusion. CNS toxicity may be mistaken for exacerbation of the primary condition. (p. 1222)

Tricyclic antidepressants commonly produce abnormalities in cardiovascular function in children and adults and there are reports of cardiac arrest and death in children. Cardiovascular function should be carefully monitored in children taking these drugs (Dulcan, 1994).

Prescribing dangerous, ineffective antidepressants for children is especially tragic because depression in children is almost always clearly a product of their environment. Helping a child overcome depressed feelings involves helping the adults attend better to the needs of the child. Children get depressed because of depressing circumstances in their life. Sometimes these circumstances may be buried in the past in the form of neglect or physical, emotional, or sexual abuse. Sometimes they are the obvious product of current circumstances.

LIKE SHINING STARS

Our children relate to us mostly through home and school, and in some families, through church, scouts, and other community organizations. In each place we need a new dedication to their basic needs rather than to treating presumed psychiatric disorders. Above all else, our children need a more caring connection with us, the adults in their lives. This link is now being forged in some school systems that have begun to abandon the large, factorylike facilities of the past in favor of "small is beautiful."

There are many advantages to smaller schools, but perhaps the most significant one is this: They allow teachers to get to know their students well enough to understand and to meet their basic educational and emotional needs. At the same time, small schools and classes meet the teachers' basic needs for a satisfying, effective professional identity. Conflict can be more readily resolved as ideally it should be—through mutually satisfying solutions—rather than suppressed through medical diagnosis and pharmacological behavior modification.

Some smaller, more child-oriented schools have shown that the DBDs can virtually disappear. There is no better evidence for how the environment powerfully shapes the behavior that results in children being psychiatrically diagnosed.

In a July 14, 1993, *New York Times* front-page report entitled "Is Small Better? Educators Now Say Yes for High School," Susan Chira reports:

> Students in schools limited to about 400 students have fewer behavior problems, better attendance and graduation rates, and sometimes higher grades and scores. At a time when more children have less support from their families, students in small schools can form close relationships with teachers.

Teachers in these schools have the opportunity for "building bonds that are particularly vital during the troubled years of adolescence."

Even students from troubled homes respond to small, more caring schools. "They are shining stars you thought were dull," said a New York City teacher. "If you're under a lot of pressure and stress, they help you through that," said a student. "They won't put you down or put you on hold."

Children respond so quickly to improvements in the way that adults relate to them that most children can be helped without being seen by a mental health consultant or therapist. Instead, the therapist can consult with the parents, teachers, and other concerned adults.

Many psychotherapists, for example, routinely practice "child therapy" without actually seeing any children. They help their adult patients become more loving or disciplined parents through the routine work of psychotherapy, indirectly transforming the lives of their children. The children ''get better'' sight unseen. These therapists, many of whom work only with adults, may not identify themselves professionally as child psychiatrists or child therapists. But they are doing far more good for children than the professionals who diagnose and medicate them.

Children aren't born with emotional disorders; they are born into emotionally disturbing conditions. I have reviewed some of the research literature linking disturbed home environments, child abuse, and other factors to emotional disturbances in children (Breggin, 1991a, 1992). A recent study by Biederman et al. (1995) confirms that there is a correlation between ''adversity'' in the child's life and a diagnosis of ADHD. Adversity includes such things as severe marital discord, low social class, large family size, foster parent placement, and mental illness or criminality in the family.

Kathleen Salyer and her colleagues (Salyer, Holmstrom, & Noshpitz, 1991) provide a discussion with citations to the literature concerning the role of environment in causing a variety of childhood disorders. The focus of their paper is learning disability (LD). They point out that families with children labeled LD are less cohesive and more chaotic, with less educational stimulation and more economic difficulties. Families with LD children tend to provide less support and less independence while emphasizing control. In the same vein, they point out that even with known biological and genetic disorders, such as brain damage, ''the psychosocial environment was found to be the most important predictor of the child's later level of functioning'' (p. 238).

Alan Green (1989) has provided a comprehensive review showing that virtually every childhood disorder can be produced by environmental trauma and stress. The whole range of childhood disorders from autistic behavior to hyperactivity and violence can be produced by the environment. The message from this seems clear cut: Adults, through their control over the environment, are in a position to provide harmful or healing alternatives to children.

When adults provide them a better environment, children tend to quickly improve their outlook and behavior. Sometimes children can benefit from learning how to help ease the conflicted situation, but it's futile to help them if the adults are not simultaneously learning the same conflict resolution approaches.

Children and teenagers can eventually become so upset, confused, and self-destructive that they internalize the pain or become compulsively rebellious—but not until years of conflict, misunderstanding, neglect, or abuse have taken their toll. At that point, they may need the intervention of a therapeutic—unconditionally caring—adult to help them overcome their inner suffering and outrage.

If children are brought into a therapy setting, they should *never* be given the idea that they are diseased or defective. They should never be told that they are the primary cause of the conflicts they are having with their schools and families. The focus of "child psychiatry" should not be children, but parents, families, schools, religious institutions, and the wider society. What's really needed is greater adult responsibility for children in all spheres of life, from the personal attention of a parent or teacher to the social reform of our family, school, religious, and social life.

Children can benefit from guidance in learning to be responsible for their own conduct; but they do not gain from being blamed for the trauma and stress that they are exposed to in the environment around them. They need empowerment, not humiliating diagnoses and mind-disabling drugs. Most of all, they thrive when adults show concern and attention to their basic needs as children. These needs include self-esteem, love, discipline, and education. They cannot be filled by adults who want to diagnose and drug the children. They can only be fulfilled by adults who are willing to open their hearts to children, and to learn new and better ways to approach troubled and troubling young people as individuals.

We have lost sight of these truths in America and become all too willing to hand over our "problem children" to experts with credentials that permit drugging. Our problem children reflect our problems as adults; it's up to us in each and every case to try harder to provide what our children need.

CHAPTER *10*

Antianxiety Drugs, Including Behavioral Abnormalities Caused by Xanax and Halcion

Antianxiety agents (anxiolytics or minor tranquilizers) are among the most commonly used drugs in both medicine and psychiatry. It is estimated that 15% of American adults use these or similar sedative/hypnotic agents during any given year, usually through a physician's prescription (Gold, Miller, Stennie, & Populla-Vardi, 1995). Almost 2% of the population may use benzodiazepines (BZs) more or less chronically (DuPont, 1986). In 1993, Xanax topped the list for frequency of use, followed by Klonopin.

Moore and Jones (1985) performed a review of all adverse drug reactions reported to the FDA from 1968 to 1982 (see chapter 11 in this book for an analysis of the FDA's system). Antibiotics ranked first with 33,959 reported adverse reactions, but "tranquilizers" were neck-and-neck with 33,720. Among the tranquilizers, diazepam (Valium), a benzodiazepine, was number one and the neuroleptic chlorpromazine was number two.

The benzodiazepines are frequently prescribed for anxiety or panic, and for sleep. They are also given to counteract the stimulating effects of the antidepressants, especially Prozac and other SSRIs. Most of the antianxiety agents, including the more potent ones, are BZs. This chapter will focus on the brain-disabling effects of BZs, especially the short-acting, high potency drugs, alprazolam (Xanax) and triazolam (Halcion). Because they produce more frequent and intensive adverse drug reactions,

184

Xanax and Halcion provide a magnifying glass for investigating the more general impact of all BZs.

With their trade names and half-lives in parenthesis (the units are hours), current BZs include: alprazolam (Xanax, 6–20 hours), chlordiazepoxide (Librium, 30–100), clonazepam (Klonopin, 18–50), clorazepate (Tranxene, 30–100 or 200), diazepam (Valium, 30–100), estazolam (ProSom, 10–24), flurazepam (Dalmane, 50–160), lorazepam (Ativan, 10–20), midazolam (Versed, 2–3), oxazepam (Serax, 3–21), prazepam (Centrax, 30–100), quazepam (Doral, 50–160), temazepam (Restoril, 8–20), and triazolam (Halcion, 1.5–5).[1]

Some BZs have been marketed as hypnotics or sleeping medications, or are more frequently prescribed for this purpose by physicians, without being substantially different in their characteristics from other BZs marketed for anxiety. As Ashton (1995, p. 159, note on chart) remarked: "The pharmacological actions of all benzodiazepines are similar; the distinction between tranquilizers and hypnotic preparations is based on commercial, not pharmacological grounds." Flurazepam, for example, is sold as a sleeping medication; but its rather lengthy half-life will produce hangover effects the following day. Temazepam, estazolam, quazepam, and clonazepam have somewhat shorter half-lives, but they are of sufficient length to cause sedation on the following day.

Xanax, and to an even greater extent, Halcion, do have a significantly different profile due to a greater capacity to bind to receptors and a shorter half-life. Halcion's very short half-life led to the hope that it would make a particularly good sleeping medication. Instead, it has proven relatively ineffective and especially dangerous.

The brain-disabling or toxic effects of the BZs can be divided into several somewhat overlapping categories:

1. The primary clinical effect of inducing sedation (tranquility) or hypnosis (sleep), which is indistinguishable from a toxic effect except in degree
2. Cognitive dysfunction, ranging from short-term memory impairment and confusion to delirium

---

[1]The data on the half-life have been compiled from varying sources and should be considered rough estimates. Half-life is the time when 50% of the drug or its active metabolite has been eliminated.

3. Disinhibition and other behavioral aberrations—including extreme agitation, psychosis, paranoia, and depression, sometimes with violence toward self or others
4. Withdrawal, in which the individual experiences a continuum of symptoms from anxiety and insomnia after routine use to psychosis and seizures after the abrupt termination of long-term, larger doses
5. Rebound, an aspect of withdrawal, in which the individual develops anxiety, insomnia, or other serious emotional reactions that are more intense than before drug treatment began (Withdrawal can take place between doses during the routine administration of BZs, especially the short-acting ones.)
6. Habituation and addiction, along a continuum from feeling dependent on the drug to compulsively organizing one's behavior in a self-destructive manner around obtaining large amounts of the agent

BRAIN DISABILITY AS
THE PRIMARY CLINICAL EFFECT

Perhaps more than most drugs, the brain-disabling effects of the BZs (or any sedative-hypnotics, including alcohol) are readily apparent. Much as for alcohol, there is a continuum of central nervous system depression from relaxation through sleep, and, in the extreme, coma. Prescribing is a matter of giving enough of the medication to the point where the patient experiences a desired effect without becoming too heavily sedated or comatose.

Neurophysiological studies show that the BZs potentiate the neuronal inhibition that is mediated by gamma-aminobutyric acid (GABA). In doses used clinically, this results in a generalized suppression of both spontaneous and evoked electrical activity of the large neurons throughout all regions of the brain and spinal cord (Ballenger, 1995).

The binding of BZs to the GABA receptors is most intense in the cerebral cortex. Some BZs, such as Xanax and Halcion, bind especially tightly, increasing their tendency to produce more intense sedation and hypnosis, and also more severe cognitive deficits, behavioral abnormalities, rebound, and withdrawal.

Some advocates of the BZs have argued for a specific antianxiety effect separate from the general sedative effect, but there's no substantial evidence for this. Rall (1990) concludes, "The question whether the so-called antianxiety effects of the benzodiazepines are the same or different from the sedative and hypnotic effects has not been resolved."

People who use BZs to calm their anxiety will frequently use alcohol and other sedatives interchangeably for the same purpose, either in combination or at different times. As they switch from drug to drug, they tend to find little or no difference in the antianxiety effect. This confirms that BZs have no specificity for anxiety in comparison to other sedative/hypnotic agents.

THE MECHANISM
FOR PRODUCING BEHAVIORAL ABNORMALITIES

There are at least two probable causes for the abnormal behavior produced by BZs. One mechanism is direct intoxication, resulting in impaired executive and cognitive function, including reduced judgment and impulse control. Fogel and Stone (1992, p. 341) observe, "Benzodiazepines, given to reduce arousal or possibly to treat a hypomanic state, may aggravate impulsive behavior by impairing the inhibition mechanism of the frontal lobes. Barbiturates may have similar effects."

Especially in regard to the BZs, a second mechanism, rebound, has been demonstrated, and is a probable cause of many more severe reactions. Rebound, or discontinuation symptoms, occur when the BZs are withdrawn or when they begin to lose their effectiveness (American Psychiatric Association, 1990a). As the BZ disappears from the GABA receptor sites, the receptors may have become down-regulated (less sensitive). The GABA system in effect becomes sluggish. Or there may be a reduction in GABA itself in response to the drug, once again leaving the GABA system relatively inactive. Without the inhibiting effects of the GABA system, the "disinhibited" brain overreacts.

Benzodiazepine disinhibition differs in some ways from alcohol disinhibition. It can occur without a noticeable sedative intoxication, such as slurred speech, lack of coordination, or impaired consciousness. Furthermore, the BZs are prescribed by a physician, often without providing the patient a warning about possible disinhibition. Unlike the experienced alcohol user, the trusting BZ user has little reason to anticipate "losing control." Expecting to be helped, and not harmed, by the drug, the patient is less able to understand or manage potentially overwhelming feelings of anger or violence, or other untoward emotional responses. Also unlike alcohol, some of the worst BZ behavioral reactions occur during withdrawal, or in between doses, adding to the patient's confusion concerning what is happening. At the time, the patient may have little idea what is driving the unfamiliar behavior, and in retrospect it may seem like a fragmented, poorly recalled nightmare.

ADVERSE REACTIONS
TO BENZODIAZEPINES AS A GROUP

Standard textbooks and reviews spanning more than two decades, as well as a variety of clinical studies, confirm widespread recognition of BZ-induced behavioral abnormalities (Arana & Hyman, 1991; Ashton, 1995; DiMascio & Shader, 1970; Kochansky, Salzman, Shader, Harmatz, & Ogeltree, 1975; Maxmen, 1991; Rosenbaum, Woods, Groves, & Klerman, 1984; Shader & DiMascio, 1977).

Salzman et al. (1974), in a placebo-controlled study, showed that volunteers taking chlordiazepoxide became more hostile when confronted with a situation of interpersonal frustration. In 1988, Dietch and Jennings reviewed the literature concerning reports about disinhibition whose "manifestations range from irritability to increased verbal hostility and frank assault." They found a variety of studies that demonstrate an increase in feelings of hostility or in verbal hostility. They did not come to a definitive conclusion concerning the existence of the phenomenon, but estimated it was probably rare.

Salzman (1992) also reviewed the literature. He too pointed out the controversial nature of BZ-induced violence, but went on to assert, "Recent observations, however, have confirmed that hostility can be seen with all benzodiazepines, including alprazolam and clonazepam" [citations omitted].

Writing in *The Pharmacological Basis of Therapeutics*, Rall (1990) summarized:

> *Adverse psychological effects*: Benzodiazepines may cause paradoxical effects. Nitrazepam frequently and flurazepam occasionally increase the incidence of nightmares, especially during the first week of use. Flurazepam

occasionally causes garrulousness, anxiety, irritability, tachycardia, and sweating. Euphoria, restlessness, hallucinations, and hypomanic behavior have been reported to occur during the use of various benzodiazepines. Antianxiety benzodiazepines have been reported to release bizarre uninhibited behavior in some users with low levels of anxiety; hostility and rage may occur in others. Paranoia, depression, and suicidal ideation occasionally also accompany the use of these agents. (p. 355)

Rall believed that "the incidence of such paradoxical reactions is extremely small." Whether or not that is true, they are extremely hazardous. They are more common in regard to the short-acting BZs.

The APA task force report on BZs (1990, p. 18) presents a table of discontinuation symptoms. The complete list of *frequent* discontinuation symptoms includes "anxiety, insomnia, restlessness, agitation, irritability, muscle tension." Among many symptoms that are *common but less frequent*, it lists "depression" and "nightmares," as well as "lethargy." Clinical experience indicates that the combination of anxiety, insomnia, restlessness, agitation, irritability, nightmares, and depression can produce a spectrum of behavioral abnormalities, including suicide and violence. Adding to the dangers, the task force's complete list of *uncommon* symptoms includes "psychosis, seizures, persistent tinnitus, confusion, paranoid delusions, hallucinations."

The Production of Mania and Rage

As the above observations confirm, reactions to benzodiazepines can reach psychotic proportions. As noted in *Drug Facts and Comparisons* (1996), the BZs in general can cause serious psychiatric problems, including "psychosis." They can disrupt central nervous system function, producing, among other things, "disorientation . . . confusion . . . delirium . . . euphoria . . . agitation." A special *Precautions* section notes "Paradoxical reactions," including "excitement, stimulation and acute rage" and "hyperexcited states, anxiety, hallucinations. . . . "

Mania, a psychosis, is a special danger in regard to Xanax. *Drug Facts and Comparisons* (p. 1440) makes a specific reference to Xanax in this regard, stating that "Anger, hostility and episodes of mania and hypomania have been noted with *alprazolam*."

The fact that mania is a particular risk with Xanax is generally recognized. As another example, Maxmen and Ward's *Psychotropic Drug*

Fast Facts (1995, p. 287) states that "manic reactions" are "most often reported with alprazolam." It also states that "rage reactions" and "violent episodes" have especially been observed with Xanax and Valium. Yet another example is the *Handbook of Psychiatric Drug Therapy* (Third edition, 1995, p. 177) by Hyman, Arana, and Rosenbaum. It singles out Xanax to observe: "Increased impulsiveness, euphoria, and frank mania have been reported with alprazolam."

Drug Facts and Comparisons, Psychotropic Drug Fast Facts, and the *Handbook of Psychiatric Drug Therapy* are intended for ready reference for physicians for the purpose of alerting them to adverse drug reactions they need to be aware of. That all three indicate that mania and uncontrollable rage are special problems with Xanax confirms my own clinical observations that this medication is more apt than many others to produce these hyperexcited, aggressive psychotic states.

The Production of Depression and Suicide

As already noted, there are reports in the clinical literature indicating that the BZs can cause depression. Some reviews mention the phenomenon but express skepticism, while nonetheless declaring it should be taken seriously. Arana and Hyman (1991), for example, stated:

> *Depression*: All benzodiazepines have been associated with the emergence or worsening of depression; whether they were causative or only failed to prevent the depression is unknown. When depression occurs during the course of benzodiazepine treatment, it is prudent to discontinue the benzodiazepine.

Ashton (1995) observed that benzodiazepines can blunt the emotions in general, producing "emotional anesthesia." He reported, "Former long-term benzodiazepine users often bitterly regret their lack of emotional response to family events during the period that they were taking the drugs." Ashton also observed that BZs can precipitate suicide in already depressed patients.

The APA task force report on BZs (1990a), in a discussion of toxicity, also observed:

> Benzodiazepines have also been reported to cause or to exacerbate symptoms of depression. This, too, is not a frequent side effect, although the depressive symptoms may be potentially serious. [citation omitted] (p. 41)

Great Britain's Committee on Safety of Medicines (1988) recommended that "benzodiazepines should not be used alone to treat depression or anxiety associated with depression. Suicide may be precipitated in such patients."

Some psychiatrists believe there is usually a predisposition toward this behavior in the affected individual, but this position lacks evidence.

Cognitive, Emotional, and Behavioral Abnormalities Caused by Halcion and Xanax

Several studies have demonstrated rebound phenomena the same night or the day following the ingestion of the short-acting BZ, triazolam (Halcion). In a controlled study, Moon, Ankier, and Hayes (1985) found: "The results support previous reports that early insomnia and an increase in daytime anxiety are problems associated with short acting benzodiazepines, such as triazolam."

De Tullio, Kirking, Zacardelli, and Kwee (1989) reviewed the charts of 72 adult male patients taking triazolam for sleep through an ambulatory Veterans Administration clinic. Thirty-nine of the patients were available for telephone interviews. Most of the patients were elderly (aged 60 or older) and almost all received 0.25 mg. Of the 39 patients interviewed, only 4 reported no adverse effects and 23 experienced more than one. The most common were dizziness, rebound insomnia, and nightmares. "Rebound insomnia was defined as waking during the night or waking too early in the morning, and having trouble falling back to sleep." As a result of the study, the VA facility modified its policies on triazolam administration: "For outpatients on chronic triazolam therapy, a switch to a longer-acting benzodiazepine was instituted with tapering if therapy was not to be continued."

We have already noted that the APA task force (1990a) on BZs described a variety of symptoms, including depression, anxiety, hostility, and paranoia, and attributed them, in part at least, to discontinuation or withdrawal. In regard to short-acting BZs, the task force made the following observations:

> Abrupt discontinuation of short half-life benzodiazepines leads to rapid drug removal from the blood and brain, rapid uncovering of the receptor site, and relatively rapid onset of post-drug discontinuation syndromes. . . . Because of the severity of symptoms related to its half-life,

short half-life benzodiazepines given for anxiety are frequently implicated in intense discontinuation syndromes. . . . With very short half-life drugs such as triazolam, rebound symptomatology has actually been described during the period of ingestion, especially when it is given nightly. [citations omitted] (pp. 39–40)

Public and professional awareness of the special dangers of Halcion began in 1978. At that time, C. van der Kroef, a psychiatrist in The Hague, Netherlands, noticed abnormal reactions to Halcion in 4 of 11 patients he treated with the drug. Here is van der Kroef's description of one of his patients:

The insomnia improved at once, but psychically she rapidly went downhill. Progressively she became paranoid. Several times she asked me what the hypnotic contained—LSD perhaps?—for she felt that she was bordering on psychosis. She felt shut off from the world; it was as if she no longer belonged to society. Her friends asked her what was happening to her, so strangely was she behaving. . . . After two months I too began to suspect, particularly in light of experience with an earlier patient, that all this might be a consequence of her taking triazolam. The drug was withdrawn and replaced with nitrazepam. Within a day she felt herself again. The people around her noticed the difference and recognized her old self again. The paranoid traits, the hypermotility urge and the hyperaesthesia disappeared in the course of two days. . . . (quoted in Dukes, 1980)

M. N. G. Dukes (1980), a physician with considerable regulatory experience, commented on van der Kroef's findings. He observed that all of the BZs, including those used to induce sleep (hypnotics), have been known to produce reactions that are "frankly psychotic." While not common, according to Dukes, "virtually every known drug in this class" has produced "hallucinations, delusions, paranoia, amnesia, delirium, hypomania—almost every conceivable symptoms of psychotic madness . . ."

According to Dukes, all the BZs used for the control of anxiety were also implicated in causing violence:

If one—to begin at an arbitrary point—looks to the literature for evidence that the benzodiazepines can unleash aggression then one will find it. More than a dozen papers in the literature speak of irritability, defiance, hostility, aggression, rage or a progressive development of hates and dislikes in certain patients treated with benzodiazepine tranquilizers; all those products which are widespread have been incriminated at one time or another. The phenomenon has been demonstrated in animal studies and it has even been proved possible to show in human volunteers that these drugs can release pent-up hostility, particularly in highly anxious or action-oriented individuals.

Until the advent of Halcion, according to Dukes, the BZs commonly used to induce sleep were not known to cause violence. We shall find his observations confirmed later on by in-house studies at the FDA indicating that Halcion—but not the older hypnotics, Dalmane or Restoril—caused a vastly increased rate of violent activities.

I have been a medical expert in criminal cases involving abnormal behavior, including theft and violence, related to Xanax intoxication. I have also been an expert in civil suits involving suicide related to Halcion.

It is, of course, extremely difficult to demonstrate drug-induced behavioral abnormalities in highly selective, short, controlled clinical trials (see chapter 11 for detailed analysis of why this is so). Nonetheless, several studies have confirmed some of the hazards associated with Halcion.

Gardner and Cowdry (1985) found an increase in "dyscontrol" in borderline patients taking alprazolam in a double-blind, placebo-controlled crossover study. The dyscontrol included the following: "Overdose, severe"; "Overdose, moderate"; "Deep neck cuts"; "Transverse wrist cuts"; "Tried to break own arm"; "Threw chair at child"; and "Arm and head banging; jumped in front of car."

Gardner and Cowdry pointed out that there are some reports of borderline patients also improving on alprazolam. They concluded, "Caution should, however, be exercised, particularly in treating individuals with a substantial history of dyscontrol."

Bayer, Bayer, Pathy, and Stoker (1986) conducted a 9-week, double-blind controlled study of triazolam and another hypnotic, chlormethiazole, in the elderly with sleep disturbances. They found daytime withdrawal effects from triazolam but not chlormethiazole. At week three, significantly more triazolam patients were rated as more restless during the day "and they also appeared more hostile, less relaxed, more irritable and more anxious." Patients on triazolam also had more adverse events related to the central nervous system, requiring 4 of 22 patients to withdraw from the study; 3 of those withdrawn recovered after terminating the medication. One patient felt the tablets were "making him nervous." The others individually developed paranoid delusions, "increasing confusion and irritability," and irrational, irritable, and uncooperative behavior.

Adam and Oswald (1989), in a double-blind, placebo-controlled study of triazolam and lormetazepam with 40 subjects in each of the three groups, found that "triazolam takers became more anxious on self-ratings, were judged more often to have had a bad response by an observer, more often wrote down complaints of distress, and suffered weight loss. After about 10 days of regular triazolam they tended to develop panics and depression, felt unreal, and sometimes paranoid." According to the authors:

> Subjects' written comments suggested that from about 10 days after starting triazolam, they became liable to panic attacks, feelings of despair and derealization. There were descriptions of panic episodes in public places in seven subjects during triazolam intake, but none during placebo or lormetazepam. . . . Several reported their family relationships were changed. . . . A number of triazolam subjects became paranoid. . . . Two men developed paranoid psychoses. [During the withdrawal period, the anxiety of the triazolam patients] fell quickly to normal levels."

Soldatos, Sakkas, Bergiannaki, and Stefanis (1986) reported on serious adverse drug reactions in all five psychiatric inpatients during a clinical trial of 0.5 mg triazolam and placebo. The patients and nurses were blind in the study, but not the physician with medical responsibility for the patients. The study consisted of 1 week of placebo baseline, 2 weeks of triazolam administration, and 1 week of withdrawal on placebo. All five patients developed severe reactions to triazolam. Case 1 developed "anxiety and hallucinations on the last two days of triazolam administration and the first withdrawal day." Case 2 had a sudden increase in anxiety and became "irritable, uncooperative, and depressed." She became withdrawn and cried, and showed "considerable impairment of memory and orientation." On withdrawal of triazolam, "she became more incoherent, expressing paranoid ideas of persecution that persisted about a week." She required Haldol to control her "delusions." Case 3 developed severe insomnia during withdrawal and "reported considerable anxiety and irritability along with an uncontrollable fear of death, which persisted to the next day when she additionally manifested a marked degree of memory impairment." Case 4, by the end of the second week of triazolam administration, "became more depressed and manifested increasingly irritability and hostility . . . ." Case 5, on the second week of triazolam administration, "experienced increasing daytime anxiety and he became, for the first time since admission, irritable, hostile, and somewhat guarded and paranoid towards the unit staff.'' The authors suggest that some of the symptoms may be related to disinhibition. They warn that these serious side effects ''may not be rare when triazolam is used in patients . . . [with] major psychiatric conditions.''

Rosenbaum et al. (1994) found that 8 of 80 patients treated with alprazolam in an outpatient clinical setting developed extreme anger or hostile behavior.

Evidence from the FDA's Spontaneous Reporting System (SRS)

In 1987, Bixler, Kales, Brubaker, and Kales, from the Sleep Research and Treatment Center and Department of Psychiatry at the Pennsylvania State University College of Medicine, reviewed adverse reactions to BZs recorded in the FDA's spontaneous reporting system (SRS). They compared triazolam with two other BZs commonly used to induce sleep, temazepam (Restoril) and flurazepam (Dalmane). They controlled the reports for the number and size of prescriptions for each of the three drugs. They found:

> In general, triazolam had much higher overall rates than did the other two drugs. Hyperexcitability and withdrawal effects were greatest for triazolam and least for flurazepam. Amnesia was reported almost exclusively with triazolam. Rates for other cognitive as well as affective and other behavior effects were also much greater for triazolam and about equal for the other two drugs.

The ''affective and other behavioral disturbances'' category of adverse drug reactions included ''Depression, Psychotic Depression, Emotional lability, Euphoria, Hostility, Personality disorder, and Decreased libido.''

Epidemiological studies at the FDA have consistently shown that alprazolam and, especially, triazolam produce more frequent and more serious adverse central nervous system effects, including drastic and life-threatening behavioral changes, than any other BZs. I have reviewed the in-house memos with detailed analyses generated by the Division of Epidemiology and Surveillance, which is responsible for the SRS. This division has consistently shown more concern about triazolam than has Paul Leber's Division of Neuropharmacological Drug Products, which originally approved the drug (see below; see chapter 11 for more about Leber and the

FDA). The data from the epidemiology studies will now be described in detail for the first time in the literature.

Robert "Bob" Wise (September 19, 1989), in a working paper for the FDA's Division of Epidemiology and Surveillance, made an "executive summary" concerning reports of hostility on triazolam. Wise addresses a syndrome that consists of "anger or rage, aggression, and some actual assaults and murders." He states:

> More such reports of this type have been received by the FDA for triazolam and alprazolam than for any other drug product regulated by the Agency. Reporting rates, which adjust for differences in the extent of each drug's utilization, reveal much higher ratios of hostility reports to drug sales for both triazolam and alprazolam than for other benzodiazepines with similar indications.
>
> The public health importance of these reactions lies in their severity, with occasionally lethal behavior unleashed, in the context of large population exposures as the popularity of both drugs continues to rise.

After a brief history of the FDA's increased focus on BZ-induced hostility, Wise explains

> Our concern with such reactions then broadened to the class of triazoloben-zodiazepines, when another Increased Frequency Report included a reaction in which a 57 year old woman fatally shot her mother two hours after taking one-half milligram of triazolam. When we looked at reports received during 1988, we found that triazolam's 1988 reporting rate for hostility reactions was more than twice as high as alprazolam's.

> In the entire SRS . . . during early August, 1989, triazolam was the suspect drug in 113 reports coded as hostility, more than any other medication. It was followed by alprazolam, which accounted for 78 reports. Only nine other drugs were suspected in more than ten cases each. Another 318 drug products had fewer hostility reports, most often one (60.4 percent of 318) or two (14.8 percent).

Three fatalities were reported to the SRS for triazolam and one for alprazolam. Five reports of alprazolam overdose were associated with assaults, including two murders. Reactions were reported across the dose range. Males (29) and females (26) were almost evenly distributed.

Four alprazolam cases showed a reduction in hostility and rage reactions with a reduction in dose, confirming the drug's role in producing the behavior.

Wise summarized, "This apparently excessive number of rage and similar reports with triazolam and alprazolam, after adjusting the differences in frequency of drug use, provides strong suspicion that a causal relationship may obtain." It should be added that the relationship to increased dosage seen in several cases further confirms causation. Wise concluded that these reports cannot "prove the presence of a causal relationship" to the drug, but that they do "imply a substantial public health importance for the potential hostility syndrome."

Wise missed an extremely important aspect of his own data. Not only were Halcion and Xanax first and second in total reports of hostility, Versed (midazolam) was third in order. Versed, like Halcion and Xanax, is a very short-acting, tightly binding benzodiazepine. It is used exclusively as an intravenous injection for preoperative sedation and memory impairment. The total numbers of reports were Halcion (112), Xanax (77), and Versed (46). Valium (34 reports) was fourth. They were followed by Symmetrel (22) and Prozac (20).

Thus, the database for all drugs in the spontaneous reporting system of the FDA—which includes all prescription drugs in the United States—shows that three short-acting, tightly binding benzodiazepines come in first, second, and third for reports of hostility as an adverse drug reaction. Furthermore, the three drugs are typically used under very different clinical conditions: Halcion orally with one daily dose at night for sleep, Xanax orally with several daily doses for daytime anxiety, and Versed intravenously for preoperative purposes, usually on one occasion only. Despite the different uses, dosage schedules, and even routes of administration, they cluster at the very top of the list for producing hostility. This is convincing and seemingly irrefutable evidence that these kinds of agents can cause violence.[2]

On April 21, 1989, Wise wrote an Increased Frequency Report for the FDA on the subject of "alprazolam and rage." Wise explained that the analysis was undertaken because "Over a 12 month period, Upjohn received six reports of rage, agitation, anger, aggression, and similar behavioral and emotional symptoms after exposures to alprazolam." All

---

[2]Attorney Michael Mosher of Paris, Texas, directed me to the significance of the Versed data.

but one involved "manifested or verbalized murderous impulses." According to Wise:

> From spontaneous reports alone, we cannot estimate the actual incidence of alprazolam-induced rage reactions. But in light of the widely acknowledged, substantial underreporting to spontaneous surveillance systems in general and to the FDA's SRS in particular, it is entirely possible that six reports of this kind of reaction within a single year might reflect sixty or more in reality. (Wise, April 21, 1989)

After reviewing all reports made to Upjohn and the FDA, Wise concluded:

> An increase in annual frequency of "rage" reports with alprazolam prompted us to compare hostility reports more generally across several anxiolytic benzodiazepines. Alprazolam appears to have an excessive reporting rate for events coded with "hostility," even after adjusting for differences in the extent of each drug's utilization. The numbers and potential gravity of these reactions and their possible relationship to dosage all appear to conflict with current labeling's brief description of "paradoxical effects" that occur only "in rare instances and in a random fashion."

On October 17, 1988, Charles Anello, Deputy Director of the Office of Epidemiology and Biostatistics, referred to an earlier FDA comparison of spontaneous reports concerning triazolam to two other BZs used to treat insomnia, temazepam (Restoril) and flurazepam (Dalmane). Anello stated that there was a proportionately increased number of reports concerning abnormal behavior in regard to triazolam. Anello reported on a further analysis comparing triazolam and temazepam, showing that for triazolam the FDA receives proportionally more adverse drug reaction reports (ADRs), more serious ADRs, and more reports of five selected "behavioral" drug reactions.

On September 12, 1989, Anello reported within the FDA on "Triazolam and Temazepam—Comparison Reporting Rates." He found that adverse drug reactions were reported 11 times more frequently with triazolam than with temazepam. The relative reporting rate was 46 to 1 for amnesia, 9 to 1 for "agitation, anxiety and nervousness," 16 to 1 for psychosis ("psychosis, hallucinations, paranoid reaction, and acute brain syndrome"), and 19 to 1 for "hostility and intentional injury."

Anello's analysis indicated that there were no convincing explanations for these differences other than actual drug effects; but he did not make a formal determination of causality. However, in a handwritten analysis attached to the document, obtained through the Freedom of Information Act, there is a summary entitled "Other Evidence in Favor of Effect of Triazolam," which we quote in full:

1. Temporal relationship of reactions to initial dose
2. Large proportion of spontaneous resolution with drug withdrawal (pos-[itive] dechallenge)[3]
3. a few reports of positive rechallenges[4]
4. reports of reactions in otherwise normal individuals
5. corroborating reports in literature (including WHO data—similar magnitude of reactions in Canada in data through 3/87)

The above note indicates some of the logical, scientific steps by which data from spontaneous reporting were used by an unidentified FDA official to confirm causality in regard to Halcion and adverse behavioral effects. (For a further discussion of the scientific process in epidemiological studies, see chapter 11.)

In 1991, Diane Wysowski and David Barash, also from the FDA's Division of Epidemiology and Surveillance, published a report in the *Archives of Internal Medicine*. A footnote stated, "This article contains the professional views of the authors and does not constitute the official position of the Food and Drug Administration." Using the FDA's spontaneous report system, the authors compared triazolam and temazepam through 1985 for "confusion, amnesia, bizarre behavior, agitation, and hallucinations." They concluded, "Considering the extent of use, reporting rates for triazolam were 22 to 99 times those for temazepam, depending upon the reaction." Echoing the handwritten remarks appended to Anello's (1990) in-house report, the authors summarize:

Factors that indicate a causal association between triazolam and adverse behavioral reactions include corroborating case reports and sleep laboratory studies in the literature, reports of reactions in otherwise normal persons, acute onset and temporal relationship to reactions with initial dose, spontaneous recoveries and return to normalcy with drug discontinuation, and occurrences of positive rechallenge. Also, the high benzodiazepine receptor

---

[3]In dechallenge, the drug is withdrawn to see if the adverse reaction then stops.
[4]In rechallenge, the drug is given again to see if the adverse reaction can be repeated.

affinity with triazolam has been postulated as a possible biological mechanism. [citations omitted]

While unable to "completely exclude the possibility that some selection factors are operating to produce higher reporting rates for triazolam," nonetheless they find that the "evidence suggests" a greater occurrence with triazolam than with temazepam. Andreadis and Schirmer (1992) responded critically for Upjohn with a letter and Wysowski and Barash (1992) were given the opportunity to try to answer their objections.

AMERICAN AND BRITISH RESPONSES DIVERGE

Finally, in November, 1991, the FDA approved new labeling for Halcion (FDA, 1992). The new label emphasizes that triazolam is indicated for short-term use, and specifies 7–10 days. Treatment lasting longer than 2 to 3 weeks requires a complete reevaluation of the patient. In addition, the label emphasizes the use of the lowest possible dose.

Here is the new warning in the Halcion label as found, for example, in the 1994 *Physicians' Desk Reference*:

A variety of abnormal thinking and behavior changes have been reported to occur in association with the use of benzodiazepine hypnotics, including HALCION. Some of these changes may be characterized by decreased inhibition, e.g., aggressiveness and extroversion that seem excessive, similar to that seen with alcohol and other CNS depressants (e.g., sedative/hypnotics). Other kinds of behavioral changes have been reported, for example, bizarre behavior, agitation, hallucinations, depersonalization. In primarily depressed patients, the worsening of depression, including suicidal thinking, has been reported in association with the use of benzodiazepines.

The warning concludes with the following:

As with some, but not all benzodiazepines, anterograde amnesia of varying severity and paradoxical reactions have (sic) been reported following therapeutic doses of HALCION. Data from several sources suggest that anterograde amnesia may occur at a higher rate with HALCION than with other benzodiazepine hypnotics.

The final label change was negotiated and approved under the authority of Paul Leber, director of the Division of Neuropharmacological Drug Products, the division responsible for Halcion's original approval. In several ways, the label seems to fall far short of conclusions generated by both the literature and the division responsible for postmarketing surveillance.

The FDA label does mention the disproportionate reporting of amnesia; but by omission it leads the reader to believe that the behavioral effects did not occur with increased frequency. Instead of linking directly to Halcion the enormously increased risk for violence, psychosis, and other extremely hazardous behavioral abnormalities, the label notes that these changes have been "reported in association with the use of benzodiazepine hypnotics, including triazolam." As we documented earlier in this chapter, Charles Anello, Deputy Director of the Office of Epidemiology and Biostatistics, compared adverse drug reaction reports for Halcion and Restoril. For Halcion versus Restoril, the relative reporting rate for "agitation, anxiety and nervousness" was 9–1; for psychosis, 16–1; and for "hostility and intentional injury," 19–1.

Great Britain took a stronger stand and ended up banning Halcion. On October 1, 1991, the Committee on the Safety of Medicines (CSM) gave notice of the withdrawal of Halcion from the market because of concerns about safety, especially in regard to causing memory loss and depression (Asscher, 1991; Brahams, 1991). On December 9, 1991, the Committee on Safety of Medicines (1991) responded to Upjohn's appeal with a definitive scientific conclusion about the dangers of Halcion (p. 1). It found what it called a clearly established causal relationship between Halcion and adverse psychiatric effects. These adverse effects occurred, in the CSM's opinion, far more frequently with Halcion than with other BZs. The CSM declared that the spontaneous reporting system data from the United States and England confirmed or strengthened the connection between Halcion and various psychiatric side effects. Concerning the FDA epidemiological data, the CSM observed that despite differences of opinion within the FDA, the U.S. data provided a signal requiring further investigation (p. 10).

Why would Great Britain take a tougher stand against Halcion? The answer lies partly in the greater power of the psychopharmaceutical complex in America and, in particular, the lavish spending of Upjohn in the maintenance of its self-avowed partnership with the American Psychiatric Association. In response to my criticism in a letter to the *New York*

Times (Breggin, 1992b), the medical director of the American Psychiatric Association (Sabshin, 1992) defended taking a gift of $1.5 million from Upjohn on the grounds that the drug company and the psychiatric association have a "responsible, ethical partnership." Upjohn confirmed the "partnership" in a letter of its own to *Clinical Psychiatry News* (Jonas, 1992). (Even after the controversy, the American Psychiatric Association continued the theme of "our partners in industry" in a mass mailing to its membership [Benedek, 1993].)

The manufacturer of Halcion, Upjohn, has been criticized in the media and in court for allegedly withholding from the FDA and the profession damaging evidence concerning the drug. Upjohn has denied allegations of intentional wrongdoing and has attributed errors in reporting adverse effects to innocent mistakes. The controversy continues in the FDA, the media, and in the courts (Breggin, 1996; Carey & Weber, 1996; Kolata, 1992; controversy summarized from a legal viewpoint in Moch, Borja, & O'Donnell, 1995).

OTHER RISKS IN BENZODIAZEPINE USE

BZs As Instruments of Suicide

Some of the tricyclic antidepressants and barbiturates are probably more lethal than BZs taken alone. But when BZs are combined with other drugs, such as alcohol, their lethality is increased. Overall, the BZs account for many more suicides than most physicians probably realize.

A survey in Britain covering the decade of the 1980s demonstrated large numbers of successful suicides using BZs, either alone or in combination with alcohol (Serfaty & Masterton, 1993; also see Buckley, Dawson, White, & O'Connell, 1995). Serfaty and Masterton found 891 fatalities with BZs alone and 591 in combination with alcohol. The total of all poisonings attributed to BZs was 1,576 during the 10-year period, putting them ahead of aspirin/salicylates at 1,308 as well as amitriptyline (1,083) and dothiepin at 981. (The latter two drugs accounted for over half the fatal poisonings attributed to antidepressants.)

Among the BZs, two commonly prescribed for sleep, flurazepam (Dalmane) and temazepam (Restoril), had the most deaths per million prescriptions (15.0 and 11.9, respectively). They were more dangerous than about half the antidepressants surveyed by the same methods. Triazolam (Halcion) had far fewer deaths per million prescriptions (5.1) than Dalmane or Restoril; but it was still above the mean for anxiolytic BZs (3.2).

In estimated deaths per million patients, the rank order among all BZs in Britain was dominated by the hypnotics. Dalmane (90 per million) was first; Restoril (71) was second; the British hypnotic, flunitrazepam (Rohypnol) (49), was third; and Halcion was fourth (30). Another British hypnotic, nitrazepam (Mogadon and others; 26) was fifth.

In deaths per million patients, among the antianxiety drugs, prazepam (Centrax; 25) and alprazolam (Xanax; 24) were close behind triazolam and nitrazepam.

Benzodiazepine-Induced Cognitive Dysfunction

Cognitive impairment, including memory impairment and confusion, is a well-known phenomenon in association with BZs (APA, 1990a; Ashton, 1995; Golombok, Moodley, & Lader, 1988; Hommer, 1991). Xanax and Halcion are especially prone to produce cognitive deficits. Individuals who take Halcion to sleep on an airplane, for example, may end with a blank in their memories for the period surrounding the trip. Students who take BZs before exams in order to relax or to get sleep are in danger of losing some of the material they have been studying. Triazolam produced more sedation and greater impairment of psychomotor performance at the same dose in healthy elderly persons than in healthy young persons (Greenblatt et al., 1991).

Effects on Sleep and the EEG

The effects of the BZs on the EEG resemble those of other sedative-hypnotic agents, including decreased alpha activity and increased low-voltage fast activity, especially beta activity (Rall, 1990). Their effects on sleep are also similar to those of other CNS depressants, and provide a window into the dysfunctions they produce (Rall, 1990).

Before the brain rebounds after one or more doses, the BZs decrease sleep latency (the time it takes to fall asleep) and reduce the number of awakenings. The overall time in REM sleep is usually shortened, but the number of cycles of REM may be increased later in sleep. Total sleep duration is usually increased. There are complex effects on the dream process.

Within a short time of starting Halcion, rebound begins to dominate the clinical picture, and insomnia worsens. Nishino, Mignot, and Dement (1995) observe that short-acting BZs were initially preferred for elderly patients. They remark, "However, it has since been found that short-acting benzodiazepines induce rebound insomnia (a worsening of sleep beyond baseline levels on discontinuation of a hypnotic), rebound anxiety, anterograde amnesia, and even paradoxical rage."

In general, the usefulness of BZs in insomnia is temporary at best. They do not provide for normal sleep, but rather for a disruption in various aspects of the normal cycle.

The Probability of Permanent Brain Damage

There have been relatively few studies on the persistence of cognitive deficits following termination of BZ treatment. Despite the analogy with alcohol-induced cognitive dysfunction and dementia, most review articles and book chapters do not raise the issue. As I have previously noted (1991a), patients on high doses of BZs develop chronic cognitive impairments (Golombok et al., 1988; Lucki, Rickels, & Geller, 1986). There is little literature concerning these effects.

At least two reports indicate brain atrophy in association with long-term BZ use (Lader & Petursson, 1984; Schmauss & Krieg, 1987). There seem to be no follow-up studies concerning these critical questions.

Ashton (1995) is among the few reviewers to show concern about the possibility of BZ-induced persistent cognitive deficits or brain damage. She notes the lack of studies and comments, "It remains possible that subtle, perhaps reversible, structural changes may underlie the neuropsychological impairments shown in long-term benzodiazepine users."

Dependence and Withdrawal

Alcohol-like withdrawal symptoms from the long-term use of excessively high doses of BZs are well established. Withdrawal can take 2 to 20 days to develop after abrupt termination of the drug, depending on the duration of activity of the particular BZ. The first signs may be insomnia, irritability, and nervousness. A subsequent stage can include abdominal cramps, muscle cramps, nausea or vomiting, trembling, sweats, hyperarousal and hypersensitivity to environmental stimuli, confusion, depersonalization, loss of impulse control, anxiety and obsessional states, psychosis and organic brain syndrome, and seizures. Occasional case reports suggest that even slow withdrawal may not obviate serious withdrawal symptoms. It is unclear if gradual withdrawal merely extends the process over time rather than avoiding it (Noyes, 1992). Many symptoms can take weeks or months to fully subside, leaving the patient with prolonged anxiety or depression (Ashton, 1995). I have seen patients who felt they had not regained their predrug condition many months or years later.

Kales et al. (1991), in a placebo-controlled sleep lab study, showed that even under "brief, intermittent administration and withdrawal" of triazolam (and, to a lesser extent, temazepam), patients experienced rebound insomnia, "thereby predisposing to drug-taking behavior and increasing the potential for drug dependence."

There are estimates that 50% or more of patients taking BZs in therapeutic doses over a year will become physically dependent, developing withdrawal symptoms on abrupt cessation (Ashton, 1995; Noyes, 1992). Among the BZs used primarily for the treatment of anxiety or panic, alprazolam seems to have an especially bad record. In the field of drug addiction, Xanax is the most frequently implicated psychiatric drug (Breggin, 1991a). Often it occurs in cross-addiction with alcohol and other sedatives. Withdrawal problems and rebound increases in anxiety and panic were so extreme in key studies used for FDA approval of Xanax for panic disorder that many or most patients had more frequent or severe symptoms at the end of the studies than before they took the drug (reviewed in Breggin, 1991a).

Some patients can find it difficult to withdraw from as little as 0.5 mg clonazepam each night for sleep. Even motivated patients have sometimes developed such a fear of trying to go to sleep without BZs that they cannot undertake a serious effort. The fear is in part psychological. But it is also based on the frightening experience of rebound insomnia.

Physicians erroneously prescribe BZs in ever-increasing doses, mistakenly thinking that their patient's anxiety was spontaneously increasing rather than rebounding from the drug. Even if the ultimate dose remains within the recommended range, patients can "roller-coaster" with anxiety or other mental aberrations through each day between doses. The patients' lives can become devoted to "finding the right drug" and "taking it at the right time."

It requires a physician's patience and understanding, and often a period of many months, in order to wean some individuals from the BZs. At the end of the weaning, patients may discover that nearly all of their symptoms were drug induced. The general principles of drug withdrawal in outpatient practice are discussed in greater detail in *Talking Back to Prozac* (Breggin & Breggin, 1994a). Patients taking large doses of BZs need detoxification in a hospital setting.

Patients who have not been properly monitored by physicians may end up taking large doses of BZs for prolonged periods of times. Their daily lives may cycle from periods of excessive sedation when they appear ''drunk'' to periods of hyperarousal and anxiety as they undergo partial withdrawal. Friends and family may attribute their symptoms to ''mental illness'' until, for example, the patient begins to stumble about in a drunken manner or collapses in a stupor after one alcoholic drink during a holiday dinner. In retrospect, it will be apparent that the patient was, for months, too intoxicated to properly evaluate his or her own condition or to exercise judgment in regard to the drug effects. Often the patient's memory for the period of time will be severely impaired. Sometimes he or she will have committed irresponsible and even illegal acts.

SUMMARY

The benzodiazepines are frankly brain-disabling drugs. Much like alcohol, their clinical effect is no different from their toxic effect—a continuum of suppression of neuronal function, leading eventually to sleep or coma. Benzodiazepines can produce a wide variety of abnormal mental responses and very hazardous behavioral abnormalities: rebound anxiety, insomnia, psychosis, paranoia, violence, antisocial acts, depression, and suicide. They impair cognition, especially memory, and can cause confusion. They probably can cause brain atrophy. They are habit forming and addictive, and when taken in large doses for a period of time, severe withdrawal syndromes can develop on termination of the drug. Mixed with alcohol and other sedatives, their hazards multiply, and unintentional fatalities are possible. Successful suicides involving BZs, especially those drugs prescribed as sleeping medications—Halcion, Dalmane, and Restoril—are much more frequent than commonly realized by physicians.

Halcion and Xanax so commonly produce a variety of potentially disastrous adverse reactions that they should not be prescribed by physicians. If a physician or patient decides to use another of the BZs, the drug should be prescribed in the smallest possible dose for the shortest possible time, usually no more than a week at a time. The physician, the patient, and the family or close friends should be alert for possible adverse drug reactions.

CHAPTER 11

Drug Companies and the Food and Drug Administration: Failed Mandates

By now the reader may be asking, "How does the FDA allow such dangerous and often ineffective psychiatric drugs to reach the market?" In fact the FDA has been subject to considerable criticism and scrutiny over the years from the U.S. Congress and the media (summarized in Shulman, Hewitt, & Manocchia, 1995), including allegations that the FDA is becoming more protective of drug companies in recent years (Skrzychi, 1996).

Much of the tightening of FDA regulations over the years has resulted from disasters and tragedies. For example, in 1937, over one hundred people, mostly children, died due to poisoning with an organic solvent used in the liquid form of the antibiotic sulfanilamide. In the following year, Congress passed the federal Food, Drug, and Cosmetic Act. The early legislation made requirements for safety but not for efficacy.

In the early 1960s, thalidomide, a sleeping medication with no special advantages in regard to efficacy, caused an epidemic of birth defects. In 1962, the Kefauver-Harris amendment strengthened the FDA drug approval process to include controlled trials to demonstrate clinical efficacy. The amendment also required manufacturers to submit proof of efficacy for all drugs marketed between 1938 and 1962. In *The Therapeutic Nightmare*, Mintz (1965) provides a critical analysis of FDA functioning up to this period of time.

Gaining Approval To Market the Drug

The FDA has evolved a complex plan for each drug application, beginning with animal experimentation and proceeding through four "phases" of human experimentation (Food & Drug Administration, 1977; Jorgensen & Harris, 1992). Phase 1 and Phase 2 involve experimentation with animals and human volunteers, and early clinical testing to determine if more expansive trials are warranted or safe.

In Phase 3, controlled clinical trials are used to compare the drug to placebo and to previously approved, similar medications. At least two of the controlled studies must show a statistically significant positive effect from the drug. Four thousand or more patients may be involved in the total database developed during the psychiatric drug approval process, but this number is misleading. It includes almost everyone who has taken even one dose of the drug. Only a few hundred patients may be involved in the Phase 3 controlled clinical trails that the FDA finds adequate for evaluating efficacy and many of these subjects have usually dropped out before completion of the trials (Breggin & Breggin, 1994a).

The entire drug development process in the past could easily take 10 to 12 years, giving the public and the profession the misleading impression that the actual clinical studies were themselves very lengthy. Most of these years were spent completing various FDA requirements that did not directly pertain to clinical studies. Several years were often spent by the FDA itself in evaluating the company's New Drug Application (NDA),[1] a process the FDA is now speeding up (see DiMasi, Seibring, & Lasagna, 1994). But the actual clinical trials for psychiatric drugs usually last a mere 4–6 weeks.

Demonstrating Efficacy before the Drug Is Marketed

All of the studies involved in the FDA approval process are designed completely by the drug companies and conducted by physicians hired and paid for by them. Would physicians be rehired if they regularly failed to churn out positive results? In complex studies involving human beings, statistics can of course be endlessly massaged until a seemingly significant result is generated. To prove a drug is an effective antidepressant, for

---

[1]The NDA is conducted under the Code of Federal Regulations, Title 21, Part 314.

example, the company needs only to develop two positive studies, even if innumerable others are entirely negative. This is not consistent with the canons of statistical analysis.

The main concern of this book is safety rather than efficacy, but the flaws in these trials (see below) will obviously affect both.

Creating the Label for the Drug

The FDA approval process is about creating and obtaining a label for the marketing of the drug. The approval of the label by the FDA is the final step in the process before the drug goes to market.

Before approval of the label, the FDA negotiates with the pharmaceutical company concerning its contents. After approval, the label appears in package inserts. It is published by the drug companies in the *Physicians' Desk Reference* (*PDR*), a commercial book sent free to all practicing physicians and found in most treatment facilities. A shortened form of the label with emphasis on adverse effects must be included in advertising and promotional materials.

The FDA-approved drug label is very important, especially in regard to defining dangerous side effects. Physicians often use the *PDR* to alert themselves to the dangers of drugs. Too often, it's the first place physicians look when they have a question about a drug. Reviews in the literature are frequently based on it as well.

Phase 4, spanning the period after the drug has been approved and entered the market, focuses on monitoring for newly discovered drug hazards. In my interviews with FDA officials in recent years, they agreed that this crucial process tends to be given relatively low priority compared to the approval process. They attribute this to congressional and consumer priorities (also see Government Accounting Office, 1990).

Monitoring after Drug Approval

After the drug has been marketed, the FDA remains responsible for reacting to new information. It can remove a drug from the market if it proves too hazardous. It can also require a drug manufacturer to add newly recognized adverse drug reactions to a label or to strengthen the information concerning known adverse reactions.

After initial approval of the drug, the FDA does not routinely require the companies to conduct any further tests for safety; and the companies almost never choose to do so on their own. Even when companies are pressed to conduct postmarketing studies, I have seen them procrastinate and protest until the FDA has dropped its demand. When reports begin to suggest dangerous outcomes, the companies almost never sponsor research to confirm the possibility.

The American Medical Association (AMA) lobbied Congress to make sure that after a drug is approved, physicians are not legally bound to follow the FDA guidelines. In the case of Prozac, for example, physicians quickly began giving it to children, even though it is not approved for them. Doctors can legally prescribe the drug for problems that have nothing to do with depression; Prozac has been prescribed for children who fight with their parents, skip school, or run away from home.

Continuing Drug Company Responsibilities

After the FDA approves a drug, the companies have continuing responsibility to inform the FDA about adverse drug reactions discovered after marketing of the drug. The drug companies are also required to monitor the literature concerning their medications and to report adverse drug reactions found in that source as well.

In some product liability cases in which I have been a medical expert for the plaintiff, there has been a tendency for drug companies to claim that the FDA holds ultimate responsibility for the information that the company places in its label and, in particular, that the drug company cannot make changes in a drug's label without prior FDA approval. This is not true. Every pharmaceutical company is empowered by law to make changes in its drug labels without prior FDA approval provided that the changes will "add or strengthen a contraindication, warning, precaution, or adverse reaction" or "add or strengthen a statement about drug abuse, dependence, or overdosage." The company can also "delete false, misleading, or unsupported indications for use or claims for effectiveness" without prior FDA approval (*Code of Federal Regulations*, 1995, 314.70c, p. 124). Thus, each drug company retains responsibility for making sure that its drug labels are as current and accurate as possible concerning risks and hazards, even to taking unilateral action to upgrade safety aspects of its labels without prior FDA approval.

Testing Safety before the Drug Is Marketed

Too much faith can be placed in premarketing clinical trials as a method of detecting adverse drug reactions. For example, it can be mistakenly assumed that controlled clinical trials are the paradigm of scientific investigation. In my forensic experience, drug companies have defended themselves in product liability cases by arguing that only a controlled clinical trial can prove the existence of an adverse drug reaction. This is a mistaken interpretation of the nature of science and scientific conclusions. (For an extensive review of drug product liability issues, including FDA–manufacturer relationships and responsibilities, see Dixon, 1995.)

In reality, proving safety in clinical trials for FDA approval is an even more flawed process than proving efficacy. Often serious and even fatal reactions will not be detected in the controlled studies and other clinical trials used for drug approval.

The FDA (1995) itself has become increasingly vocal about the flaws in premarketing testing and in the importance of the postmarketing spontaneous reporting system. The agency has recently stepped up its efforts to inform physicians and other members of the health community that drug approval by no means guarantees that all serious side effects have been detected. The FDA has distributed a dramatic white on black poster with the following point emblazoned on it:

> When a drug goes to market, we
> know everything about its safety.
> Wrong.

The FDA's June, 1995, publication, "A MEDWatch Continuing Education Article," replicates the poster, and makes the following points in a section subtitled "Limitations of Premarketing Clinical Trials":

Short duration—effects that develop with chronic use or those that have a long latency period are impossible to detect

Narrow population—generally don't include special groups, (e.g., children, elderly), to a large degree and are not always representative of the population that may be exposed to the drug after approval

Narrow set of indications—those for which efficacy is being studied and don't cover actual evolving use

Small size (generally include 3,000 to 4,000 subjects)—effects that occur rarely are very difficult to detect.

The FDA (1995) makes the following point concerning the probability of detecting an adverse reaction:

> **Clinical trials are effective tools primarily designed for assessing efficacy and risk-benefit ratio, but in most cases they are neither large enough nor long enough to provide all information on a drug's safety.** At the time of approval for marketing, the safety database for a new drug will often include 3,000 to 4,000 exposed individuals, an insufficient number to detect rare adverse events. For example, in order to have a 95% chance of detecting an adverse event with an incidence of 1 per 10,000 patients, an exposed population of 30,000 patients would be required.

The director of the FDA's new MEDWatch program, Dianne Kennedy, wrote:

> The safety profile of a drug continually evolves over time. Clinical trials that precede product approval typically include safety data on only a few thousand patients. New information is expected to be discovered as a drug is used in larger and larger populations, in subgroups not studied during the clinical trials (e.g., pregnant women, the elderly), or in patients with numerous medical conditions taking multiple other medications. (Kennedy & McGinnis, 1993)

Writing in the *Journal of the American Medical Association* on behalf of the FDA, Commissioner David Kessler (1993) declared:

> Even the large, well-designed clinical trials that are conducted to gain premarket approval cannot uncover every problem than can come to light once a product is widely used. . . . If an adverse event occurs in perhaps one in 5000 or even in 1000 users, it could be missed in clinical trials but pose a serious safety problem when released to the market.

Writing in *The Pharmacologic Basis of Therapeutics*, Alan Nies (1996) makes a similar point:

> Since only a few thousand patients are exposed to experimental drugs in more or less controlled and well-defined circumstances during drug development, adverse drug effects that occur as frequently as 1 in 1,000 may not be detected prior to marketing. Postmarketing surveillance of drug usage is thus imperative to detect infrequent but significant adverse effects. (p. 57)

To pursue Kessler and Nies's point, assume as a hypothetical example that Prozac causes suicide in 1 in 1,000 patients. If this were true, among the first 5 million patients to take the drug, 5,000 would die by suicide. Yet the problem could have gone wholly undetected in the trials. This, of course, gives even more weight to the actual finding of Prozac-induced suicidality in the controlled clinical trials (chapter 6).

Paul Leber (1992), director of the FDA's Division of Neuropharmacological Drug Products, has himself addressed the limitations of premarket testing and the importance of postmarketing surveillance. He points out that "even the best designed and well-executed premarketing evaluation programs may fail to detect risks that can have extremely serious consequences for the public health." Again using the illustration of a drug testing program involving 1,000 patients, he observes "There remains a 5% chance that the drug, upon marketing, might regularly cause serious, even fatal, injury to one in every 333 or so patients treated."

Thomas Laughren (1992), the group leader of the psychiatric drugs section in Leber's division, summarized the drug approval process—the New Drug Application (NDA). He reviewed the standards (Center for Drug Evaluation and Research, 1988) and limitations or problems inherent in using clinical trials to determine adverse drug effects (also see Castle, 1986; Leber, 1992; Peace, 1987).

After describing the small size and short duration of the premarketing clinical trials, Laughren (1992) concluded:

> It is important to acknowledge this limitation of the typical development programs and to recognize that careful postmarketing surveillance is the most feasible method for detecting the more infrequent adverse events occurring with the use of a new drug.

Because the trials err toward missing adverse reactions, Laughren suggested that the FDA should lean toward assuming a drug connection when adverse events occur in association with it.

Paul Leber (1992) also points out that the risks may be even greater than a statistical analysis indicates. Additional factors include:

1. The patients and volunteers in the study are not likely to represent a true sample of the people who will be treated once the drug is marketed.
2. The studies are quite brief.
3. There may be differences in postmarketing dosing.

4. The "unique combination of concomitant illness, polypharmacy, and compromised physiological status" of real-life patients treated after the drug is approved cannot be anticipated.

In regard to the final point, Leber states:

> In any event, whatever the reasons, it is likely that Phase III testing ordinarily fails to reproduce the conditions of illness and polypharmacy that occur in actual clinical practice with market drugs, and this may generate a misleadingly reassuring picture of a drug's safety in use.

Leber concludes, "In sum, at the time a new drug is first marketed, a great deal of uncertainty invariably remains about the identity, nature, and frequency of all but the most common and acutely expressed risks associated with its use."

Karl E. Peace (1987), Director, Research Statistics, SmithKline and French Laboratories, points out that "it is frequently impossible to design trials to provide definitive information about safety—particularly about adverse events." He describes occasions when it has been possible to design adequate safety studies, but concludes, "However, for most new drugs in clinical development it is not possible."

More Subtle Difficulties in Evaluating Clinical Trial Data

There are other difficulties that further compromise the clinical trials used for FDA approval. While several thousands of drug patients may be involved in the overall studies—what FDA calls the database—the individual trials may be relatively small. One principal investigator, for example, may supervise a project involving only a few dozen patients. He then sends in a report to the drug company which takes on the ultimate task of looking over the entire database in search of patterns of adverse drug reactions.

If an unexpected adverse reaction were to appear in one of the smaller projects, its significance might easily be missed by the local clinical investigator. He might not even bother to report it. For example, worsening of depression might easily be attributed to the patient's illness rather than to the antidepressant drug, and go unreported as an adverse drug reaction. A seemingly bizarre abnormal movement may be attributed to the patient's schizophrenia rather than to a drug-induced neurological disorder, and again go unreported.

Individual projects and investigators will also vary in their approach to evaluating adverse reactions. The ultimate database is not drawn from one consistent source, but from the variable efforts of different investigators often operating under somewhat different experimental protocols and with markedly different subjective perceptions.[2]

Leber (1992) addresses some of these issues when he states:

> Finally, of course, clinical testing during premarket development may fail to detect drug associated risks for any number of commonplace reasons: poor or careless technique, uncooperative patients, incompetent professional staff, clerical mistakes, etc. Indeed, even in closely monitored inpatient environments, it would be naive to believe that every adverse event that occurs is observed. Further, even if an untoward clinical event is observed, there is no certainty that it will be recognized as drug related, or if it is, that it will be subsequently recorded and/or reported.

Even in the smaller clinical trials, the patients are not taking the drug at the same time, making it more difficult for the investigators to have an overview of what's going on. Patients are included in the trial as they become available over a period of weeks or months. Some are starting the trial long after others have finished it. The principal investigator and associates are therefore not able to survey the group altogether or all at once, but must rely on memory and on records in order to discern patterns of adverse drug reactions. They must do this over an extended period of time while preoccupied with many other unrelated professional activities.

Especially for individuals who have not been exposed to scientific research, the phrase "controlled trials" is likely to conjure up something much more rigorous than individual patients signing up at various times in a doctor's office or in a clinic for an opportunity to participate in a project. These research subjects are not sequestered on a hospital ward. They return home to their everyday lives, including whatever undisclosed psychological or physical problems they may harbor, and including any legal or illegal drugs which they may take without informing the investigator.

---

[2]A protocol is a series of clinical trials conducted under the same rules. One protocol—that is, one model for conducting studies—may be used at several centers during the drug approval process. Numerous different protocols are utilized in the overall NDA.

Clinical experience and various studies have shown that patient compliance is spotty in regard to taking drugs at home. Rarely can the investigator be sure that the patient is taking the drug in question at all, let alone in the prescribed fashion. Efforts are seldom made to detect the drug in the subject's blood or urine.

The pool of individuals who sign up for drug testing has not been given adequate consideration in evaluating the usefulness of clinical trials. Often the subjects are obtained from newspaper advertisements that invite members of the public to sign up for a clinical trial for a new drug for anxiety, depression, phobia, or some other named disorder. Sometimes flyers for the trial are distributed at meetings or conferences of patients who suffer chronically from these disorders. The individuals to whom these promotions will appeal may be desperate for money, desperate for therapeutic relief, or both. Why else would they go into an unfamiliar setting in order to risk taking an experimental drug whose safety and efficacy have not been demonstrated? Their need to be in the experiment may influence what these subjects tell the investigators about their past histories, as well as their responses to the drugs. Their hope for a cure or their desire to please the doctors may influence their own perceptions and communications (see ahead for recent pertinent disclosures).

The placebo control does not ensure that either patients or doctors will remain blind to what the patients are getting. A drug like Prozac, for example, has such specific stimulating side effects that it is easy to determine which patient is taking it rather than taking a more sedative tricyclic antidepressant or an inert placebo. Fisher and Greenberg (1989) have made the point that there are very few truly blind studies, even when controls are carefully implemented. The failure to keep the study blind may easily play into the patient's or the investigator's need to make a positive evaluation of the drug in regard to both safety and efficacy.

Since the individual drug trials are too small, too short, and otherwise inadequate to the task, it remains the ultimate responsibility of the drug company to go through the complete database in search of patterns of adverse drug reactions. Even if drug companies were properly motivated, there is no foolproof way to oversee the entire group of several thousand patients.

Controlled clinical trials are not inevitably scientific. They may meet the canons of science or they may not, depending on their structure and on how they are carried out. But even if they are performed to a high standard, they do not by themselves prove anything. Their data must be scientifically interpreted—that is, subjected to reasoned analysis.

As the FDA has made clear, a reasoned analysis discloses that the controlled clinical trials used in the FDA process have grave limitations in regard to the detection of adverse drug effects. The FDA came to this conclusion without discussing some of the more subtle issues I have raised in this chapter.

Other Neglected Areas in the FDA Approval Process

There are some obvious oversights in the FDA requirements imposed on drug companies, including some specific areas that are wholly neglected.

First, the FDA does not require drug manufacturers to demonstrate through animal (or human) research that the brain recovers from any of the various biochemical imbalances and other malfunctions produced by every psychiatric medication. Information is frequently provided to the FDA concerning the impact of the drug on neurotransmitters and other brain functions in animals, while no information is provided concerning the potential for recovery. All of the neuroleptics and antidepressants, as well as lithium, produce profound changes in brain function during treatment; but to this day, there has been little research on the recovery of these functions (see chapter 6 in regard to Prozac; also Breggin & Breggin, 1994a).

Second, the FDA does not require intensive neuropsychological testing of human subjects to document cognitive impairment or other brain dysfunction associated with drug treatment. There is no follow-up to determine if cognitive and other functions return to normal after termination of drug treatment. For example, it took independent postmarketing studies to show that antidepressants (chapter 6) and lithium (chapter 7) can impair cognition.

Third, the FDA does not require the drug company to show that any patients actually recover from their psychiatric disorders as a result of drug treatment. Instead, all measures aim at demonstrating relative degrees of improvement in comparison to placebo or other medications. To get into an antidepressant study, subjects typically must be shown to suffer from major depression, and to get into a neuroleptic study, they must be shown to suffer from schizophrenia. However, they are not usually evaluated at the end of the study to determine whether or not they have partially, largely, or fully recovered from depression or schizophrenia. Instead, improvement on a few items on a symptom check list is usually sufficient to determine a positive outcome. Thus the drug companies avoid asking potentially embarrassing questions about actual recovery.

Fourth, for a drug to be approved, there is no requirement that the patients rate themselves improved as a result of it. Checklist ratings by outside observers are sufficient evidence for FDA approval, even if the patients rate themselves no more improved on the drug than on placebo.

Fifth, where there are known and even extreme risks in association with a particular class of drugs, the FDA does not require that the drug company specifically determine the new drug's risk in regard to these known dangers. For example, neuroleptics cause tardive dyskinesia (TD) and neuroleptic malignant syndrome (NMS). Yet during the approval process of new neuroleptics, the companies are not required to demonstrate the specific risk that the new drug poses in regard to TD or NMS. A class warning may be required, for example, for TD or NMS; but there will be no requirement to test for the possibility of an increased risk with the new agent.

Finally, the FDA does not conduct any drug studies on its own. It relies entirely on research produced, monitored, and financed by the pharmaceutical companies. In *Talking Back to Prozac* (Breggin & Breggin, 1994a), we have documented the far-reaching negative consequences of the FDA's dependency on data generated by drug companies.

THE PROFIT MOTIVE

While the FDA has procedures for monitoring the drug companies during their application for new drug approval, the validity of the process nonetheless rests on the ethical and scientific integrity of the corporations. Drug companies have a strong financial incentive not to focus their attention on discovering or reporting adverse drug reactions that might threaten the approval of their product or cause future legal liability. They often fight hard against the passage of tougher FDA regulations and sometimes try to evade them after they are put into effect.

In reading drug company in-house communications and depositions, it is apparent that the overriding concern is to market a drug that makes a profit. When an adverse drug reaction becomes a public scandal, for example, the tendency is to campaign against the "bad image," instead of evaluating the actual danger. A researcher, marketing representative, publicist, attorney, or CEO does not overnight become devoted to the public good simply because he or she takes a job with a drug company. Some product liability attorneys have told me, to the contrary, that the pharmaceutical industry seems especially self-protective.

For example, in reviewing an NDA for a product liability suit against a drug manufacturer, I discovered that a company official had written a memo recommending a comparative study between the company's drug and an older one. In the hope that his company's drug was safer, he wanted to compare the frequency with which the two drugs caused the same serious side effect. Penciled into one corner of his memo was a note from another company executive stating that it was a bad idea to ask questions whose answers might prove embarrassing. The study was never done.

Bias may affect a drug company's overall analysis of the patterns of adverse reports from the clinical trials. In my forensic experience, the methodology of the analyses may deviate drastically from the scientific process. In addition, if the conclusions seem to threaten the future of the drug, the conclusions may be modified or kept secret (see chapter 6).

Monitoring Safety after the Drug Is Marketed

By 1969, the Food and Drug Administration developed a systematic approach to collecting and maintaining adverse drug reactions after marketing. For many years, it was called the "spontaneous reporting system." The regulations were updated in 1985 and the system has been recently renamed MEDWatch (for the basic regulations, see Johnson & Barash, 1991; for critiques see the various citations below). Anyone, including patients, can initiate an adverse report by writing to the drug company or the FDA. The vast majority come from physicians and from hospital pharmacists.

Unlike England, in America there is no formal requirement or readily available mechanism for health professionals to make these postmarketing reports. Goodman and Gilman's *The Pharmacological Basis of Therapeutics* (Nies, 1991) estimates that over 40% of doctors don't know they can report adverse effects directly to the FDA.

In addition to the larger numbers of patients involved and the longer treatment periods, the postmarketing spontaneous reporting system has a number of advantages over the premarketing clinical trials.

First of all, most of the pharmacists and physicians making the reports from the field, unlike those conducting the clinical trials, are not being directly paid by the drug companies. They are likely to have much less vested interest in retaining the drug company's goodwill.

Second, the largest portion of those who send in spontaneous reports are hospital pharmacists. They are working in institutional settings where they can overview hundreds of patient experiences with the drug. They are in an especially good position to spot something requiring scrutiny.

Third, spontaneous reports are sent in by professionals who are evaluating the drug under more "natural" field conditions. Many of the patients are receiving other drugs, suffering from physical illnesses, or taking large, and sometimes excessive, dosages of the drug. Adverse drug reactions are more likely to show up under these conditions. For example, adverse drug reactions typically occur more frequently at doses in excess of those used in the clinical trials. Reactions to excessive dosages can provide a signal that these reactions are in all probability occurring at more standard doses as well, although less frequently or less intensively. Age and infirmity, usually untested factors in clinical trials, are likely to be encountered in general practice, and can be bellwethers. Tricyclic antidepressants, for example, will cause life-threatening cardiovascular problems much more frequently in the elderly; but they cause similar if less frequent or intense reactions among healthy young people as well. Similarly, neuroleptics cause tardive dyskinesia much more frequently among the elderly, but the rate is still high among younger patients as well. Because the spontaneous reporting system includes a larger variety of patients taking a broader spectrum of doses, it is much more likely to disclose adverse reactions than a controlled clinical trial for the NDA.

Fourth, the professionals making the reports have been alerted through their own experience and through reports in the literature concerning initially unexpected adverse reactions. They have the benefit of increased clinical awareness, as well as hindsight, in identifying adverse drug reactions.

The Impact of the Spontaneous Reporting System

In describing the impact of the spontaneous reporting system, the FDA's Kessler (1993) said:

> In response to voluntary reports from physicians to the FDA or the manufacturer, the FDA has issued warnings, made label changes, required manufac-

turers to conduct postmarketing studies, and ordered product withdrawals that have ultimately prevented patient deaths and suffering.

The 1995 FDA MEDWatch publication makes clear that the spontaneous reporting system is the most important source of postmarketing information on adverse drug reactions. It frequently leads to scientific determinations for the need to modify drug labels or to withdraw drugs from the market. According to a 1990 Government Accounting Office (GAO) report, more than 50% of all drugs approved by the FDA between 1976 and 1985 were found during postmarketing to have previously undetected "serious" side effects, sometimes requiring removal from the market. Fifteen psychopharmaceuticals were approved during this period, nine of which turned out to have serious risks during postmarketing, leading in one case to removal from the market (GAO, 1990, pp. 25, 74–78). Since then, yet another drug from that era has been withdrawn from the market. The antidepressant nomifensine was found to cause massive intravascular hemolytic anemia—but only after it had been on the market worldwide for 8 or 9 years (Leber, 1992, p. 6).

I have reviewed the entire list of serious adverse reactions to psychiatric drugs detected during the postmarketing period in the GAO study. It seems probable that every one of them was discovered and confirmed through a combination of the spontaneous reporting system and general clinical experience. As far as I can ascertain, not one of these adverse reactions was primarily, if at all, identified by means of a controlled clinical trial. As a result of postmarket discoveries, alprazolam (Xanax) had rage added to the label as a paradoxical reaction and amoxapine (Asendin) had neuroleptic malignant syndrome added.

Drawing Scientific Conclusions from the Spontaneous Reporting System

There are a number of approaches that can be used to confirm from spontaneous reports that a drug is actually causing the adverse reaction. Chapter 10 described how several FDA officials went about confirming for themselves a possible or probable causal relationship between Halcion (and Xanax) and various behavioral abnormalities, including violence. To confirm causality, some of the following factors are useful:

1. a disproportionately high frequency of reporting or disproportionately large number of reports in comparison to other drugs, especially in the same or similar class of medications
2. a meaningful or strong enough association as reflected in epidemiological and clinical data
3. an absence of alternative explanations for the increased frequency or number of reports
4. reports indicating a temporal relationship between the adverse reactions and initial doses of the drug or increased doses of the drug
5. reports of dose-dependent reactions, that is, increased frequency or numbers of adverse reactions with higher dosages
6. reports of resolution of the adverse reaction following drug withdrawal
7. reports of positive rechallenges—the adverse reaction is provoked once again by resuming the drug
8. reports of adverse reactions in individuals with no predrug history of similar symptoms
9. corroborating clinical experience (published and unpublished)
10. data from clinical trials, including controlled trials
11. a rational medical and/or neurochemical explanation for a causal connection between the drug and the adverse reaction, and the corresponding absence of a better explanation

The Federal Judicial Center (Bailey, Gordis, & Green, 1994) has proposed a series of criteria that compact many of the points I have made. The difference in approach is in part due to their epidemiological emphasis in contrast to my clinical emphasis. Drawing on Koch's postulates, they state that "seven factors should be considered when an epidemiologist determines whether the association between an agent and a disease is causal." Put in the form of questions, they list the following factors:

1. How strong is the association between the exposure and the disease?
2. Is there a temporal relationship?
3. Is the association consistent with other research?
4. Is the association biologically plausible?
5. Have alternative explanations been ruled out?
6. Does the association exhibit specificity?
7. Is there a dose-response relationship?
   (pp. 161–164)

None of the above individual criteria is an absolute requirement for coming to a scientific conclusion. One must weigh the best available evidence and come to as sound a conclusion as possible. Commonly or even typically, decisions with a high degree of probability will be made with an incomplete set of data.

While it would be helpful to have confirmation from controlled clinical trials, it is typically impossible to obtain it, even in regard to known or proven adverse drug reactions. As we have already seen, negative findings from controlled clinical trials involving a drug cannot be used to rule out a causal connection between a drug and an adverse reaction. To illustrate this, we turn in the next section to the stories of neuroleptic malignant syndrome and tardive dyskinesia.

FOUR APPROVAL SYSTEM FAILURES

Failure to Recognize Neuroleptic Malignant Syndrome

Neuroleptic malignant syndrome (NMS) (see chapter 4) provides an example of how a devastating, common disorder can be wholly missed in the clinical trials during the approval process. It also illustrates how long it can take drug companies and the FDA to give formal recognition to such a disorder.

Neuroleptic malignant syndrome is a potentially fatal reaction to neuroleptic drugs. It occurs at a relatively high rate, developing in somewhere from 1.4% to 2.4% of patients exposed to neuroleptics (chapter 4). A reaction that occurs 1/100 times is considered common or frequent by FDA standards. This particular reaction is extremely dramatic and therefore not easily overlooked. Yet NMS was entirely missed in one study after another conducted by drug companies when applying for FDA approval of neuroleptic drugs.

The failure to detect NMS in clinical trials cannot be attributed to the need for longer studies, since an estimated 80% of NMS reactions develop within the first few weeks of treatment (Davis, Janicak, & Khan, 1991). Nor can the failure be forgiven on the basis of inadequate knowledge about the disorder. Suggestions of its existence began soon after the neuroleptic drugs went into use and it was clearly identified in the English-language literature by 1968 (chapter 4).

In 1986, nearly two decades after NMS had become an identifiable syndrome, the FDA at last began to force the drug companies to add the adverse drug reaction to their neuroleptic labels. Since the disease is fatal in approximately 20% of cases when it goes unrecognized and untreated, the failure to properly inform physicians probably cost many lives and untold suffering.

There are important lessons from the history of NMS. First, for many years neither the FDA nor the drug companies came close to fulfilling their ethical and legal obligations by warning physicians and by adding the disorder to the neuroleptic label. The drug companies did almost nothing until forced to act by the FDA. Both the FDA and the drug companies were much too late, causing unnecessary death and suffering. Second, the history confirms that clinical trials cannot be relied upon by themselves to identify even common, obvious hazards, such as NMS.

The FDA Caves in to Industry on Tardive Dyskinesia

Tardive dyskinesia occurs with extreme frequency in neuroleptic-treated patients (chapter 4). In relatively young, physically healthy adults, 4%–7% per year will develop the disease. After a total of 5 years' exposure, approximately one-third will develop this largely irreversible, disfiguring, and potentially disabling movement disorder. In older patients, the rate may exceed an astronomical 20% per year. Patients taking the drug for a lifetime will approach a 100% risk. Why is there nothing in the current FDA-required warning label to alert a physician or patient about the extraordinarily high risk?

The neuroleptic drugs were in widespread use by 1954 and TD was documented within the first few years (chapter 4). Yet for nearly 20 additional years, the drug companies and the FDA failed to provide an appropriate warning in the label of neuroleptic drugs. In the early 1970s, the agency finally forced a very weak uniform label statement about TD on the drug companies. It gave no hint about the frequency of the disorder, mentioning only that "some patients" might get it.

As the tragic news about TD accumulated, the drug companies did little or nothing to update their labels. Then on February 24, 1984, Paul Leber called a meeting of the FDA's Psychopharmacologic Drugs Advisory Committee (FDA, 1984) to discuss the agency's proposal for an updated uniform class warning label for all neuroleptics.[3] Leber explained to the committee that public pressure about TD had been generated by a CBS-TV Dan Rather report. I had given CBS an advanced manuscript copy of my 1983 book on psychiatric drugs. It inspired the Dan Rather show and I consulted on planning the program.

In the 1984 meeting, Leber proposed a version of the label that included specific numerical estimates to underscore the very high rates. Seven expert drug consultants confirmed the need for mentioning actual numbers, and an eighth sent in a report taking the same viewpoint. Based on the 1980 APA task force report, some of the experts recommended citing a 20% risk in routine neuroleptic exposure. Others suggested a figure of 15% in the first 4 years. Leber himself observed that extrapolating from the data indicated that over a lifetime, "100% of patients may in fact develop the disorder" (1984, p. 54). These are most extraordinary estimates for the rate of contracting a drug-induced, irreversible, and potentially severe disorder.

Approximately 5 months after the meeting, in the summer of 1984, Leber sent a formal letter to all neuroleptic manufacturers, suggesting a revision of the proposed class warning label. By then, almost surely in response to industry pressure, the proposed language had already been watered down. Without mentioning any figures, Leber's proposed label stated that TD would develop in a "substantial portion of patients treated with neuroleptics" (Leber, 1984, p. 3). The meaning of "substantial" was left up to interpretation.

The FDA's Pharmacologic Drugs Advisory Committee met a second time on January 31, 1985, to discuss TD. Leber again mentioned the impact of the "clamor from the press" in the fall of 1983—the date of Dan Rather's TV report and the simultaneous publication of my book.

Leber told the assembled representatives of the drug companies that he would not act without their endorsement or approval. He stated he'd been through "a year and a half of trying to bring about change in the labeling of neuroleptic products that would be fair and that would be *acceptable to everyone . . .* " [italics added] (FDA, 1985).

Leber described to the meeting the elaborate back and forth negotiating that had already gone on between the FDA and industry. He said that one of his aims was to obtain "equitable labeling that *did not cause injury*

---

[3]This is probably the first time that the history of the FDA's handling of its proposed class warning label on TD has been told.

to industry, as much as it also should not cause injury to patients or physicians who have to use neuroleptics under trying circumstances'' (FDA, 1985, p. 9, italics added).

Can the FDA perform a watchdog function without biting industry? Without even growling at them? If the process of identifying dangerous drug effects were painless to industry (''should not cause injury to industry''), industry would not need the FDA to regulate it. A properly functioning FDA would at times have to ''cause injury to industry'' through diminished revenues and other sanctions related to marketing dangerous drugs. The neuroleptics were being prescribed with too little regard for their devastating adverse effects; if the new warning label had done its job, neuroleptic sales would of necessity have dropped. There's nothing in the FDA legislation that urges the agency to protect industry. It's supposed to protect patients, with sometimes painful results for industry.

By this second meeting, Leber and the FDA had surrendered to industry. The somewhat ominous phrase ''substantial proportion'' was replaced by the entirely innocuous phrase ''some patients,'' implying a minimal risk. Ironically, it was the same phrase that appeared on the outdated 1973 label. No change had been made.

Ultimately, ''some patients'' was also dropped. The warning in the current neuroleptic label states that TD ''may develop in patients'' treated with neuroleptics—not even a hint of a serious risk, let alone an astronomical one, with millions of victims. In the critical arena of TD rates, the class warning label is possibly weaker than the old one.

Partly due to the persistently inadequate label, too many ill-informed physicians and their patients continue to believe that the risk of TD is insignificant. Leber succeeded in causing little or no injury to industry— but at what cost to patients, their families, and the health care system?

The story of the FDA's handling of warning labels for NMS and TD leads to a dismal conclusion. When it comes to warning about the dangers of psychiatric drugs, the FDA is more responsive to the profit needs of industry than to the safety needs of patients.

Massaged Data: The Prozac Approval Process

In *Talking Back to Prozac*, I examined the overall FDA approval process in regard to Prozac. It reconfirmed that in regard to psychiatric drugs, the FDA is more concerned about industry goodwill than the public good. What follows is a small taste of what went wrong in the Prozac approval process.

While several thousand patients were involved in studies of various kinds, I counted only 286 who actually finished the three placebo-controlled protocols (groups of studies) used for approval. Many patients dropped out because of adverse stimulant reactions. Prozac seldom proved any better than placebo and was not as good as the older antidepressants. It was so stimulating that sedatives were often given along with it.

In perhaps the most important study, called Protocol 27, the results indicated that Prozac by itself had no efficacy. To get a positive result, the FDA had to allow the drug companies to include all the patients who, against the rules, were also given sedative and tranquilizing medications with their Prozac.

Protocol 27 was conducted by several separate investigators at sites in different cities. The individual study sites could not show that Prozac was any better than placebo; so the FDA allowed the negative results to be pooled and manipulated until a positive result was barely achieved.

The FDA's Laughren (1992), in a recent analysis of the NDA process, observed, "Pooling of effectiveness data from independent studies is not standard and must be done with great care." Protocol 27 was not only made up of independent studies conducted at separate centers, but almost all of them had negative results. Furthermore, in the pooling process, one center was dropped entirely, eliminating 25% of the original data.

Lilly employees Stark and Hardison (1985) eventually published Protocol 27 in the *Journal of Clinical Psychiatry*. They did so without mentioning (a) that four of the five individual centers produced negative results before the data were pruned and pooled, (b) that the pooled data were negative when Prozac patients taking sedatives and tranquilizers were excluded, (c) that the FDA had many criticisms of the study and its practices, or (d) that the success of the drug was marginal. The publication by Stark and Hardison claims that Prozac was "comparable to" Tofranil in efficacy—a myth that gained considerable currency in the profession—when in fact the older tricyclic outperformed Prozac most of the time.

Falling behind European Standards: Zoloft

The general perception in America is that the FDA is far more tough on drug companies than comparable European authorities. If that were ever true, it's not any more, at least in the arena of psychiatric drugs.

On December 10, 1991, Thomas Laughren, Group Leader for Psychiatric Drug Products, wrote a memo concerning Zoloft's upcoming approval. Laughren listed a series of concerns about the drug expressed by several European nations as well as by FDA advisors. These included "failure to provide data on depressed inpatients, severely depressed patients, 'major depression,' etc; failure to provide long term data, relapse efficacy, etc.; failure to provide comparative data, i.e., for alternative antidepressant agents." Despite these problems with Zoloft, he concluded, "the data were sufficiently persuasive to justify approval of this product."

Spurred on by Laughren's critique, an exchange of memos occurred between Paul Leber and his boss, Robert Temple, Director, Office of Drug Evaluation I. The continuing subject was the approval of Zoloft, whose efficacy as an antidepressant remained in doubt up to the last minute. Temple noted that Zoloft was not being approved in some European countries because of its "lack of robustness" in the efficacy trials. Zoloft often failed to do any better than placebo in studies in the United States and never did as well as the older antidepressant, amitriptyline. Despite the failures, one positive study and two supportive studies were found sufficient to earn approval.

On December 24—a mere 6 days before the official approval letter was written for Zoloft—Leber responded to Temple's concerns about approving the drug. About the tougher standards in the European countries, Leber wrote:

This turn of events may seem somewhat surprising in view of the fact that the agency is traditionally more conservative than its European counterparts. Obviously, changes are underway throughout western Europe, perhaps in response to EEC's [European Economic Community] harmonization initiatives. In any case, with the exception of the UK's [drug approval authority], standards for antidepressant drug product approval seem to be becoming more demanding in regard to 1) the duration of controlled trials serving as sources of evidence of efficacy, 2) the need to document efficacy in hospitalized depressed patients (because these are presumed, arguably, to be more severely depressed), 3) the need to show efficacy in maintaining remission, 4) the need to show efficacy in preventing relapse in euthymic [normal mood] patients with a history of recurrent episodes of affective illness, and 5) a need to establish equivalency and/or superiority of a new antidepressant to already marketed products.

Having outlined these standards, Leber acknowledged their merit, but stated they could not be implemented in America's current political climate:

Many of these foreign regulatory initiatives have potential merit, but, given the perceived urgency we express as an institution for expediting the public's access to new, potentially promising drugs, I do not believe we can successfully introduce similar, more demanding, requirements domestically, at least until there is a significant 'sea change' in our society's collective attitude toward Federal regulation of new drugs.

Leber believed that Zoloft, despite its relative ineffectiveness, had met the FDA's official requirements for approval. He then concluded his memo with the following warning:

Approval [of Zoloft] may, however, for the reasons enumerated above, come under attack by constituencies that do not believe the agency is as demanding as it ought to be in regard to its standard for establishing the efficacy of antidepressant drug products.

It is striking that these concerns and misgivings are being expressed less than a week before final approval of the drug. Temple did not respond for another week, until December 31, 1991—one day *after* the date on the final approval letter. He agreed that the drug should be approved but concluded, "I would, however, strongly encourage formal thinking, in which I would be pleased to participate, about whether we should modify the advice we give to companies to assure that they examine aspects of their drug's effectiveness that are not being well enough studied . . . "

A significant portion of the public believes that the FDA moves too slowly and places too many barriers in the way of new drug products. Despite all the bureaucratic time it wastes, in the arena of psychiatric drugs the FDA is nowhere near thorough enough. The approval of a psychiatric drug does not in reality demonstrate either its efficacy or safety. The postmarketing surveillance is equally flawed. Not only is the system too haphazard, the division responsible for psychiatric drugs often fails to make an appropriate response to the most extreme drug-induced reactions, such as neuroleptic malignant syndrome and tardive dyskinesia produced by drugs like Haldol and Prolixin, and destructive behavior caused by drugs like Prozac and Halcion.

Recently Breaking News

Three controversies involving Eli Lilly & Co., the maker of Prozac, have raised further questions concerning pharmaceutical industry adherence to ethical practices and FDA standards. In a developing story, the media and the FDA have begun investigating Eli Lilly's use of homeless alcoholics as "normal" experimental subjects in Phase 1 studies (Associated Press, 1996; Cohen, 1996). This is not an acceptable practice, according to the FDA. Because homeless, addicted people might feel compelled by the offer of large sums of money and a safe place to stay, they are not capable of freely consenting to experiments. The use of homeless, alcoholic people could also compromise the research results. Confused by their pre-existing drug problems, they might fail to detect adverse reactions to the experimental drug. They might also be unwilling to report adverse effects for fear of being dropped from the study and left penniless back on the streets.

A recent advertising campaign by Eli Lilly has raised the specter of unleashing more widespread adverse drug reactions on the public before these dangers can be detected or appreciated by doctors. Writing in the *Wall Street Journal*, physician Philip R. Alper (1996) asked, "Who to Trust: Drug Companies or Your Doctor?" Alper criticizes Eli Lilly's promotion of a new, expensive form of insulin, Humalog, directly to the public through two-page ads in *People* magazine. The aim of these "market blitzes," according to Alper, "is to create consumer demand even before the doctor would be willing to use the drug spontaneously. Call it an end-run around the doctor, arm-twisting, manipulation, or whatever. The result is the same." These promotional tactics, Alper warns, will cause patients to press doctors to prescribe new drugs before their safety has been sufficiently demonstrated.

Before drug companies advertised directly to the public, the introduction of drugs into the marketplace was more gradual and hence safer. Many prudent doctors would wait to observe the results with new drugs before prescribing them to their own patients. Serious or life-threatening adverse effects might be detected before the drug was widely prescribed.

Alper (1996) expresses concern that Humalog and other drugs could meet the same fate as Lilly's earlier medication, Oraflex, which, he says, was among the first to be promoted directly to the public. It caused fatalities and was taken off the market in 1982. Lilly pleaded guilty to criminal charges in regard to Oraflex (Food and Drug Administration Quarterly Activities Report, 1985; Shenon, 1985). Alper laments bygone days when Eli Lilly was a "bastion of the ethical drug industry." He attributes the problem to a general decay within the pharmaceutical industry.

In a third controversy, National Institute of Health (NIH) researchers were conducting Phase 1 studies for a new Eli Lilly investigational drug, called FIAU (fialuridine), as a treatment for liver disease (Newsday, 1994). The FDA accused Lilly of "serious violations" by failing to inform volunteers of all the risks and by failing to report severe drug reactions, including fatalities, until months and even a year afterward (Associated Press, 1994). An NIH panel attempted to defend the institute from FDA accusations (Altman, 1994; Schwartz, 1994a; Thompson, 1994). The FDA (Food and Drug Administration, 1994; Schwartz, 1994b) issued new proposed regulations which cite the failures of Lilly in regard to its FIAU research.

BETTER THAN NOTHING?

Goodman and Gilman's textbook of pharmacology (Nies, 1996, p. 57) warns that patients are unaware that FDA approval does not protect them from "even relatively common risks of new drugs." In this way, the FDA misleads the public, lulling them into an unrealistic sense of safety. The watchdog role of the Division of Psychopharmacologic Drug Products in particular is so diluted by its friendly relationship with industry that it may be doing more harm than good by lulling the mental health profession and the consumer into a false sense of security in regard to the safety and efficacy of psychiatric drugs.

The problem in regard to psychiatric drugs is compounded by the ideology of biological psychiatry. Approving a drug for the treatment of a proven physical disease, such as pneumonia or diabetes, is very different from approving the use of specific drugs for expressions of human suffering that are psychological and social in origin. By giving its official imprimatur to the use of drugs for the control of "mental illness" or "mental disorders," the FDA takes sides in the conflict between biological and psychosocial psychiatry. It gives official government support to biopsychiatry and to brain-disabling therapies.

What's needed? To begin with, mental health professionals, physicians, and the public must become more skeptical, perhaps even cynical, and certainly more sophisticated about what psychiatric drugs and electroshock really do to the mind and brain. Awareness of the brain-disabling principles of psychiatric treatment is key to this understanding. Psychiatric drugs do not cure mental disorders. Instead, their primary or essential effect is to cause brain dysfunction and to compromise mental and emotional acuity.

Drug companies, the Food and Drug Administration, organized psychiatry, and other interest groups try to promote biopsychiatric interventions as grounded in good science. Instead, their widespread use defies both science and common sense, and inflicts brain dysfunction and damage on millions of individuals.

Bibliography

Abrahamson, I. (1935). *Lethargic encephalitis*. New York: privately published.

Abrams, R. (1988). *Electroconvulsive therapy*. New York: Oxford University Press.

Adam, K., & Oswald, I. (1989). Can a rapidly-eliminated hypnotic cause daytime anxiety? *Pharmakopsychiatrie, 22,* 115–119.

Adams, C., & Essali, M. (1991). Working with Clozaril. *Psychiatric Bulletin, 15,* 336–338.

Adams, R., & Victor, M. (1989). *Principles of neurology* (4th ed.). New York: McGraw-Hill.

Addington, D., Toews, J., & Addington, J. (1995, October). Risperidone and tardive dyskinesia: A case report. *Journal of Clinical Psychiatry, 56,* 484–485.

Addonizio, G., Susman, V., & Roth, S. (1986). Symptoms of neuroleptic malignant syndrome in 82 consecutive inpatients. *American Journal of Psychiatry, 143,* 1587–1590.

Alarcon, R., & Carney, M. W. P. (1969). Severe depressive mood changes following slow-release intramuscular fluphenazine injection. *British Medical Journal, 3,* 564–567.

Alexander, P. E., Van Kammen, D. P., & Bunney, W. E. (1979). Antipsychotic effects of lithium in schizophrenia. *American Journal of Psychiatry, 136,* 283–287.

Alexopoulos, G. S. (1979). Lack of complaints in schizophrenics with tardive dyskinesia. *Journal of Nervous and Mental Diseases, 167,* 125–127.

Alheid, F., Heimer, L., & Switzer, R. (1990). Basal ganglia. In S. Paxinos (Ed.), *The human nervous system* (pp. 483–582). New York: Academic Press.

Altman, L. (1994, June 3). Panel clears fatal studies of new drug: Contradicts F.D.A. on hepatitis report. *New York Times*, p. A20.

Alper, P. R. (1996, December). Who to trust: Drug companies or your doctor? *Wall Street Journal*, p. A18.

American College of Neuropsychopharmacology/Food and Drug Administration Task Force. (1973). A special report: Neurological syndromes associated with antipsychotic drug use. *Archives of General Psychiatry*, *28*, 463–467.

American Psychiatric Association (APA). (1975). The current status of lithium therapy: Report of the APA Task Force. *American Journal of Psychiatry*, *132*, 997–1001.

American Psychiatric Association. (1978). *Electroconvulsive therapy: A task force report*. Washington, DC: Author.

American Psychiatric Association. (1980). *Task force report: Tardive dyskinesia*. Washington, DC: Author.

American Psychiatric Association. (1985). *Task force on tardive dyskinesia: Letter to the membership of the Association* [Direct mailing to membership].

American Psychiatric Association. (1987). *Diagnostic and statistical manual of mental disorders* (3rd ed., rev.). Washington, DC: Author.

American Psychiatric Association. (1989). *Treatments of psychiatric disorders: A task force report of the American Psychiatric Association*. Washington, DC: Author.

American Psychiatric Association. (1990a). *Benzodiazepine dependence, toxicity and abuse: A task force report*. Washington, DC: Author.

American Psychiatric Association. (1990b). *The practice of electroconvulsive therapy: A task force report*. Washington, DC: Author.

American Psychiatric Association. (1992). *Tardive dyskinesia: A task force report*. Washington, DC: Author.

American Psychiatric Association. (1994). *Diagnostic and statistical manual of mental disorders* (4th ed.). Washington, DC: Author.

American Psychological Association National Task Force on Women and Depression. (1990). *Women and depression: Risk factors and treatment issues*. Washington, DC: Author.

Ananth, J. (1978). Side effects in the neonate from psychotropic agents excreted through breast-feeding. *American Journal of Psychiatry*, *135*, 801–805.

Anderson, E., & Powers, P. (1991). Neuroleptic malignant syndrome associated with clozapine use. *Journal of Clinical Psychiatry, 52*, 102–104.

Andreadis, N. A., & Schrimer, R. G. (1992). Use of spontaneous reporting system data. *Archives of Internal Medicine, 152*, 1527–1528.

Andreasen, N. (1984). *The broken brain: The biological revolution in psychiatry.* New York: Harper & Row.

Andreasen, N. (1988). Brain imaging: Applications in psychiatry. *Science, 239*, 1381–1388.

Andreasen, N., Rezai, K., Alliger, R., Swayze, V., Flaum, M., Kirchner, P., Cohen, G., & O'Leary, D. (1992). Hypofrontality in neuroleptic-naive patients and in patients with chronic schizophrenia. *Archives of General Psychiatry, 49*, 943–958.

Anello, C. (1988, October 17). Memorandum to Director, Division of Neuropharmacological Drugs. Subject triazolam (Halcion). FDA Office of Epidemiology and Biostatistics. Obtained through the Freedom of Information Act.

Anello, C. (1989, September 12). Memorandum: Triazolam and temazepam—Comparison reporting rates. FDA Center for Drug Evaluation and Research, Office of Epidemiology and Biostatistics. Obtained through the Freedom of Information Act.

Antipsychotic drug therapy poses hazards for elderly. (1988, June). *Drug Utilization Review, 4*(6), 73–84.

Anton-Stephens, D. (1954). Preliminary observations on the psychiatric uses of chlorpromazine (Largactile). *Journal of Mental Science, 100*, 543–557.

Antonuccio, D. O., Danton, W. G., & DeNelsky, G. Y. (1994). Psychotherapy: No stronger medicine. *Scientist Practitioner, 4*(1), 2–18.

Antonuccio, D. O., Danton, W. G., & DeNelsky, G. Y. (1995). Psychotherapy versus medication for depression: Challenging the conventional wisdom with data. *Professional Psychology: Research and Practice, 26*, 574–585.

Appleton, W. S. (1982). Fourth psychoactive drug usage guide. *Journal of Clinical Psychiatry, 43*, 12–27.

Arai, N., Amano, N., Iseki, E., Yokoi, S., Saito, A., Takekawa, Y., & Micugi, K. (1987). Tardive dyskinesia with inflated neurons of the cellular dentate nucleus. *Acta Neuropathologica (Berlin), 73*, 38–42.

Arana, G., & Hyman, S. (1991). *Handbook of psychiatric drug treatment* (2nd ed.). Boston: Little, Brown.

Arieti, S. (1959). Schizophrenia: Other aspects; psychotherapy. In S. Arieti (Ed.), *American handbook of psychiatry* (Vol. I, pp. 455–484). New York: Basic Books.

Armstrong, L. (1993). *And they call it help: The psychiatric policing of America's children*. New York: Addison-Wesley.

Ashton, H. (1995). Toxicity and adverse consequences of benzodiazepine use. *Psychiatric Annals, 25*, 158–165.

Asscher, A. W. (1991, October 1). Dear Doctor/Dentist/Pharmacist: Withdrawal of triazolam [Letter]. Committee on Safety of Medicines, London, England.

Associated Press (1994, May 14). Hepatitis drug trials broke rules, FDA says. *Washington Post*, p. A8.

Associated Press (1996, December 26). NIH queries university on use of homeless in tests. *Washington Post*, p. A13.

Aubree, J. C., & Lader, M. H. (1980). High and very high dosage antipsychotics. *Journal of Clinical Psychiatry, 14*, 341–350.

Avery, D., & Winokur, G. (1976). Mortality in depressed patients treated with electroconvulsive therapy and antidepressants. *Archives of General Psychiatry, 33*, 1029–1037.

Avery, D., & Winokur, G. (1977). The efficacy of electroconvulsive therapy and antidepressants in depression. *Biological Psychiatry, 12*, 507–523.

Avorn, J., Dreyer, P., Connelly, K., & Soumerai, S. (1989). Use of psychoactive medication and the quality of care in rest homes. *New England Journal of Medicine, 320*, 227–232.

Ayd, F. J. (1974). Once-a-day dosage of tricyclic antidepressant drug therapy: A survey. *Diseases of the Nervous System, 35*, 475–480.

Ayd, F. J. (1975). The depot fluphenazines: A reappraisal after 10 years' clinical experience. *American Journal of Psychiatry, 132*, 491–500.

Ayd, F. J. (1992, May). Triazolam 0.25 mg: A reappraisal. *International Drug Therapy Newsletter, 27*(5), 17–24.

Baastrup, P. C., & Schou, M. (1967). Lithium as a prophylactic agent. *Archives of General Psychiatry, 16*, 162–172.

Babayan, E. (1985). *The structure of psychiatry in the Soviet Union*. New York: International Universities Press.

Babigian, H., & Guttmacher, L. (1984). Epidemiologic considerations in electroconvulsive therapy. *Archives of General Psychiatry, 41*, 246–253.

Bailey, L., Gordis, L. & Green, M. (1994). Reference guide on epidemiology. In *Federal Judicial Center's Reference Manual on Scientific Evidence* (pp. 122–179). St. Paul, MN: West.

Baker, B. (1995, March). Though data lacking, antidepressants used widely in children. *Clinical Psychiatry News*, p. 16.

Baker, B. (1996, September). Risperidone cuts symptoms of dementia in elderly. *Clinical Psychiatry News*, p. 19.

Baldessarini, R. J. (1977). Schizophrenia. *New England Journal of Medicine, 297*, 988–995.

Baldessarini, R. J. (1978). Chemotherapy. In A. Nicholi (Ed.), *The Harvard guide to modern psychiatry*. Cambridge: Harvard University Press.

Baldessarini, R. J., & Marsh, E. (1990, February). Fluoxetine and side effects. *Archives of General Psychiatry, 47*, 191–192.

Baldessarini, R., & Frankenburg, F. (1991, March 14). Clozapine: A novel antipsychotic agent. *New England Journal of Medicine, 324*, 746–754.

Ballenger, J. (1995). Benzodiazepines. In A. Schatzberg & C. Nemeroff (Eds.), *The American Psychiatric Press textbook of psychopharmacology*. Washington, DC: American Psychiatric Press.

Balter, M. (1977, May 2). [Response to request for information from Congressman Obey of Wisconsin.] Unpublished memorandum from Special Studies Section, Psychopharmacology Research Branch, National Institute of Mental Health, Rockville, Maryland.

Baribeau, J., Laurent, J-P., & Décary, A. (1993, September). Tardive dyskinesia and associated cognitive disorders: A convergent neuropsychological and neurophysiological approach. *Brain and Cognition, 23*(1), 40–55.

Barkley, R. (1981). *Hyperactive children: A handbook for diagnosis and treatment*. New York: Guilford.

Barnes, T. (1992). Neuromuscular effects of neuroleptics: Akathisia. In J. Kane & J. Lieberman (Eds.), *Adverse effects of psychotropic drugs*. New York: Guilford.

Baron, B. M., Ogden, A-M., Siegel, B. W., Stegeman, J., Ursillo, R. C., & Dudley, M. W. (1988). Rapid down regulation of B-adrenoreceptors by coadministration of desipramine and fluoxetine. *European Journal of Pharmacology, 154*, 125–134.

Bartels, M., & Themelis, J. (1983). Computerized tomography in tardive dyskinesia. Evidence of structural abnormalities in the basal ganglia system. *Archive für Psychiatrie and Nervenkrankheiten, 231*, 371–379.

Bassuk, E. L., & Schoonover, S. C. (1977). *The practitioner's guide to psychoactive drugs*. New York: Plenum.

Batoosingh, K. (1995, June). Ritalin prescriptions triple over last 4 years. *Clinical Psychiatry News*, p. 1.

Battaglia, G., Yeh, S. Y., O'Hearn, E., Molliver, M. E., Kuhar, M. J., & De Souza, E. B. (1987). 3,4-Methylenedioxyamphetamine destroy serotonin terminals in rat brain: Quantification of neurodegeneration by measurement of [³H]paroxetine-labeled serotonin uptake sites. *Journal of Pharmacology and Experimental Therapeutics, 242,* 911–916.

Baughman, Jr., F. A. (1993, May 12). Treatment of attention-deficit hyperactivity disorder. *Journal of the American Medical Association, 269,* 2368.

Baughman, F. (1996, February 14). Personal Communication to Peter R. Breggin.

Bayer, A. J., Bayer, E. M., Pathy, M. S. J., & Stoker, M. J. (1986). A double-blind controlled study of chlormethiazole and triazolam as hypnotics in the elderly. *Acta Psychiatrica Scandinavica, 73*(Supp. 329), 104–111.

Beasley, C. (1994a, May 17). Deposition, Volume I, in Fentress et al. v. Shea Communications et al., Jefferson Circuit Court, Division One, No. 90-Cl-6033.

Beasley, C. (1994b, August 30). Deposition, Volume II, in Fentress et al. v. Shea Communications et al., Jefferson Circuit Court, Division One, No. 90-Cl-6033.

Beitman, B. D. (1978). Tardive dyskinesia reinduced by lithium carbonate. *American Journal of Psychiatry, 135,* 1229–1230.

Belmaker, R., & Wald, D. (1977). Haloperidol in normals. *British Journal of Psychiatry, 131,* 222–223.

Benedek, E. (1993, February 8). Letter to Peter Roger Breggin, M.D., as a part of a mass mailing soliciting funds for the American Psychiatric Foundation.

Benes, F., Sunderland, P., Jones, B., LeMay, M., Cohen, B. M., & Lipinski, J. F. (1982). Normal ventricles in young schizophrenics. *British Journal of Psychiatry, 141,* 90–93.

Bergen, J. A., Eyland, E. A., Campbell, J. A., Jenkings, P., Kellehear, K., Richards, A., & Beaumont, J. V. (1989). The course of tardive dyskinesia in patients on long-term neuroleptics. *British Journal of Psychiatry, 154,* 523–528.

Bergsholm, P., Larsen, J. L., Rosendahl, K., & Holsten, F. (1989). Electroconvulsive therapy and cerebral computed tomography. *Acta Psychiatrica Scandinavica, 80,* 566–572.

Bergstromm, R. F., Peyton, A. L., & Lemberger, L. (1992). Quantification and mechanism of fluoxetine and tricyclic antidepressant interaction. *Clinical Pharmacology and Therapeutics, 51,* 239–248.

Bernat, J., & Vincent, F. (1987). (Eds.). *Neurology: Problems in primary care.* Oradell, NJ: Medical Economics.

Besson, J., Corrigan, F., Cherryman, F., & Smith, F. (1987). Nuclear magnetic resonance brain imaging in chronic schizophrenia. *British Journal of Psychiatry, 150,* 161–163.

Biederman, J., Milberger, S., Faraone, S. V., Kiely, K., Guite, J., Mick, E., Ablon, S., Warburton, R., & Reed, E. (1995, June). Family-environment risk factors for attention-deficit hyperactivity disorder: A test of Rutter's indicators of adversity. *Archives of General Psychiatry, 52,* 464–470.

Bishop, K. (1989, March 13). Studies find drugs still overused to control nursing home elderly. *The New York Times,* p. A8.

Bixler, E. O., Kales, A., Brubaker, B. H., & Kales, J. D. (1987). Adverse reactions to benzodiazepine hypnotics: Spontaneous reporting system. *Pharmacology, 35,* 286–300.

Black, D., Winokur, G., Mohandoss, E., Woolson, R., & Nasrallah, A. (1989). Does treatment influence mortality in depressives? A follow-up of 1076 patients with major affective disorders. *Annals of Clinical Psychiatry, 1,* 165–173.

Blakeslee, T. (1983). *The right brain: A new understanding of the unconscious mind and its creative powers.* New York: Berkeley.

Bleuler, E. (1924). *The textbook of psychiatry.* New York: Macmillan.

Bleuler, M. (1978). *The schizophrenic disorders: Long-term patient and family studies.* New Haven: Yale University Press.

Block, S., & Reddaway, P. (1977). *Psychiatric terror.* New York: Basic Books.

Boodman, S. (1996, September 24). Shock therapy: It's back. *Washington Post Health,* pp. 14–20.

Booth, N. H. (1977). Psychotropic agents. In L. M. Jones, N. H. Booth, & L. E. McDonald (Eds.), *Veterinary pharmacology and therapeutics* (4th ed.). Ames, IA: Iowa State University Press.

Booth, W. (1993, October 7). U.S. accused of sedating deportees. *Washington Post,* p. A1.

Bost, R. O., & Kemp, P. M. (1992, March/April). A possible association between fluoxetine use and suicide. *Journal of Analytical Toxicology, 16,* 142–145.

Boyle, G. (1986, November). Concussion of the brain with electroconvulsive shock therapy (ECT): An appropriate treatment for depression and suicidal ideation? *Australian Clinical Psychology*, pp. 21–27.

Bracha, H. S., & Kleinman, J. E. (1986). Postmortem neurochemistry in schizophrenia. *Psychiatric Clinics of North America, 9*, 133–141.

Bradley, W., Daroff, R., Fenichel, G., & Marsden, C. (Eds). (1991). *Neurology in clinical practice*. Boston: Butterworth-Heinemann.

Brahams, D. (1991, October 12). Triazolam suspended. *Lancet, 338*, 938.

Branchey, M., Charles, J., & Simpson, G. (1976). Extrapyramidal side effects in lithium maintenance therapy. *American Journal of Psychiatry, 133*, 444–445.

Breeding, J. (1996). *The wildest colts make the best ponies: The truth about Ritalin, ADHD, and other 'Disruptive Behavior Disorders.'* Austin, TX: Bright Books.

Breggin, P. R. (1964). Coercion of voluntary patients in an open hospital. *Archives of General Psychiatry, 10*, 173–181.

Breggin, P. R. (1975). Psychosurgery for political purposes. *Duquesne Law Review, 13*, 841–862.

Breggin, P. R. (1979). *Electroshock: Its brain-disabling effects*. New York: Springer.

Breggin, P. R. (1980). Brain-disabling therapies. In E. Valenstein (Ed.), *The psychosurgery debate: Scientific, legal and ethical perspectives* (pp. 467–505). San Francisco: Freeman.

Breggin, P. R. (1981a). Disabling the brain with electroshock. In M. Dongier & D. Wittkower (Eds.), *Divergent views in psychiatry*. Hagerstown, MD: Harper & Row.

Breggin, P. R. (1981b). Psychosurgery as brain-disabling therapy. In M. Dongier & D. Wittkower (Eds.), *Divergent views in psychiatry*. Hagerstown, MD: Harper & Row.

Breggin, P. R. (1983a). *Psychiatric drugs: Hazards to the brain*. New York: Springer.

Breggin, P. R. (1983b). Iatrogenic helplessness in authoritarian psychiatry. In R. F. Morgan (Ed.), *The iatrogenics handbook*. Toronto: IPI.

Breggin, P. R. (1986). Neuropathology and cognitive dysfunction from ECT. [Presented at the Consensus Development Conference on Electroconvulsive Therapy, sponsored by NIMH and NIH, 1985.] *Psychopharmacology Bulletin, 22*, 476–479.

Breggin, P. R. (1989a). Addiction to neuroleptics? (letter). *American Journal of Psychiatry, 146*, 560.

Breggin, P. R. (1989b). Addiction to neuroleptics: Dr. Breggin replies (letter). *American Journal of Psychiatry, 146,* 1240.

Breggin, P. R. (1990). Brain damage, dementia and persistent cognitive dysfunction associated with neuroleptic drugs: evidence, etiology, implications. *Journal of Mind and Behavior, 11,* 425–464.

Breggin, P. R. (1991a). *Toxic psychiatry: Why therapy, empathy and love must replace the drugs, electroshock and biochemical theories of the 'new psychiatry.'* New York: St. Martin's.

Breggin, P. R. (1991b, Spring). San Francisco Board of Supervisors passes resolution against shock [Report from the Center for the Study of Psychiatry]. *Rights Tenet: Newsletter of the National Association for Rights Protection and Advocacy (NARPA),* p. 3.

Breggin, P. R. (1991c, Summer). More on the California shock controversy [Report from the Center for the Study of Psychiatry]. *Rights Tenet: Newsletter of the National Association for Rights Protection and Advocacy (NARPA),* p. 3.

Breggin, P. R. (1992a). *Beyond conflict: From self-help and psychotherapy to peacemaking.* New York: St. Martin's.

Breggin, P. (1992b, February 11). The president's sleeping pill [Halcion] and its makers (letter). *New York Times,* p. A24.

Breggin, P. (1992c). A case of fluoxetine-induced stimulant side effects with suicidal ideation associated with a possible withdrawal syndrome ("Crashing"). *International Journal of Risk and Safety in Medicine, 3,* 325–328.

Breggin, P. R. (1993). Parallels between neuroleptic effects and lethargic encephalitis: The production of dyskinesias and cognitive disorders. *Brain and Cognition, 23,* 8–27.

Breggin, P. R. (1994, October 17–19). Testimony in *Joyce Fentress et al. vs. Shea Communications et al. ["The Wesbecker Case"]* Jefferson Circuit Court, Division 1, Louisville, Kentucky. No. 90-CI-06033. Volume XVI.

Breggin, P. R. (1995, September). Prozac 'hazardous' to children (letter). *Clinical Psychiatry News,* p. 10.

Breggin, P. (1996, July 8). The FDA was agitated over Halcion (letter). *Business Week,* p. 12.

Breggin, P. R. (1997). *The heart of being helpful.* New York: Springer.

Breggin, P. R., & Breggin, G. (1994a). *Talking back to Prozac: What doctors aren't telling you about today's most controversial drug.* New York: St. Martin's.

Breggin, P. R., & Breggin, G. (1994b). *The war against children: The government's intrusion into schools, families and communities in search of a medical "cure" for violence.* New York: St. Martin's.

Breggin, P. R., & Breggin, P. L. (1974, June). Psychiatric oppression of prisoners. *Psychiatric Opinion.*

Breggin, P., & Stern, E. M. (Eds.). (1996). *Psychosocial approaches to deeply disturbed patients.* NY: Haworth. Also published as *The Psychotherapy Patient,* Volume 9, Numbers 3/4, 1996.

Breier, A., Buchanan, R., Elkashef, A., Munson, R., Kirkpatrick, B., & Gellad, F. (1992). Brain morphology and schizophrenia. *Archives of General Psychiatry, 49,* 921–926.

Brill, H. (1959). Postencephalitic psychiatric conditions. In S. Arieti (Ed.), *American handbook of psychiatry* (pp. 1163–1174). New York: Basic Books.

Brill, H. (1975). Postencephalitic states or conditions. In S. Arieti (Ed.), *American handbook of psychiatry* (2nd ed.). New York: Basic Books.

Brodal, A. (1969). *Neurological anatomy.* New York: Oxford University Press.

Brooks, G. W. (1959). Withdrawal from neuroleptic drugs. *American Journal of Psychiatry, 115,* 931–932.

Brown, P., & Funk, S. C. (1986). Tardive dyskinesia: Barriers to the professional recognition of an iatrogenic disease. *Journal of Health and Social Behavior, 27,* 116–132.

Brown, R., Colter, N., Corsellis, J., Crow, T. J., Frith, C. D., Jagoe, R., Johnstone, E. C., & Marsh, L. (1986). Postmortem evidence of structural brain changes in schizophrenia. *Archives of General Psychiatry, 43,* 36–42.

Bruun, R. (1988). Subtle and underrecognized side effects of neuroleptic treatment in children with Tourette's Disorder. *American Journal of Psychiatry, 145,* 621–624.

Buchsbaum, M., Ingvar, D. H., Kessler, R., Waters, R. N., Cappelletti, J., van Kammen, D. P., King, A. C., Johnson, J. L., Manning, R. G., Flynn, R. W., Mann, L. S., Bunney, W. E., & Sokoloff, L. (1982). Cerebral glucography with positron tomography. *Archives of General Psychiatry, 39,* 251–259.

Buchsbaum, M., Haier, R., Potkin, S., Nuechterlein, K., Bracha, S., Katz, M., Lohr, J., Wu, J., Lottenberg, S., Jerabek, P., Trenary, M., Tafalla, R., Reynolds, C., & Bunney, W. (1992). Frontostriatal disorder of cerebral metabolism in never-medicated schizophrenics. *Archives of General Psychiatry, 49*, 935–942.

Buckley, N. A., Dawson, A. H., Whyte, I. M., & O'Connell, D. L. (1995). Relative toxicity of benzodiazepines in overdose. *British Medical Journal, 310*, 219–220.

Burke, R., Fahn, S., Jankovic, J., Marsden, C. D., Lang, A. E., Gollomp, S., & Ilson, J. (1982). Tardive dystonia: Late-onset and persistent dystonia caused by antipsychotic drugs. *Neurology, 32*, 1335–1346.

Burke, R., & Kang, U. J. (1988). Tardive dystonia: Clinical aspects and treatment. In J. Jankovic & E. Tolosa (Eds.), *Facial dyskinesias: Advances in neurology, 49* (pp. 199–210). New York: Raven.

Burke, W., Rubin, E., Zorumski, C., & Wetzel, R. (1987). The safety of ECT in geriatric psychiatry. *Journal of the American Geriatrics Society, 35*, 516–521.

Burstow, B., & Weitz, D. (Eds.). *Shrink resistant: The struggle against psychiatry in Canada.* Vancouver, BC: New Star Books.

Byck, R. (1975). Drugs and the treatment of psychiatric disorders. In L. S. Goodman & A. Gilman, *The pharmacological basis of therapeutics* (5th ed.). New York: Macmillan.

Byerly, M. J., Greer, R. A., & Evans, D. L. (1995). Behavioral stimulation associated with risperidone initiation. *American Journal of Psychiatry, 152*(7), 1096–1097.

Cade, J. F. J. (1949). Lithium salts in the treatment of psychotic excitement. *Medical Journal of Australia, 2*, 349–352.

Caine, E., Grossman, H., & Lyness, J. (1995). Delirium, dementia, and amnestic and other cognitive disorders and mental disorders due to a general medical condition. In H. Kaplan & B. Sadock (Eds.), *Comprehensive textbook of psychiatry.* New York: Williams & Wilkins.

Calloway, S. P., Dolan, R. J., Jacoby, R. J., & Levy, R. (1981). ECT and cerebral atrophy. *Acta Psychiatrica Scandinavica, 64*, 442–445.

Cameron, D. G. (1994, Winter/Spring). ECT: Sham statistics, the myth of convulsive therapy and the case for consumer misinformation. *Journal of Mind and Behavior, 15*, 177–198.

Cameron, D. E., Lohrenz, J., & Handcock, K. (1962). The depatterning treatment of schizophrenia. *Comprehensive Psychiatry, 3*, 67–71.

Campbell, H., & Harthoorn, A. M. (1963). The capture and anaesthesia of the African lion in his natural environment. *Veterinary Record, 75*, 275–276.

Caplan, P. (1995). *They say you're crazy: How the world's most powerful psychiatrists decide who's normal.* New York: Addison-Wesley.

Carey, J., & Weber, J. (1996, June 17). How the FDA let Halcion slip through: It admits it didn't adequately examine Upjohn's data. *Business Week*, p. 38.

Casey, D. E. (1993). Neuroleptic-induced acute extrapyramidal syndromes and tardive dyskinesia. *Psychiatric Clinics of North America, 3*, 589–610.

Castellano, M. (1995, May 15). Kentucky fried verdict up for grabs. *New Jersey Law Journal*, p. 39.

Castle, W. M. (1986). Problems in assessing drug safety: A plea for improved methodology and a possible route. *Drug Information Journal, 20*, 323–326.

Cauchon, D. (1995, December 6). Shock treatment: Controversy and questions. *USA Today*, p. 1A.

Center for Drug Evaluation and Research, Food and Drug Administration [FDA]. (1988, July). Guidelines for the format and content of the clinical and statistical sections of an application. Rockville, MD: FDA.

CH.A.D.D. (1992, October 15–17). Program for the Fourth Annual Conference: Pathways to Progress, Chicago.

CH.A.D.D. (undated). *CH.A.D.D.: Children with attention deficit disorders—Hyperactive?, inattentive?, impulsive?.* Available from CH.A.D.D., 499 N.W. 70th Avenue, Suite 308, Plantation, FL 33317.

Chamberlin, J. (1978). *On our own: Patient-controlled alternatives to the mental health system.* New York: Hawthorn.

Chard, F., Sharon, D., & Myslobodsky, M. (1986). *Anosognosia and disturbances of emotions in TD patients.* Unpublished paper. Cited in Myslobodsky (1993).

Chengappa, K. N. R., Shelton, M. D., Baker, R. W., Schooler, N. R., Baird, J., & Delaney, J. (1994). The prevalence of akathisia in patients receiving stable doses of clozapine. *Journal of Clinical Psychiatry, 55*(4), 142–145.

Chiodo, L. A., & Bunney, B. S. (1983). Typical and atypical neuroleptics: Differential effects of chronic administration on the activity of A9 and A10 midbrain dopaminergic neurons. *Journal of Neuroscience, 3*, 1607–1619.

Chira, S. (1993, July 14). Is small better? Educators now say yes for high school. *New York Times*, p. 1.

Chouinard, G., Annable, L., Mercier, P., & Ross-Chouinard, A. (1986). A five-year follow-up study of tardive dyskinesia. *Psychopharmacology Bulletin, 22*, 259–263.

Chouinard, G., Annable, L., Ross-Chouinard, A., & Nestoros, J. N. (1979). Factors related to tardive dyskinesia. *American Journal of Psychiatry, 136*(1), 79–83.

Chouinard, G., & Jones, B. (1980). Neuroleptic-induced supersensitivity psychosis: Clinical and pharmacologic characteristics. *American Journal of Psychiatry, 137*, 16–21.

Chouinard, G., & Jones, B. (1982). Neuroleptic-induced supersensitivity psychosis, the 'hump course,' and tardive dyskinesia. *Journal of Clinical Psychopharmacology, 2*, 143–144.

Chouinard, G., Jones, B., & Annable, L. (1978). Neuroleptic-induced supersensitivity psychosis. *American Journal of Psychiatry, 135*, 1409–1410.

Chouinard, G., & Steiner, W. (1986). A case of mania induced by high-dose fluoxetine treatment. *American Journal of Psychiatry, 143*, 686.

Christensen, E., Moller, J. E., & Faurbye, A. (1970). Neuropathological investigation of 28 brains from patients with dyskinesia. *Acta Psychiatrica Scandinavica, 46*, 14–23.

Cleghorn, J. M., Garnett, E. S., Nahmias, C., Firnau, G., Brown, G. M., Kaplan, R., Szechtman, H., & Szechtman, B. (1989). Increased frontal and reduced parietal glucose metabolism in acute untreated schizophrenia. *Psychiatry Research, 28*, 119–133.

Clozapine withdrawal syndrome. (1994, February). *Psychiatric Times*, p. 33.

Code of federal regulations: Food and drugs. (1995, April 1). 21:Parts 300–499. Washington, DC: Office of the Federal Register, National Archives and Records Administration.

Coffey, C. E., Weiner, R. D., Djand, W. T., Fiegel, G. S., Soady, S. A. R., Patterson, L. J., Holt, P. D., Spritzer, C. E., & Wilkinson, W. E. (1991). Brain anatomic effects of electroconvulsive therapy: A prospective magnetic resonance imaging study. *Archives of General Psychiatry, 48*, 1013–1021.

Cohen, D., & Cohen, H. (1986). Biological theories, drug treatments, and schizophrenia: A critical assessment. *Journal of Mind and Behavior, 7*, 11–36.

Cohen, D., & McCubbin, M. (1990). The political economy of tardive dyskinesia: Asymmetries in power and responsibility. *Journal of Mind and Behavior, 11*, 465–488.

Cohen, D. (Editor) (1990). Challenging the therapeutic state: Critical perspectives on psychiatry and the mental health system. *Journal of Mind and Behavior, 11*, 3 & 4.

Cohen, H., & Cohen, D. (1993, September). What may be gained from neuropsychological investigations of tardive dyskinesia? *Brain and Cognition, 23*(1), 1–7.

Cohen, P. (1996, November 14). To screen new drugs for safety, Lilly pays homeless alcoholics. *Wall Street Journal*, p. A1.

Cohen, W. J., & Cohen, N. H. (1974). Lithium carbonate, haloperidol, and irreversible brain damage. *Journal of the American Medical Association, 230*, 1283–1287.

Colbert, T. (1995). *Broken brains or wounded hearts: What causes mental illness.* Santa Ana, CA: Kevco.

Cole, J. O. (1960). Behavioral toxicity. In L. Uhr & J. G. Miller (Eds.), *Drugs and behavior.* New York: Wiley.

Coleman, L. (1974, June). Prisons: The crime of treatment. *Psychiatric Opinion*, p. 5.

Coles, G. (1987). *The learning mystique: A critical look at 'learning disabilities'.* New York: Pantheon.

Coln, E. J. (1975). Long-lasting changes in cerebral neurons induced by drugs. *Biological Psychiatry, 10*, 227–264.

Committee on Safety of Medicines. (1988). Benzodiazepines, dependence and withdrawal symptoms. *Current Problems, 21*, 1–2.

Committee on Safety of Medicines. (1991). Triazolam: Assessor's Report. Appeal by Upjohn against revocation of product license. London, England.

Consensus Conference: Electroconvulsive Therapy. (1985). *Journal of the American Medical Association, 245*, 2103–2108.

Coons, D. J., Hillman, F. J., & Marshall, R. W. (1982). Treatment of neuroleptic malignant syndrome with dantrolene sodium: A case report. *American Journal of Psychiatry, 139*, 943–945.

Corcoran, A. C., Taylor, R. D., & Page, I. H. (1949). Lithium poisoning from the use of salt substitutes. *Journal of the American Medical Association, 139*, 685–688.

Crane, G. (1973). Clinical psychopharmacology in its 20th year. *Science, 181*, 124–128.

Crane, G. (1977). Prevention of tardive dyskinesia. In J. Masserman (Ed.), *Current Psychiatric Therapies 17.* New York: Grune & Stratton.

Crews, E. L., & Carpenter, A. E. (1977). Lithium-induced aggravation of tardive dyskinesia. *American Journal of Psychiatry*, *134*, 933.

Crow, T., & Johnstone, E. (1986). Controlled trials of electroconvulsive therapy. *Annals of the New York Academy of Sciences*, *462*, 12–29.

Csernansky, J., & Hollister, L. E. (1982). Probable case of supersensitivity psychosis. *Hospital Formulary*, *17*, 395–399.

Damluji, N., & Ferguson, J. (1988). Paradoxical worsening of depressive symptomatology caused by antidepressants. *Journal of Clinical Psychopharmacology*, *8*, 347–349.

Daniel, W., Crovitz, H., Weiner, R., & Rogers, H. (1982). The effects of ECT modifications on autobiographical and verbal memory. *Biological Psychiatry*, *17*, 919–924.

DasGupta, K., & Young, A. (1991). Clozapine-induced neuroleptic malignant syndrome. *Journal of Clinical Psychiatry*, *52*(3), 105–107.

Dave, M. (1995). Two cases of risperidone-induced neuroleptic malignant syndrome. *American Journal of Psychiatry*, *152*(8), 1233–1234.

Davies, R. K., Tucker, G. J., Harrow, M., & Detre, T. P. (1971). Confusional episodes and antidepressant medication. *American Journal of Psychiatry*, *128*, 95–99.

Davis, J. M. (1980). The antipsychotic drugs. In H. I. Kaplan, A. M. Freedman, & B. J. Sadock (Eds.), *Comprehensive textbook of psychiatry* (3rd ed.). Baltimore: Williams & Wilkins.

Davis, J. M., & Cole, J. O. (1975). Antipsychotic drugs. In A. M. Freedman, H. I. Kaplan, & B. J. Sadock (Eds.), *Comprehensive textbook of psychiatry* (2nd ed.). New York: Grune & Stratton.

Davis, J., Janicak, P., & Khan, A. (1991). Neuroleptic malignant syndrome. In D. Dunner (Ed.), *Current psychiatric therapy* (pp. 170–175). Philadelphia: Saunders.

Dawson, E. B., Moore, T. D., & McGanity, W. J. (1970). The mathematical relations of drinking water, lithium, and rainfall to mental hospital admissions. *Diseases of the Nervous System*, *31*, 811–820.

Debattista, C., & Schatzberg, A. (1995). Physical symptoms associated with paroxetine withdrawal (letter). *American Journal of Psychiatry*, *152*, 1235–1236.

Delay, J., & Deniker, P. (1952). Le traitement des psychoses par une méthode neurolytique dérivée de l'hybernothérapie. In *Congrès des Médecins Aliénistes et Neurologistes de France*, *50*, 497–502.

Delay, J., & Deniker, P. (1968). Drug-induced extrapyramidal syndromes. In P. J. Vinken & G. W. Bruyn (Eds.), *Handbook of clinical neurology: Vol. 6. Diseases of the basal ganglia* (pp. 248–266). New York: Wiley.

Demers, R. G., & Davis, L. S. (1971). The influence of prophylactic lithium treatment on the marital adjustment of manic-depressives and their spouses. *Comprehensive Psychiatry, 12,* 348–353.

Demers, R. G., & Heninger, G. R. (1971). Visual-motor performance during lithium treatment—A preliminary report. *Journal of Clinical Pharmacology, 11,* 274–279.

DeMeyer, M. K., Gilmore, R., DeMeyer, W. E., Hendrie, H., Edwards, M., & Franco, J. N. (1984). Third ventricle size and ventricular/brain ratio in treatment-resistant psychiatric patients. *Journal of Operational Psychiatry, 15,* 2–8.

DeMeyer, M. K., Gilmore, R., Hendrie, H., DeMeyer, W. E., & Franco, J. N. (1984). Brain densities in treatment resistant schizophrenic and other psychiatric patients. *Journal of Operational Psychiatry, 15,* 9–16.

Dempsey, G. M., & Herbert, M. L. (1977). Lithium toxicity: A review. In L. Roizen, H. Shiraki, & N. Grčević, *Neurotoxicology.* New York: Raven.

Deniker, P. (1970). Introduction to neuroleptic chemotherapy into psychiatry. In F. Ayd & B. Blackwell (Eds.), *Discoveries in biological psychiatry* (pp. 155–164). Philadelphia: Lippincott.

Deniker, P. (1971, October 6). Deniker recounts to symposium discovery of chlorpromazine. *Psychiatric News,* p. 6.

DeToma v. Brohamer. (1991, January 16). No. 86-20906 CT, P.155 Broward County (FL) Circuit Court, 17th Judicial District.

De Tullio, P. L., Kirking, D. M., Zacardelli, D. K., & Kwee, P. (1989). Evaluation of long-term triazolam use in an ambulatory veterans administration medical center population. *DICP, The Annals of Pharmacotherapy, 23,* 290–293.

Devanand, D. P., Dwork, A. J., Hutchinson, E. R., Bolwig, T. G., & Sackeim, H. A. (1994). Does ECT alter brain structure? *American Journal of Psychiatry, 151*(7), 957–970.

DeVeaugh-Geiss, J. (1979). Informed consent for neuroleptic therapy. *American Journal of Psychiatry, 136,* 959–962.

DeWolfe, A. S., Ryan, J. J., & Wolf, M. E. (1988). Cognitive sequelae of tardive dyskinesia. *Journal of Nervous and Mental Disease, 176,* 270–274.

DiBella, G. A. W. (1979). Educating staff to manage paranoid patients. *American Journal of Psychiatry, 136,* 333–335.

Dietch, J. T., & Jennings, R. K. (1988). Aggressive dyscontrol in patients treated with benzodiazepines. *Journal of Clinical Psychiatry*, *49*(5), 184–187.

DiMascio, A. (1970). Behavioral toxicity. In A. DiMascio & R. Shader (Eds.), *Clinical handbook of psychopharmacology*. New York: Science House.

DiMascio, A., & Shader, R. I. (1970). *Clinical handbook of psychopharmacology*. New York: Science House.

DiMasi, J. A., Seibring, M. A., & Lasagna, L. (1994). New drug development in the United States from 1963 to 1992. *Clinical Pharmacology and Therapeutics*, *55*(6), 609–622.

Dionne, E. J. (1978, July 11). Levitt reports on misuse of drugs by three state mental hospitals. *New York Times*, p. B8.

Division of Epidemiology & Surveillance, Office of Epidemiology & Biostatistics. (1990, March 20). Memorandum: Increased Frequency Report: triazolam deaths, interaction with alcohol, and CNS depression. Rockville, MD: FDA Center for Drug Evaluation and Research. Obtained through the Freedom of Information Act.

Dixon, M. G. (1995). *Drug product liability* (Vol. 1, rev. ed). New York: Bender.

Donlon, P., Hopkin, J., & Tupin, J. (1979). Overview: Efficacy and safety of the rapid neuroleptization method with injectable haloperidol. *American Journal of Psychiatry*, *136*, 273–278.

Drug Enforcement Administration (DEA). (1995a, October 20). *Methylphenidate: DEA Press Release*. Washington, DC: DEA.

Drug Enforcement Administration (DEA). (1995b, October). Methylphenidate (A background paper). Washington, DC: Drug and Chemical Evaluation Section, Office of Diversion Control, DEA. Obtained through the Freedom of Information Act.

Drug facts and comparisons. (1996). St. Louis: Facts and Comparisons.

Drugs and psychiatry: A new era. (1979, November 12). *Newsweek*, pp. 98–102.

Dukes, M. N. G. (1980). The van der Kroef syndrome. *Side Effects of Drugs Annual*, *4*, v–ix.

Dulcan, M. (1994). Treatment of children and adolescents. In R. Hales, S. Yudofsky, & J. Talbott (Eds.), *The American Psychiatric Press textbook of psychiatry* (2nd ed.) (pp. 1209–1250). Washington, DC: American Psychiatric Press.

Dulcan, M. & Popper, C. (1991). *Concise guide to child and adolescent psychiatry*. Washington, DC: American Psychiatric Press.

Dupont, R. (1986). Substance abuse. *Journal of the American Medical Association, 256,* 2114–2115.

DuPont, R. L. (1993, October 7). "Dear Doctor" letter, accompanied by a two-page publication, *Clinical Trials Today,* edited by Elizabeth DuPont Spencer (Fall, 1993). Rockville, MD: Institute for Behavior and Health, Inc.

Dwight, M., Keck, P., Stanton, S., Strakowski, S., & McElroy, S. (1994, August 20). Antidepressant activity and mania associated with risperidone treatment of schizoaffective disorder. *Lancet, 344,* 554–555.

Dyson, W. L., & Mendelson, M. (1968). Recurrent depressions and the lithium ion. *American Journal of Psychiatry, 125,* 544–548.

Editorial. (1995, June). *Archives of General Psychiatry, 52,* 422–423.

Edwards, H. (1970). The significance of brain damage in persistent oral dyskinesia. *British Journal of Psychiatry, 116,* 271–275.

Edwards, J. G. (1995). Suicide and antidepressants. *British Medical Journal, 310,* 205–206.

Einbinder, E. (1995). Fluoxetine withdrawal? (letter). *American Journal of Psychiatry, 152,* 1235.

Electroshock: Key element in personality-changing therapy. (1972, November 15.) *Roche Report: Frontiers in Psychiatry, 2*(19), 1–2. [pharmaceutical company bulletin]

Eli Lilly. (circa late 1987). *Other events observed during the premarketing evaluation of Prozac.* Undated submission to the FDA, edited by the FDA, with a cover letter (December 28, 1987) from R. Temple, Director, Office of Drug Research Review, FDA, to Director (Paul Leber), Division of Neuropharmacological Drug Products, FDA, subject "Fluoxetine Labeling." Rockville, Maryland: Food and Drug Administration. Obtained through the Freedom of Information Act.

Ellinwood, Jr., E. H., & Kilbey, M. M. (Eds.). (1977). *Cocaine and other stimulants.* New York: Plenum.

Emerich, D., & Sanberg, P. (1991). Editorial: Neuroleptic dysphoria. *Biological Psychiatry, 29,* 201–203.

Espinosa, S. (1993, January 26). Women prisoners allege drugging during trials. *San Francisco Chronicle,* p. 1.

Excerpts from statement by dissident on his detention in Soviet mental hospital (1976, February 4). *New York Times,* p. 8C.

Famuyiwa, O. O., Eccleston, D., Donaldson, A. A., & Garside, R. F. (1979). Tardive dyskinesia and dementia. *British Journal of Psychiatry, 135,* 500–504.

Fann, W. E., Smith, R. C., Davis, J. M., & Domino, E. F. (Eds.). (1980). *Tardive dyskinesia.* New York: SP Medical and Scientific Books.

Fann, W. E., Sullivan, J. L., & Richman, B. W. (1977). Dyskinesia associated with tricyclic antidepressants. *British Journal of Psychiatry, 128,* 490–493.

Farde, L., Wiesel, F-A., Halldin, C., & Sedvall, G. (1988). Central D2-dopamine receptor occupancy in schizophrenic patients treated with antipsychotic drugs. *Archives of General Psychiatry, 45,* 71–76.

Farkas, T., Wolf, A. P., Jaeger, J., Brodie, J. D., Christman, D. R., & Fowler, J. S. (1984). Regional brain glucose metabolism in chronic schizophrenia. *Archives of General Psychiatry, 41,* 293–300.

Fasnacht, B. (1993, September 3). Child and adolescent disorders get fine-tuning in DSM-IV. *Psychiatric News,* p. 8.

Faurbye, A. (1970). The structural and biochemical basis of movement disorders in treatment with neuroleptic drugs and in extrapyramidal diseases. *Comprehensive Psychiatry, 11,* 205–225.

Faurbye, A., Rasch, P-J., Petersen, P. B., Brandborg, G., & Pakkenberg, H. (1964). *Acta Psychiatrica Scandinavica, 40*(1), 10–27.

Fava, M., & Rosenbaum, J. (1991, March). Suicidality and fluoxetine: Is there a relationship? *Journal of Clinical Psychiatry, 52,* 108–111.

Fentress et al. vs. Shea Communications et al. ["The Wesbecker Case"]. (1994). Jefferson Circuit Court, Division One, Louisville, KY: NO. 90-CI-06033. Volume XVI.

Ferraro, A., & Roizin, L. (1949). Cerebral morphologic changes in monkeys subjected to a large number of induced convulsions (32–100). *American Journal of Psychiatry, 106,* 278–284.

Ferraro, A., Roizin, L., & Helfand, M. (1946). Morphologic changes in the brain of monkeys following convulsions electrically induced. *Journal of Neuropathology and Experimental Neurology, 5,* 285–308.

Fieve, R. R. (1989). *Mood swing.* New York: Morrow.

Figiel, G., Coffey, C., Djang, W., Hoffman, G., & Doraiswamy, P. (1990). Brain magnetic resonance imaging findings in ECT-induced delirium. *Neurosciences, 2,* 53–58.

Figueroa, A. (1991, February 12). SF supervisors vote against shock treatment. *San Francisco Chronicle,* p. 3.

Fink, M. (1957). A unified theory of the action of the physiodynamic therapies. *Journal of Hillside Hospital, 6,* 197–206.

Fink, M. (1966). Cholinergic aspects of convulsive therapy. *Journal of Nervous and Mental Disease, 142,* 475–484.

Fink, M. (1974). Induced seizures and human behavior. In M. Fink, S. Kety, J. McGaugh, & T. Williams (Eds.), *Psychobiology of convulsive therapy.* New York: Wiley.

Fink, M. (1979). *Convulsive therapy.* New York: Raven.

Fink, M. (1994, May). Can ECT be an effective treatment for adolescents? *Harvard Mental Health Letter, 10,* p. 8.

Fink, M. (1995, January). Reconsidering ECT in adolescents. *Psychiatric Times,* p. 18.

Fireside, H. (1979). *Soviet psychoprisons.* New York: Norton.

Fischman, M., & Smith, R. (1976). Effects of chlorpromazine on avoidance and escape responses in humans. *Pharmacology, Biochemistry and Behavior, 4,* 111–114.

Fisher, C. M. (1989). Neurological fragments. II. Remarks on anosognosia, confabulation, memory, and other topics; and an appendix on self-observation. *Neurology, 39,* 127–132.

Fisher, J. M. (1985). Cognitive and behavioral consequences of closed head injury. *Seminars in Neurology, 5*(3).

Fisher, R., & Fisher, S. (1996). Antidepressants for children: Is scientific support necessary? *Journal of Nervous and Mental Disease, 184,* 99–102.

Fisher, S., Bryant, S. G., & Kent, T. A. (1993). Postmarketing surveillance by patient self-monitoring: Trazodone versus fluoxetine. *Journal of Clinical Psychopharmacology, 13,* 235–242.

Fisher, S., & Greenberg, R. (1989). *The limits of biological treatments for psychological distress: Comparisons with psychotherapy and placebo.* Hillsdale, NJ: Erlbaum.

Fisher, S., & Greenberg, R. (1995, September/October). Prescriptions for happiness. *Psychology Today,* pp. 32–37.

5-HT blockers and all that (1990, August 11). *Lancet* (editorial) *336,* 345–346.

Fluoxetine (Prozac) revisited. (1990). *The Medical Letter: On Drugs and Therapeutics, 32,* 83–85.

Fog, R., Pakkenberg, H., Juul, P., Bock, E., Jorgensen, O. S., & Andersen, J. (1976). High-dose treatment of rats with perphenazine enanthate. *Psychopharmacology, 50,* 305–307.

Fogel, B. S., & Stone, A. B. (1992). Practical pathophysiology in neuropsy-
    chiatry: A clinical approach to depression and impulsive behavior in
    neurological patients. In S. C. Yudofsky & R. E. Hales (Eds.), *Ameri-
    can Psychiatric Press textbook of Neuropsychiatry* (pp. 329–344).
    Washington, DC: American Psychiatric Press.
Food and Drug Administration (FDA). (1977, September). General consid-
    erations for the clinical evaluation of drugs. Rockville, MD: FDA.
    Obtained through the Freedom of Information Act.
Food and Drug Administration (FDA). (1984, February 24). Transcript
    of Psychopharmacologic Drugs Advisory Committee: 26th Meeting.
    Rockville, MD. Obtained through the Freedom of Information Act.
Food and Drug Administration (FDA). (1985, January 31). Transcript of
    Psychopharmacologic Drugs Advisory Committee (Workshop): 27th
    Meeting. Rockville, MD. Obtained through the Freedom of Informa-
    tion Act.
Food and Drug Administration Quarterly Activities Report (1985, July-
    September). United States v. Eli Lilly and Company. Department of
    Health and Human Services, Public Health Administration, Food and
    Drug Administration, Rockville, MD, p. 2. Obtained through the
    Freedom of Information Act.
Food and Drug Administration (FDA). (1990, September 5). Neurological
    devices; proposed rule to reclassify the electroconvulsive device in-
    tended for use in treating severe depression. 21 CFR Part 882 [Docket
    No. 82P-0316]. *Federal Register, 55*(172), 36578-36590.
Food and Drug Administration (FDA). (1991, September 20). Transcript
    of Psychopharmacologic Drugs Advisory Committee: 34th Meeting.
    Rockville, MD: Department of Health and Human Services, Public
    Health Service, Food and Drug Administration. Obtained through the
    Freedom of Information Act.
Food and Drug Administration (FDA). (1992). New Halcion labeling.
    Medical Bulletin, 22(1), 7.
Food and Drug Administration (FDA). (1993, January 23). Summary of
    post-marketing reports on Prozac from the Spontaneous Reporting
    System of the FDA. Rockville, MD: FDA. Obtained through the
    Freedom of Information Act.
Food and Drug Administration (1994, October 27). Adverse experience
    reporting requirements for human drug and licensed biological prod-
    ucts; proposed rule. *Federal Register* 21 CFR Parts, 20, 310, 312,
    314, and 600.

Food and Drug Administration (FDA). (1995, June). *A MEDWatch contin-uing education article.* Rockville, MD: Staff College, Center for Drug Evaluation and Research, Food and Drug Administration.

Foote, S. (1983, June 1). Reclassification of electroconvulsive therapy device (ECT). Memo from Professor Susan Bartlett Foote, Consumer Representative, Respiratory and Nervous System Device Panel, Neu-rological Section, to Dockets Management Branch (HFA-305), Food and Drug Administration, Rockville, MD. Obtained through the Free-dom of Information Act.

Forrest, F. M., Forrest, I. S., & Roizin, L. (1963). Clinical, biochemical and post mortem studies on a patient treated with chlorpromazine. *Revue Agressologie, 4,* 259–265.

Fowler, M. (1992). *Educators manual: A project of the CH.A.D.D. Na-tional Education Committee.* Plantation, FL: CH.A.D.D.

Frank, L. (Ed.). (1978). *A history of shock treatment.* Available from L. Frank, 2300 Webster Street, San Francisco, CA 94115.

Frank, L. (1979, May). Gleanings. *On the Edge,* p. 11.

Frank, L. (1980, November). San Francisco conference. *On the Edge,* p. 1.

Frank, L. (1990). Electroshock: death, brain damage, memory loss, and brainwashing. *Journal of Mind and Behavior, 11,* 489–512.

Frank, L. (1991, Winter). The Center for the Study of Psychiatry feature report: San Francisco puts electroshock on public trial. *Rights Tenet: Newsletter of the National Association of Rights Protection and Advo-cacy (NARPA),* pp. 3–5.

Freeman, C., & Kendell, R. (1986). Patients' experience of and attitudes to electroconvulsive therapy. *Annals of the New York Academy of Sciences, 462,* 341–352.

French, A. (1989). Dangerous aggressive behavior as a side effect of alprazolam. *American Journal of Psychiatry, 146,* 276.

Freyhan, F. A. (1980, December). Medication compliance. *International Committee for Prevention and Treatment of Depression Bulletin,* p. 3.

Friedberg, J. (1976). *Electroshock is not good for your brain.* San Fran-cisco: Glide.

Friedberg, J. (1977). Shock treatment, brain damage, and memory loss: A neurological perspective. *American Journal of Psychiatry, 134,* 1010–1014.

Friedman, M. J., Culver, C. N., & Ferrell, R. B. (1977). On the safety of long-term treatment with lithium. *American Journal of Psychiatry, 134,* 1123–1126.

From couch to coffee shop: A new personality via 'psychosynthesis.' (1972, November 1). *Roche Report: Frontiers in Psychiatry, 2*(18), 1–2. [pharmaceutical company bulletin]

Fudge, J. L., Perry, P. J., Garvey, M. J., & Kelly, M. W. (1990). A comparison of the effect on fluoxetine and trazodone on the cognitive functioning of depressed outpatients. *Journal of Affective Disorders, 18*, 275–280.

Fuller, R. (1994, April 14). Deposition, Volume I., in Fentress, et al. v. Shea Communications et al., Jefferson Circuit Court, Division One, No. 90-Cl-6033.

Fuller, R. W., Perry, K. W., & Molloy, B. B. (1974). Effect of an uptake inhibitor on serotonin metabolism in rat brain. *Life Sciences, 15*, 1161–1171.

Gaines, D. (1992). *Teenage wasteland: Suburbia's dead end kids.* New York: Harper Perennial.

Gardner, D. L., & Cowdry, R. W. (1985). Alprazolam-induced dyscontrol in borderline personality disorder. *American Journal of Psychiatry, 142*, 98–100.

Gelman, S. (1984). Mental hospital drugs, professionalism, and the constitution. *Georgetown Law Journal, 72*, 1725–1784.

Gerbino, L., Oleshansky, M,, & Gershon, S. (1978). Clinical use and mode of action of lithium. In M. A. Lipton, A. DiMascio, & K. F. Killman, *Psychopharmacology: A generation of progress.* New York: Raven.

Gerlach, J. (1975). Long-term effect of perphenazine on the substantia nigra in rats. *Psychopharmacologia (Berlin), 45*, 51–54.

Gibeaut, J. (1996, August). Mood-altering verdict. *American Bar Association Journal*, p. 18.

Giedd, J. N., Castellanos, F. X., Casey, B. J., Kozuch, P., King, A. C., Hamburger, S. D., & Rapoport, J. L. (1994). Quantitative morphology of the corpus callosum in attention deficit hyperactivity disorder. *American Journal of Psychiatry, 151*, 665–669.

Gillis, J. S. (1975). Effects of chlorpromazine and thiothixene on acute schizophrenic patients. In K. R. Hammond & C. R. B. Joyce (Eds.), *Psychoactive drugs and social judgment* (pp. 109–120). New York: Wiley.

Gitlin, M., Swendsen, J., Heller, T., & Hammen, C. (1995). Relapse and impairment in bipolar disorder. *American Journal of Psychiatry, 152*, 1635–1640.

Glazer, W., Morgenstern, H., & Doucette, J. (1993). Predicting the long-term risk of tardive dyskinesia in outpatients maintained on neuroleptic medications. *Journal of Clinical Psychiatry, 54,* 133–139.

Glazer, W. M., Morgenstern, H., Schooler, N., Berkman, C. S., & Moore, D. C. (1990). Predictors of improvement in tardive dyskinesia following discontinuation of neuroleptic medication. *British Journal of Psychiatry, 157,* 585–592.

Glue, P., Nutt, D., Cowen, P., & Broadbent, D. (1987). Selective effect of lithium on cognitive performance in man. *Psychopharmacology, 91,* 109–111.

Goetz, C. G., Dysken, M. W., & Klawans, A. L. (1980). Assessment and treatment of drug-induced tremor. *Journal of Clinical Psychiatry, 41,* 310–315.

Goetz, K. L., & van Kammen, D. P. (1986). Computerized axial tomography scans and subtypes of schizophrenia: A review of the literature. *Journal of Nervous and Mental Disease, 174,* 31–41.

Gold, M., Miller, N., Stennie, K., & Populla-Vardi, C. (1995). Epidemiology of benzodiazepine use and dependence. *Psychiatric Annals, 25,* 146–148.

Goldberg, E. (1985). Akinesia, tardive dysmentia, and frontal lobe disorder in schizophrenia. *Schizophrenia Bulletin, 11,* 255–263.

Goldberg, T. E., Weinberger, D. R., Berman, K. F., Pliskin, N. H., & Podd, M. H. (1987). Further evidence for dementia of the prefrontal type in schizophrenia. *Archives of General Psychiatry, 44,* 1008–1014.

Golden, C. J., Moses, J. A., Zelazowski, M. A., Graber, B., Zatz, L. M., Horvath, T. B., & Berger, P. A. (1980). Cerebral ventricular size and neuropsychological impairment in young chronic schizophrenics. *Archives of General Psychiatry, 37,* 619–623.

Golden, G. S. (1991). Role of attention deficit hyperactivity disorder in learning disabilities. *Seminars in Neurology, 11*(1), 35–41.

Golombok, S., Moodley, P., & Lader, M. (1988). Cognitive impairment in long-term benzodiazepine users. *Psychological Medicine, 18,* 365–374.

Gomez, G., & Gomez, E. (1990). The special concerns of neuroleptic use in the elderly. *Journal of Psychosocial Nursing, 28*(1), 7–14.

Goodman, A. G., Rall, T. W., Nies, A. S., & Taylor, P. (1991). *The pharmacological basis of therapeutics* (8th ed.). New York: Pergamon.

Goodwin, F. K., & Ebert, M. H. (1977). Specific antimanic-antidepressant drugs. In M. E. Jarvik (Ed.), *Psychopharmacology in the practice of medicine.* New York: Appleton-Century-Crofts.

Goodwin, F., & Jamison, K. (1990). *Manic-depressive illness.* New York: Oxford University Press.

Gorham, D. R., & Sherman, L. J. (1961). The relation of attitude toward medication to treatment outcomes in chemotherapy. *American Journal of Psychiatry, 117,* 830–831.

Government Accounting Office (GAO). (1990, April). *FDA Drug Review: Postapproval Risks 1976–1985.* (Report to the Chairman, Subcommittee on Human Resources and Intergovernmental Relations, Committee on Government Operations, House of Representatives). GAO/PEMD-90-15.

Grahame-Smith, D. G., & Aronson, J. K. (1992). *Oxford textbook of clinical pharmacology and drug therapy.* Oxford: Oxford University Press.

Grant, I., Adams, K. M., Carlin, A. S., Rennick, P. M., Judd, L. L., & Schooff, K. (1978). *The collaborative neuropsychological study of polydrug users.* Unpublished paper delivered at the International Neuropsychological Association Conference, Minneapolis.

Grant, I., Adams, K. M., Carlin, A. S., Rennick, P. M., Judd, L. L., Schooff K., & Reed, R. (1978). Organic impairment in polydrug users: Risk factors. *American Journal of Psychiatry, 135,* 178–184.

Grant, I., Adams, K. M., Carlin, A. S., Rennick, P. M., Lewis, J. L., & Schooff, K. (1978). The collaborative neuropsychological study of polydrug users. *Archives of General Psychiatry, 135,* 1063–1074.

Gratz, S., Levinson, D., & Simpson, G. (1992). Neuroleptic malignant syndrome. In J. Kane & J. Lieberman (Eds.), *Adverse effects of psychotropic drugs.* New York: Guilford.

Green, A. (1989). Physical and sexual abuse of children. In H. Kaplan & B. Sadock (Eds.), *Comprehensive textbook of psychiatry* (pp. 1962–1970). Baltimore: Williams and Wilkins.

Greenberg, H. R., & Blank, H. R. (1973). Serious side effects from routine doses of nonMAO inhibitor antidepressants. *New York State Journal of Medicine, 73,* 1676–1680.

Greenberg, L. B., & Gujavarty, K. (1985). The neuroleptic malignant syndrome: Review and report of three cases. *Comprehensive Psychiatry, 26*(1), 63–70.

Greenberg, R., & Fisher, S. (1989). Examining antidepressant effectiveness: Findings, ambiguities, and some vexing problems. In S. Fisher & R. Greenberg (Eds.), *The limits of biological treatments for psychological distress* (pp. 1–37). Hillsdale, NJ: Erlbaum.

Greenblatt, D. J., Harmatz, J. S., Shapiro, L., Engelhardt, N., Gouthro, T. A., & Shader, R. I. (1991). Sensitivity to triazolam in the elderly. *New England Journal of Medicine, 324,* 1691–1698.

Greenhouse, L. (1979, January 6). Paralyzed convict gets $518,000 award. *New York Times,* p. 6.

Grobe, J. (Ed.) (1995). *Beyond Bedlam: Contemporary women psychiatric survivors speak out.* Chicago: Third Side Press.

Gross, H., & Kaltenback, E. (1968). Neuropathological findings in persistent hyperkinesia after neuroleptic long-term therapy. In A. Cerletti & F. J. Bove (Eds.), *The present status of psychotropic drugs* (pp. 474–476). Amsterdam: Excerpta Medica.

Growe, G. A., Crayton, J. W., Klass, D. B., Evans, H., & Strizich, M. (1979). Lithium in chronic schizophrenia. *American Journal of Psychiatry, 136,* 454–455.

Gualtieri, C. T. (1993). The problem of tardive akathisia. *Brain and Cognition, 23*(1), 102–109.

Gualtieri, C. T., & Barnhill, L. J. (1988). Tardive dyskinesia in special populations. In M. E. Wolf and A. D. Mosnaim (Eds.), *Tardive dyskinesia: Biological mechanisms and clinical aspects* (pp. 135–154). Washington, DC: American Psychiatric Press.

Gualtieri, C. T., Quade, D., Hicks, R. E., Mayo, J. P., & Schroeder, S. R. (1984). Tardive dyskinesia and other clinical consequences of neuroleptic treatment in children and adolescents. *American Journal of Psychiatry, 141,* 20–23.

Gualtieri, C. T., Schroeder, R., Hicks, R., & Quade, D. (1986). Tardive dyskinesia in young mentally retarded individuals. *Archives of General Psychiatry, 43,* 335–340.

Gualtieri, C. T., & Sovner, R. (1989). Akathisia and tardive akathisia. *Psychiatric Aspects of Mental Retardation Reviews, 8*(12), 83–87.

Gunne, L. M., & Haggstrom, J. (1985). Experimental tardive dyskinesia. *Journal of Clinical Psychiatry, 46,* 48–50.

Gur, R. E., Resnick, S. M., Alavi, A., Gur, R. C., Caroff, S., Dann, R., Silver, F. L., Saykin, A. J., Chawluk, J. B., Kushner, M., & Reivich, M. (1987). Regional brain function in schizophrenia. I: A positron emission tomography study. *Archives of General Psychiatry, 44*, 119–125.

Gur, R. E., Resnick, S. M., Gur, R. C., Alavi, A., Caroff, S., Kushner, M., & Reivich, M. (1987). Regional brain function in schizophrenia. II: Repeated evaluation with positron emission tomography. *Archives of General Psychiatry, 44*, 126–129.

Guze, B. H., & Baxter, Jr., L. R. (1985). Neuroleptic malignant syndrome. *New England Journal of Medicine, 313*, 163–164.

Guze, S. B. (1979, May). Learning, memory and mood on lithium. *Psychiatric Capsule and Comment* (Roche Laboratories Publication), p. 2.

Haase, H. J. (1959). The role of drug-induced extrapyramidal syndromes. In N. Kline (Ed.), *Psychopharmacology frontiers* (pp. 197–208). Boston: Little, Brown.

Hall, L. W. (1971). *Wright's veterinary anaesthesia and analgesia* (7th ed.). London: Tindall.

Hall, R. A., Jackson, R. B., & Swain, J. M. (1956). Neurotoxic reactions resulting from chlorpromazine administration. *Journal of the American Medical Association, 161*, 214–216.

Hansen, H., Andersen, R., Theilgaard, A., & Lunn, V. (1982). Stereotactic psychosurgery: A psychiatric and psychological investigation of the effects and side effects of the interventions. *Acta Psychiatrica Scandinavica* (Supp. 301), *66*, 1–123.

Hartelius, H. (1952). Cerebral changes following electrically induced convulsions. *Acta Psychiatrica Neurologica Scandinavica, 77*(Suppl.), 1–128.

Hartlage, L. C. (1965). Effects of chlorpromazine on learning. *Psychological Bulletin, 64*, 235–245.

Henry, J. A., Alexander, C. A., & Sener, E. K. (1995). Relative mortality from overdose of antidepressants. *British Medical Journal, 310*, 221–224.

Hersh, C. B., Sokol, M. S., & Pfeffer, C. R. (1991). Transient psychosis with fluoxetine. *Journal of the Academy of Child and Adolescent Psychiatry, 30*, 851.

Hoenig, J., & Chaulk, R. (1977). Delirium associated with lithium therapy and electroconvulsive therapy. *Canadian Medical Association Journal, 116*, 837–838.

Hogan, T. P., & Awad, A. G. (1983). Pharmacotherapy and suicide risk in schizophrenia. *Canadian Journal of Psychiatry, 28*, 277–281.

Hollister, L. E. (1961). Medical intelligence: Current concepts in therapy. Complications from psychotherapeutic drugs. I. *New England Journal of Medicine, 264*, 291–293.

Hollister, L. E. (1976). Psychiatric disorders. In G. S. Avery (Ed.), *Drug treatment*. Littleton, MA: Publishing Sciences.

Hommer, D. (1991). Benzodiazepines: Cognitive and psychomotor effects. In P. Roy-Byrne & D. Cowley (Eds.), *Benzodiazepines in clinical practice: Risks and benefits*. Washington, DC: American Psychiatric Press.

Hornykiewicz, O. (1967). Extrapyramidal side effects of neuro-(psycho-)tropic drugs. Proceedings of the European Society for the Study of Drug Toxicity, VIII, in *Excerpta Medica* (pp. 122–135), International Congress Series #118.

Hotchner, A. E. (1966). *Papa Hemingway: A personal memoir*. New York: Random House (Bantam Edition).

Huber, S. J., & Paulson, G. W. (1985). The concept of subcortical dementia. *American Journal of Psychiatry, 142*, 1312–1317.

Hudson, W. (1980, March). The mental health professional as advocate. *Advocacy Now*, pp. 12–15.

Hughes, R., & Brewin, R. (1979). *The tranquilizing of America*. New York: Harcourt, Brace, Jovanovich.

Hunt, J., Singh, H., & Simpson, G. (1988). Neuroleptic-induced supersensitivity psychosis: Retrospective study of schizophrenic inpatients. *Journal of Clinical Psychiatry, 49*, 258–261.

Hunter, R., Blackwood, W., Smith, M. C., & Cumings, J. N. (1968). Neuropathological findings in three cases of persistent dyskinesia following phenothiazine medication. *Journal of the Neurological Sciences, 7*, 263–273.

Hunter, R., Earl, C. J., & Thornicroft, S. (1964). An apparently irreversible syndrome of abnormal movements following phenothiazine medication. *Proceedings of the Royal Society of Medicine, 57*, 24–28.

Hyman, S., Arana, G., & Rosenbaum, J. (1995). *Handbook of psychiatric drug therapy* (3rd ed.). New York: Little, Brown.

Hynd, G. W., Semrud-Clikeman, M., Lorys, A. R., Novey, E. S., Eliopulos, D., & Lyytinen, H. (1991). Corpus callosum morphology in attention deficit-hyperactivity disorder: Morphometric analysis of MRI. *Journal of Learning Disabilities, 24*(3), 141–146.

Iacono, W. G., Smith, G. N., Moreau, M., Beiser, M., Fleming, J. A. E., Lin, T., & Flak, B. (1988). Ventricle and sulci size at onset of psychosis. *American Journal of Psychiatry, 145*, 820–824.

Impastato, D. J. (1957, July). Prevention of fatalities in electroshock therapy. *Diseases of the Nervous System*, *18*(7), (sect. 2), 34–74.

Inayatulla, M., & Cantor, S. (1980). Effects of thioridazine on the cognitive functioning of a hypotonic schizophrenic boy. *American Journal of Psychiatry*, *137*, 1459–1460.

Innis, R., & Malison, R. (1995). Principles of neuroimaging. In H. Kaplan & B. Sadock (Eds.), *Comprehensive textbook of psychiatry*. New York: Williams & Wilkins.

In Texas: The more lithium in tap water, the fewer mental cases. (1971, October 15). *Medical World News*, p. 18.

Inuwa, I., Horobin, R., & Williams, A. (1994, July). A TEM study of white blood cells from patients under neuroleptic therapy. *ICEM 13-Paris* [International Congress of Electron Microscopy], pp. 1091–1092.

Itil, T. M., Reisberg, B., Huque, M., & Mehta, D. (1981). Clinical profiles of tardive dyskinesia. *Comprehensive Psychiatry*, *22*, 282–290.

Ivnik, R. J. (1979). Pseudodementia in tardive dyskinesia. *Psychiatric Annals*, *9*, 211–218.

Jacobs, D. J. (1995). Psychiatric Drugging: Forty years of pseudo-science, self-interest, and indifference to harm. *Journal of Mind and Behavior*, *16*, 421–470.

Jafri, A. B., & Greenberg, W. M. (1991, September). Fluoxetine side effects. *Journal of the American Academy of Child and Adolescent Psychiatry*, *30*, 852.

Jamison, K. R., Gerner, R. H., & Goodwin, F. K. (1979). Patient and physician attitudes toward lithium. *Archives of General Psychiatry*, *36*, 866–869.

Jancin, B. (1979, January). Could chronic neuroleptic use cause psychosis? *Clinical Psychiatry News*, p. 1.

Janis, I. L. (1948). Memory loss following electroconvulsive treatments. *Journal of Personality*, *17*, 29–32.

Janis, I. L. (1950). Psychological effects of electric convulsive treatments. *Journal of Nervous and Mental Disease*, *111*, 359–397, 469–489.

Janis, I. L., & Astrachan, M. (1951). The effect of electroconvulsive treatments on memory efficiency. *Journal of Abnormal Psychology*, *46*, 501–511.

Jarvik, M. E. (1970). Drugs used in the treatment of psychiatric disorders. In L. Goodman & H. Gilman (Eds.), *The pharmacological basis of therapeutics* (4th ed.). New York: Macmillan.

Jefferson, J. (1993). Mood stabilizers: A review. In D. Dunner (Ed.), *Current psychiatric therapy* (pp. 246–254). Philadelphia: Saunders.

Jellinck, E. H. (1976). Cerebral atrophy and cognitive impairment in chronic schizophrenia. *Lancet, 2*, 1202–1203.

Jellinger, K. (1977). Neuropathologic findings after neuroleptic long-term therapy. In L. Roizin, H. Shiraki, & N. Grčević (Eds.), *Neurotoxicology* (pp. 25–45). New York: Raven.

Jenner, P., & Marsden, C. D. (1983). Neuroleptics and tardive dyskinesia. In J. T. Coyle & S. J. Enna (Eds.), *Neuroleptics: Neurochemical, behavioral and clinical perspectives* (pp. 223–254). New York: Raven.

Jensen, P., Bain, M., & Josephson, A. (circa 1989). *Why Johnny can't sit still: Kids' ideas why they take stimulants.* Unpublished manuscript.

Jernigan, T. L., Zatz, L. M., Moses, J. A., & Cardellino, J. P. (1982). Computed tomography in schizophrenics and normal volunteers. I: Fluid volume. *Archives of General Psychiatry, 39*, 765–770.

Jerome, L. (1991). Hypomania with fluoxetine. *Journal of the American Academy of Child and Adolescent Psychiatry, 30*, 850–851.

Jeste, D. V., & Caligiuri, M. P. (1993). Tardive dyskinesia. *Schizophrenia Bulletin, 19*, 303–315.

Jeste, D. V., Iager, A. C., & Wyatt, R. J. (1986). The biology and experimental treatment of tardive dyskinesia and other related movement disorders. In P. A. Berger & H. K. Brodie (Eds.), *Biological psychiatry* (pp. 535–580). New York: Basic Books.

Jeste, D. V., Lacro, J. P., Gilbert, P. L., Kline, J., & Kline, N. (1993). Treatment of late-life schizophrenia with neuroleptics. *Schizophrenia Bulletin, 19*, 817–830.

Jeste, D. V., Lohr, J., & Manley, M. (1992). Study of neuropathologic changes in the striatum following 4, 8 and 12 months of treatment with fluphenazine in rats. *Psychopharmacology, 106*, 154–160.

Jeste, D. V., Wagner, R. L., Weinberger, D. R., Reith, K. G. R., & Wyatt, R. J. (1980). Evaluation of CT scans in tardive dyskinesia. *American Journal of Psychiatry, 137*, 247–248.

Jeste, D. V., Wisniewski, A. A., & Wyatt, R. J. (1986). Neuroleptic-associated tardive syndromes. *Psychiatric Clinics of North America, 9*, 183–192.

Jeste, D. V., & Wyatt, R. J. (1981). Changing epidemiology of tardive dyskinesia: An overview. *American Journal of Psychiatry, 138*, 297–309.

Jeste, D. V., & Wyatt, R. J. (1982). *Understanding and treating tardive dyskinesia.* New York: Guilford.

Jick, S., Dean, A., & Jick, H. (1995). Antidepressants and suicide. *British Medical Journal, 310,* 215–219.

Johnson, G., Gershon, S., & Hekimian, L. J. (1968). Controlled evaluation of lithium chlorpromazine in treatment of manic states: An interim report. *Comprehensive Psychiatry, 9,* 563–573.

Johnson, M., & Barash, D. (1991). A review of postmarketing adverse drug experience reporting requirements. *Food, Drug, & Cosmetic Law Journal, 46,* 665–672.

Johnstone, E. C., Crow, T. J., Frith, C. D., Husband, J., & Kreel, L. (1976). Cerebral ventricular size and cognitive impairment in chronic schizophrenia. *Lancet, 2,* 924–926.

Johnstone, E. C., Crow, T. J., Frith, C. D., Stevens, M., Kreel, L., & Husband, J. (1978). The dementia of dementia praecox. *Acta Psychiatrica Scandinavica, 57,* 305–324.

Jonas, J. (1992, October). Dr. Jeffrey M. Jonas, director of CNS clinical development at Upjohn, replies. *Clinical Psychiatry News,* p. 5.

Jones, B. D. (1985). Tardive dysmentia: Further comments. With commentary by S. Mukherjee & R. M. Bilder. *Schizophrenia Bulletin, 11,* 87–190.

Jorgensen, H., & Harris, J. S. (1992). The drug research process. *Dermatology Nursing, 4*(6).

Judd, L. L. (1979). Effect of lithium on mood, cognition, and personality function in normal subjects. *Archives of General Psychiatry, 36,* 860–865.

Judd, L. L., Hubbard, B., Janowsky, D. S., Huey, L. Y., & Attewell, P. A. (1977). The effect of lithium carbonate on affect, mood, and personality of normal subjects. *Archives of General Psychiatry, 34,* 346–351.

Judd, L. L., Hubbard, B., Janowsky, D. S., Huey, L. Y., & Takahashi, K. I. (1977). The effect of lithium carbonate on the cognitive function of normal subjects. *Archives of General Psychiatry, 34,* 355–357.

Judd, L., Squire, L., Butters, N., Salmon, D., & Paller, K. (1987). Effects of psychotropic drugs on cognition and memory in normal humans and animals. In H. Y. Meltzer (Ed.), *Psychopharmacology: The third generation of progress* (pp. 1467–1475). New York: Raven.

Juhl, R. P., Tsuang, M. T., & Perry, P. J. (1977). Concomitant administration of haloperidol and lithium carbonate in acute mania. *Diseases of the Nervous System, 38,* 675–676.

Kahn, R., Fink, M., & Weinstein, E. (1956). Relation of amobarbital test to clinical improvement in electroshock. *Archives of Neurology and Psychiatry, 76,* 23–29.

Kales, A. (1991, September). An overview of safety problems of triazolam. *International Drug Therapy Newsletter, 26*(7), 25–28.

Kales, A., Bixler, E. O., & Vgontzas, A. N. (1993). The evidence against is extensive and consistent. *British Medical Journal, 307,* 626.

Kales, A., Manfedi, R. L., Vgontzas, A. N., Bixler, E. O., Vela-Bueno, A., & Fee, E. C. (1991). Rebound insomnia after only brief and intermittent use of rapidly eliminated benzodiazepines. *Clinical Pharmacology and Therapeutics, 49,* 468–476.

Kales, A., Scharf, M. B., & Kales, J. D. (1978). Rebound insomnia: A new clinical syndrome. *Science, 201,* 1039–1041.

Kales, A., Soldatos, C. R., Bixler, E. O., & Kales, J. D. (1983). Rebound insomnia and rebound anxiety: A review. *Pharmacology, 26,* 121–137.

Kalinowsky, L. (1959). Convulsive shock treatment. In S. Arieti (Ed.), *American handbook of psychiatry, Vol. II.* New York: Basic Books.

Kalinowsky, L. (1973). Attempt at localization of psychological manifestations observed in various psychosurgical procedures. In L. Laitinen & K. Livingston (Eds.), *Surgical approaches to psychiatry* (pp. 18–21). Baltimore: University Park Press.

Kalinowsky, L. (1975). The convulsive therapies. In A. M. Freedman, H. I. Kaplan, & B. J. Sadock (Eds.), *Comprehensive textbook of psychiatry.* Baltimore: Williams and Wilkins.

Kalinowsky, L., & Hippius, H. (1969). *Pharmacological, convulsive and other somatic treatments in psychiatry.* New York: Grune and Stratton.

Kane, J., & Lieberman, J. (1992). Tardive dyskinesia. In J. Kane & J. Lieberman (Eds.), *Adverse effects of psychotropic drugs.* New York: Guilford.

Kane, J., Rifkin, A., Quitkin, F., & Klein, D. (1978). Extrapyramidal side effects with lithium treatment. *American Journal of Psychiatry, 135,* 851–853.

Kane, J. M., Safferman, A. Z., Pollack, S., Johns, C., Szymanski, S., Kronig, M., & Lieberman, J. A. (1994). Clozapine, negative symptoms and extrapyramidal side effects. *Journal of Clinical Psychiatry, 55*(9) (supp. B), 74–77.

Kapit, R. M. (1986, March 28). Safety review of NDA 18-936 [Prozac]. Internal document of the Department of Health and Human Services, Public Health Service, Food and Drug Administration, Center for Drug Evaluation and Research. Obtained through the Freedom of Information Act.

Kapit, R. M. (1986, October 17). Safety Update. NDA 18-936. Internal document of the Department of Health and Human Services, Public Health Service, Food and Drug Administration, Center for Drug Evaluation and Research. Obtained through the Freedom of Information Act.

Kapit, R. M. (1986, December 17). Response to Dr. Laughren's Q's regarding Review of Safety Update, Memo #3. NDA 18-936. Internal document of the Department of Health and Human Services, Public Health Service, Food and Drug Administration, Center for Drug Evaluation and Research. Obtained through the Freedom of Information Act.

Kapit, R. M. (1987, December 10). Review and evaluation of clinical data. NDA 18-936. Internal document of the Department of Health and Human Services, Public Health Service, Food and Drug Administration, Center for Drug Evaluation and Research. Obtained through the Freedom of Information Act.

Kapit, R. M. (1988, March 4). Memorandum: Revision of Clinical Portion of Prozac SBA. NDA 18-936. Internal document, Department of Health and Human Services, Public Health Service, Food and Drug Administration, Center for Drug Evaluation and Research. Obtained through the Freedom of Information Act.

Karel, R. (1994, January 7). Federal agency blamed for serious shortage of Ritalin. *Psychiatric News*, p. 14.

Karon, B., & Vandenbos, G. (1981). *The psychotherapy of schizophrenia: The treatment of choice*. New York: Aronson.

Kaufman, E. (1980). The violation of psychiatric standards of care in prison. *American Journal of Psychiatry, 137*, 566–570.

Kelso, Jr., J. R., Cadet, J. L., Pickar, D., & Weinberger, D. R. (1988). Quantitative neuroanatomy in schizophrenia: A controlled magnetic resonance imaging study. *Archives of General Psychiatry, 45*, 533–541.

Kennedy, D. L., & McGinnis, T. (1993, September). Monitoring adverse drug reactions: The FDA's new MedWatch program. Rockville, MD:

Food and Drug Administration. Obtained through the Freedom of Information Act.

Kessler, D. (1993). Introducing MEDWatch: A new approach to reporting medication and device adverse effects and product problems. *Journal of the American Medical Association, 269,* 2765–2768.

Kielholz, P. (1980, December). Side effects of antidepressants. *International Committee for the Prevention and Treatment of Depression Bulletin 4,* pp. 4–5.

King, R. A., Riddle, M. A., Chappell, P. B., Hardin, M. T., Anderson, G. M., Lombroso, P., & Scahill, L. (1991). Emergence of self-destructive phenomena in children and adolescents during fluoxetine treatment. *Journal of the American Academy of Child and Adolescent Psychiatry, 30,* 695.

Kinross-Wright, V. (1955). Complications of chlorpromazine treatment. *Diseases of the Nervous System, 16,* 114–119.

Kirk, A., & Kutchins, H. (1992). *The selling of DSM: The rhetoric of science in psychiatry.* New York: Aldine De Gruyter.

Kirkpatrick, B., Alphs, L., & Buchanan, R. (1992). The concept of super-sensitivity psychosis. *Journal of Nervous and Mental Diseases, 180,* 265–270.

Klawans, H. L. (1973). The pharmacology of tardive dyskinesias. *American Journal of Psychiatry, 130,* 82–87.

Klerman, G. L., & Cole, J. O. (1965). Clinical pharmacology of imipramine and related antidepressant compounds. *Pharmacological Reviews, 17,* 101–141.

Kochansky, G. E., Salzman, C., Shader, R. I., Harmatz, J. S., & Ogeltree, A. M. (1975). The differential effects of chlordiazepoxide and oxazepam on hostility in a small group setting. *American Journal of Psychiatry, 132,* 861–863.

Kolata, G. (1991, January 23). Nursing homes are criticized on how they tie and drug some patients. *New York Times,* p. A13.

Kolata, G. (1992, January 20). Maker of sleeping pill [Halcion] hid data on side effects, researchers say. *New York Times,* p. 1.

Kolb, L. (1977). *Modern clinical psychiatry* (9th ed.). Philadelphia: Saunders.

Korczyn, A. D., & Goldberg, G. J. (1976). Extrapyramidal effects of neuroleptics. *Journal of Neurology, Neurosurgery and Psychiatry, 39,* 866–869.

Koshino, Y., Hiramatsu, H., Isaki, K., & Yamaguchi, N. (1986). An electroencephalographic study of psychiatric inpatients with antipsychotic-induced tardive dyskinesia. *Clinical Electroencephalography*, *17*, 30–35.

Kostowski, W. (1978). Effects of sedatives and major tranquilizers in aggressive behavior. *Modern Problems in Pharmacopsychiatry*, *13*, 1–12.

Kramer, J. C. (1970). Introduction to amphetamine abuse. In E. H. Ellinwood & S. Cohen (Eds.), *Current concepts on amphetamine abuse: Proceedings of a workshop, Duke University Medical Center, June 5–6, 1970*. Rockville, MD: National Institute of Mental Health.

Kramer, J. C., Lipton, M., Ellinwood, Jr., E. H., & Sulser, F. (Chairpersons). (1970). Discussion of part II. In E. H. Ellinwood & S. Cohen (Eds.), *Current concepts on amphetamine abuse: Proceedings of a workshop, Duke University Medical Center, June 5–6, 1970*. Rockville, MD: National Institute of Mental Health.

Krishnan, K. R. R., Ellinwood, Jr., E. H., & Rayasam, K. (1988). Tardive dyskinesia: Structural changes in the brain. In M. E. Wolf & A. D. Mosnaim (Eds.), *Tardive dyskinesia: Biological mechanisms and clinical aspects* (pp. 165–178). Washington, DC: American Psychiatric Press.

Kroessler, D., & Fogel, B. (1993). Electroconvulsive therapy for major depression in the oldest of old. *American Journal of Geriatric Psychiatry*, *1*, 30–37.

Kroph, D., & Müller-Oerlinghausen, B. (1979). Changes in learning, memory, and mood during lithium treatment. *Acta Psychiatrica Scandinavica*, *59*, 97–124.

Kruesi, M., Hibbs, E., Zahn T., Keysor, C., Hamburger, S., Bartko, J., & Rapoport, J. (1992, June). A 2-year prospective follow-up study of children and adolescents with disruptive behavior disorders: Prediction by cerebrospinal fluid 5-hydroxyindoleacetic acid, homovanillic acid, and autonomic measures? *Archives of General Psychiatry*, *49*, 429–435.

Kruse, W. (1960). Persistent muscular restlessness after phenothiazine treatment: A report of three cases. *American Journal of Psychiatry*, *117*, 152–153.

Kuehnel, T. G., & Slama, K. M. (1984). Guidelines for the developmentally disabled. In K. M. Tardiff (Ed.), *The psychiatric uses of seclusion and restraint* (pp. 87–102). Washington, DC: American Psychiatric Press.

Lacro, J. P., Gilbert, P. L., Paulsen, J. S., Fell, R., Bailey, A., Juels, C., Caligiuri, M., McAdams, L. A., Harris, M. J., & Jeste, D. V. (1994). Early course of new-onset tardive dyskinesia in older patients. *Psychopharmacology Bulletin, 30,* 187–191.

Lader, M. (1993). Neuroleptic-induced deficit syndrome. *Journal of Clinical Psychiatry, 54,* 493–500.

Lader, M., & Petursson, H. (1984). Computed axial brain tomography in long-term benzodiazepine users. *Psychological Medicine, 14,* 203–206.

Laporta, M., Chouinard, G., Goldbloom, D., & Beauclair, L. (1987). Hypomania induced by sertraline, a new serotonin reuptake inhibitor. *American Journal of Psychiatry, 144,* 1513–1514.

Laughren, T. (1991, December 10). Zoloft NDA Approval Action Recommendation. Memorandum to File. Internal document of the Department of Health and Human Services, Public Health Service, Food and Drug Administration, Center for Drug Evaluation and Research. Obtained through the Freedom of Information Act.

Laughren, T. (1992). Premarketing safety evaluation of new drugs. In J. Kane & J. Lieberman (Eds.), *Adverse effects of psychotropic drugs.* New York: Guilford.

Lavin, M., & Rifkin, A. (1992). Neuroleptic-induced parkinsonism. In J. Kane & J. Lieberman (Eds.), *Adverse effects of psychotropic drugs.* New York: Guilford.

Lawson, W. B., Waldman, I. N., & Weinberger, D. R. (1988). Schizophrenic dementia: Clinical and computed axial tomography correlates. *Journal of Nervous and Mental Disease, 176,* 207–212.

Lebegue, B. (1987). Mania precipitated by fluoxetine. *American Journal of Psychiatry, 144,* 1620.

Leber, P. (1984, summer). Untitled letter from the Director, Division of Neuropharmacological Drug Products, Office of Drug Research and Review, Center for Drugs and Biologics, the Food and Drug Administration, Rockville, Maryland, to all manufacturers of neuroleptics concerning the proposed new class label for neuroleptics. Obtained through the Freedom of Information Act.

Leber, P. (1988). The emperor's clothes revisited. In *Proceedings of the American Statistical Association, Biopharmaceuticals Section* (pp. 9–14). Alexandria, VA: ASA (New Orleans).

Leber, P. (1991, December 24). Recommendation to Approve NDA 19-839 (Zoloft; sertraline). Memorandum to Robert Temple. Internal document of the Department of Health and Human Services, Public Health Service, Food and Drug Administration, Center for Drug Evaluation and Research. Obtained through the Freedom of Information Act.

Leber, P. (1992). Postmarketing surveillance of adverse drug effects. In J. Kane & J. Lieberman (Eds.), *Adverse effects of psychotropic drugs* (pp. 3–12). New York: Guilford.

Lehmann, H. E. (1955). Therapeutic results with chlorpromazine (Largactile) in psychiatric conditions. *Canadian Medical Association Journal, 72,* 91–99.

Lehmann, H. E. (1970). The philosophy of long-acting medication in psychiatry. *Diseases of the Nervous System, 31*(Suppl.), 7–9.

Lehmann, H. E. (1975, Summer). Psychopharmacological treatment of schizophrenia. *Schizophrenia Bulletin,* pp. 25–45.

Lehmann, H. E., & Hanrahan, G. C. (1954). Chlorpromazine, a new inhibiting agent for psychomotor excitement and manic states. *Archives of Neurology and Psychiatry, 71,* 227–237.

Leipzig, R. M., & Saltz, B. (1992). Adverse reactions to psychotropics in geriatric patients. In J. Kane & J. Lieberman (Eds.), *Adverse effects of psychotropic drugs* (pp. 447–469). New York: Guilford.

Levenson, J. L. (1985). Neuroleptic malignant syndrome. *American Journal of Psychiatry, 142,* 1137–1145.

Liberman, R. (1961). A criticism of drug therapy in psychiatry. *Archives of General Psychiatry, 4,* 131–136.

Lidbeck, W. L. (1944). Pathologic changes in the brain after electric shock: An experimental study on dogs. *Journal of Neuropathology and Experimental Neurology, 3,* 81–86.

Lidz, T. (1981). Psychoanalysis, schizophrenia, and the art of book reviewing [letter]. *American Journal of Psychiatry, 138,* 854.

Linnoila, M., Saario, I., & Maki, M. (1974). Effect of treatment with diazepam or lithium and alcohol on psychomotor skills related to driving. *European Journal of Clinical Pharmacology, 7,* 337–342.

Lipinski, Jr., J. F., Mallaya, G., Zimmerman, P., & Pope, Jr., H. G. (1989, September). Fluoxetine-induced akathisia: Clinical and theoretical implications. *Journal of Clinical Psychiatry, 50,* 339–352.

Logan, J. (1976). *Josh: My up and down, in and out life.* New York: Delacorte.

Lohr, J. B., & Bracha, H. S. (1988). Association of psychosis with movement disorders in the elderly. *Psychiatric Clinics of North America, 11*, 61–68.

Louie, A., Lannon, R., & Ajari, L. (1994). Withdrawal reaction after sertraline discontinuation (letter). *American Journal of Psychiatry, 151*, 450–451.

Lucki, I., Rickels, K., & Geller, A. (1986). Chronic use of benzodiazepines and psychomotor and cognitive test performance. *Psychopharmacology, 88*, 426–433.

Lund, D. S. (1989, May). Tardive dyskinesia lawsuits on increase. *Psychiatric Times*, p. 1.

Lyon, K., Wilson, J., Golden, C. J., Graber, B., Coffman, J. A., & Bloch, S. (1981). Effects of long-term neuroleptic use on brain density. *Psychiatric Research, 5*, 33–37.

Mackiewicz, J., & Gershon, S. (1964). An experimental study of the neuropathological and toxicological effects of chlorpromazine and reserpine. *Journal of Neuropsychiatry, 5*, 159–169.

"Madhouse" brainwashing—The Soviets' method. (1976, February 16). *U.S. News and World Report*, p. 30.

Mahendra, D. (1995). Two cases of risperidone-induced neuroleptic malignant syndrome [one of the two cases] (letter). *American Journal of Psychiatry, 152*, 1233–1234.

Maletzky, B. M. (1981). *Multiple-monitored electroconvulsive therapy.* Boca Raton, FL: CRC Press.

Mandel, M. R., Madsen, J., Miller, A. L., & Baldessarini, R. J. (1980). Intoxication associated with lithium and ECT. *American Journal of Psychiatry, 137*, 1107–1109.

Marcus, L., Plasky, P., & Salzman, C. (1988). Effects of psychotropic drugs on memory: Part I. *Hospital and Community Psychiatry, 39*, 255–256.

Marini, J. L., & Sheard, M. H. (1977). Antiaggressive effect of lithium ion in man. *Acta Psychiatrica Scandinavica, 55*, 269–285.

Marsden, C. D. (1976). Cerebral atrophy and cognitive impairment in chronic schizophrenia. *Lancet, 2*, 1079.

Marsden, C., & Obeso, J. (1994). The functions of the basal ganglia and the paradox of stereotaxic surgery in Parkinson's disease. *Brain, 117*, 877–897.

Marsden, C. D., & Parkes, J. D. (1977). Success and problems of long-term levodopa therapy in Parkinson's disease. *Lancet, 1*, 345–349.

Marshall, R., Printz, D., Cardenas, D., & Liebowitz, M. (1995). Adverse events in PTSD patients taking fluoxetine (letter). *American Journal of Psychiatry, 152,* 1238–1239.

Marvel, D. (1993, March 15). Letter to Peter R. Breggin from the Clinical Research Administrator, Drug Epidemiology Unit, Lilly Research Laboratories, a Division of Eli Lilly and Company, Indianapolis, IN.

Matheson Commission (1939). *Epidemic encephalitis.* New York: Columbia University Press.

Matsubara, T., & Hagihara, B. (1968). Action mechanism of phenothiazine derivatives on mitochondrial respiration. *Journal of Biochemistry, 63,* 156–164.

Maxmen, J. S. (1991). *Psychotropic drugs fast facts.* New York: Norton.

Maxmen, J., & Ward, N. (1995). *Psychotropic drugs fast facts.* New York: Norton.

May, R. (1959). Catatonic-like states following phenothiazine therapy. *American Journal of Psychiatry, 115,* 1119–1120.

Mayerhoff, D., & Lieberman, J. (1992). Behavioral effects of neuroleptics. In J. Kane & J. Lieberman (Eds.), *Adverse effects of psychotropic drugs.* New York: Guilford.

Mayfield, D., & Brown, R. G. (1966). The clinical and electroencephalographic effects of lithium. *Journal of Psychiatric Research, 4,* 207–219.

McCabe, M. S. (1977). ECT in the treatment of mania: A controlled study. *American Journal of Psychiatry, 133,* 88–91.

McClelland, R. J., Fenton, G. W., & Rutherford, W. (1994). The postconcussional syndrome revisited. *Journal of the Royal Society of Medicine, 87,* 508–510.

McCready, K. (1995, Summer). What heals human beings? Technology or humanity—there is a choice [Report from the Center for the Study of Psychiatry and Psychology]. *Rights Tenet: Newsletter of the National Association for Rights Protection and Advocacy (NARPA),* p. 3.

McDonald, M. C. (1979, April 20). Damages awarded in drug misuse case. *Psychiatric News,* p. 1.

McEvoy, J. (1987). A double-blind crossover comparison of antiparkinsonism drug therapy: Amantadine versus anticholinergics in 90 normal volunteers, with an emphasis on differential effects on memory function. *Journal of Clinical Psychiatry, 48*(Supp.), 20–23.

McGuinness, D. (1989). Attention deficit disorder: The emperor's new clothes, animal "pharm," and other fiction. In S. Fisher & R. P.

Greenberg (Eds.), *The limits of biological treatments for psychological distress* (pp. 151–188). Hillsdale, NJ: Erlbaum.

McKeith, I., Fairbairn, A., Perry, R., Thompson, P., & Perry, E. (1992). Neuroleptic sensitivity in patients with senile dementia of Lewy body type. *British Medical Journal, 305,* 673–678.

McMahon, T. C. (1986). A clinical overview of syndromes following withdrawal from antidepressants. *Hospital and Community Psychiatry, 37,* 883–884.

Meeks, J. E. (1975). Child psychiatry: Behavior disorders of childhood and adolescence. In A. M. Freedman, H. I. Kaplan, & B. J. Sadock (Eds.), *Comprehensive textbook of psychiatry* (2nd ed.). Baltimore: Williams and Wilkins.

Meerloo, J. A. M. (1955). Medication into submission: The danger of therapeutic coercion. *Journal of Nervous and Mental Diseases, 122,* 353–360.

Meldrum, B. S., & Brierley, J. B. (1973, January). Prolonged epileptic seizures in primates: Ischemic cell change and its relation to ictal physiological events. *Archives of Neurology, 28,* 10–17.

Meldrum, B. S., Horton, R. W., & Brierley, J. B. (1974). Epileptic brain damage in adolescent baboons following seizures induced by allylglycine. *Brain, 97,* 407–418.

Meldrum, B. S., Vigouroux, R. A., & Brierley, J. B. (1973). Systematic factors and epileptic brain damage: Prolonged seizures in paralyzed, artificially ventilated baboons. *Archives of Neurology, 29,* 82–87.

Meltzer, H. Y. (1995, March). Neuroleptic withdrawal in schizophrenic patients: An idea whose time has come. *Archives of General Psychiatry, 52,* 200–202.

Meltzer, H. Y., Young, M., Metz, J., Fang, V. S., Schyve, P. M., & Arora, R. C. (1979). Extrapyramidal side effects and increased serum prolactin following fluoxetine, a new antidepressant. *Journal of Neural Transmission, 45,* 165–175.

Merritt, H. (1979). *A textbook of neurology* (6th ed.). Philadelphia: Lea & Febiger.

Metoclopramide-induced movement disorders "severely underestimated." *Clinical Psychiatry News,* p. 4.

Micer, V., & Lynch, D. M. (1974). Effect of lithium on disturbed severely mentally retarded patients. *British Journal of Psychiatry, 125,* 110.

Millett, K. (1990). *The loony-bin trip.* New York: Simon and Schuster.

Milstein, V., Small, J. G., Small, I. F., & Green, G. E. (1986). Does electroconvulsive therapy prevent suicide? *Convulsive Therapy, 2*, 3–6.

Mintz, M. (1965). *The therapeutic nightmare.* Boston: Houghton Mifflin.

Mirsky, A. F. (1970). An overview of neuroelectrophysiologic studies of central-acting drugs. In A. DiMascio & R. Shrader, *Clinical handbook of psychopharmacology.* New York: Science House.

Mirsky, A. F., Primac, D. W., & Bates, R. (1959). The effects of chlorpromazine and secobarbital on the CPT. *Journal of Nervous and Mental Diseases, 129*, 12–17.

Mitford, J. (1973). *Kind and usual punishment.* New York: Knopf.

Moch, J., Borja, A., & O'Donnell, J. (1995). *Pharmacy law: Litigating pharmaceutical cases.* Tucson, AZ: Lawyers & Judges.

Modrow, J. (1992). *How to become a schizophrenic: The case against biological psychiatry.* Seattle: Apollyon Press.

Moon, C. A. L., Ankier, S. I., & Hayes, G. (1985, September). Early morning insomnia and daytime anxiety—A multicentre general practice study comparing loprazolam and triazolam. *British Journal of Clinical Practice*, 352–358.

Moore, S., & Jones, J. (1985). Adverse drug reaction surveillance in the geriatric population: A preliminary review. In S. Moore & T. Teal (Eds.), *Geriatric drug use—Clinical & social perspectives* (pp. 70–77). New York: Pergamon.

Morgan, T. (1974, February 17). Entombed. *New York Times Magazine.*

Morrison, S. D., Erwin, C. W., Gionturco, D. T., & Gerber, C. J. (1973). Effect of lithium on combative behavior in humans. *Diseases of the Nervous System, 34*, 186–189.

Mosher, L. R., & Burti, L. (1989). *Community mental health: Principles and practice.* New York: Norton.

Mukherjee, S. (1984). Tardive dysmentia. A reappraisal. *Schizophrenia Bulletin, 10*, 151–152.

Mukherjee, S., & Bilder, R. M. (1985). Commentary. *Schizophrenia Bulletin, 11*, 189–190.

Müller-Oerlinghausen, B., Bauer, H., Girke, W., Kanowski, S., & Goncalves, N. (1977). Impairment of vigilance and performance under lithium treatment: Studies in patients and normal volunteers. *Pharmakopsychiatrie Neuro-psychopharmakologie, 10*, 67–68.

Murray, M. J., & Hooberman, D. (1993, January). Fluoxetine and prolonged erection. *American Journal of Psychiatry, 150*, 167–168.

Myslobodsky, M. S. (1986). Anosognosia in tardive dyskinesia: "Tardive dysmentia" or "tardive dementia"? *Schizophrenia Bulletin, 12,* 1–6.

Myslobodsky, M. S. (1993, September). Central determinants of attention and mood disorder in tardive dyskinesia ("tardive dysmentia"). *Brain and Cognition, 23*(1), 88–101.

Myslobodsky, M. S., Tomer, R., Holden, T., Kempler, S., & Sigol, M. (1985). Cognitive impairment in patients with tardive dyskinesia. *Journal of Nervous and Mental Disease, 173,* 156–160.

Nasrallah, H. A., Loney, J., Olson, S. C., McCalley-Whitters, M., Kramer, J., & Jacoby, C. G. (1986). Cortical atrophy in young adults with a history of hyperactivity in childhood. *Psychiatry Research, 17,* 241–246.

National Institute of Mental Health. (1970). *Lithium in the treatment of mood disorders* (National Clearinghouse for Mental Health Publication No. 5033). Rockville, MD: Department of Health, Education, and Welfare.

Neuroleptics to carry FDA class warning. (1985, May 17). *Psychiatric News,* p. 1.

A new old treatment. (1973, July 9). *Newsweek.*

Newsday (1994, October 29). FDA tightens testing rules in response to Lilly drug. *Fort Wayne Journal-Gazette, p. 3A.*

Nicholi, A. M. (Ed.). (1978). The Harvard guide to modern psychiatry. Cambridge, MA: Belknap.

Nicholi, A. M. (Ed.). (1988). *The new Harvard guide to psychiatry.* Cambridge, MA: Belknap.

Nielsen, E. G., & Lyon, M. (1978). Evidence for cell loss in corpus striatum after long-term treatment with a neuroleptic drug (flupenthixol) in rats. *Psychopharmacology, 59,* 85–89.

Nies, A. S. (1996). Principles of therapeutics. In A. G. Goodman, T. W. Rall, A. S. Nies, & T. Palmer (Eds.), *The pharmacological basis of therapeutics* (9th ed.) (pp. 63–86). New York: Pergamon.

Nishino, S., Mignot, E., & Dement, W. (1995). Sedative-hypnotics. In A. Schatzberg & C. Nemeroff (Eds.), *The American Psychiatric Press textbook of psychopharmacology* (pp. 405–416). Washington, DC: American Psychiatric Press.

Nitenson, N. C., Kando, J. C., Frankenburg, F. R., & Zanarini, M. C. (1995). Fever associated with clozapine administration. *American Journal of Psychiatry, 152,* 1102.

Nolan, L., & O'Malley, K. (1988). Prescribing for the elderly: Part I: Sensitivity of the elderly to adverse drug reactions. *Journal of the American Geriatrics Society, 36,* 142–149.

Noyes, A. P., & Kolb, L. C. (1958). *Modern clinical psychiatry* (5th ed.). Philadelphia: Saunders.

Noyes, R. (1992, February). Discontinuing benzodiazepine use in anxiety disorder patients. *Psychiatric Times,* p. 39.

Nyback, H., Weisel, F-A., Berggren, B-M., & Hindmarsh, T. (1982). Computed tomography of the brain in patients with acute psychoses and healthy volunteers. *Acta Psychiatrica Scandinavica, 65,* 403–414.

O'Donovan, M. C., & McGuffin, P. (1993, April 10). Short acting benzodiazepines. *British Medical Journal, 306,* 945–946.

Ogilvie, J. (1992, fall). Drugging for time: Medicating the pretrial detainee. *The California Prisoner,* p. 14.

Opton, E. M. (1974). Psychiatric violence against prisoners: When therapy is punishment. *Mississippi Law Journal, 45,* 605–655.

Oregon State Prisoner. (1971, December 24). Con's punishment by drugs laid out. *Berkeley Barb,* p. 1.

Oswald, I. (1991). Safety of triazolam. *Lancet, 338,* 516–517.

Pakkenberg, H., Fog, R., & Nilakantan, B. (1973). The long-term effect of perphenazine enanthate on the rat brain. Some metabolic and anatomical observations. *Psychopharmacologia (Berlin), 29,* 329–336.

Pande, A. C., Grunhaus, L. J., Aisen, A. M., & Haskett, R. F. (1990). A preliminary magnetic resonance imaging study of ECT-treated depressed patients. *Biological Psychiatry, 27,* 102–104.

Patient may not be cognizant of his dyskinetic manifestations. (1982, July). *Clinical Psychiatry News,* p. 14.

Patients, public need full story on shock therapy (editorial). (1995, December 8). *USA Today,* p. 12A.

Pauker, N. E. (1981). Trimipramine: A safe, effective antidepressant. *Psychiatric Annals, 11,* 375–378.

Paulsen, J., Heaton, R., & Jeste, D. (1994). Neuropsychological impairment in tardive dyskinesia. *Neuropsychology, 8,* 227–241.

Paulson, G. M. (1959). Phenothiazine toxicity, extrapyramidal seizures, oculo-gyric crises. *Journal of Mental Science, 105,* 798–802.

Peace, K. E. (1987). Design, monitoring, and analysis issues relative to adverse events. *Drug Information Journal, 21,* 21–28.

Peach, M. J. (1975). Cations: calcium, magnesium, barium, lithium, and ammonium. In S. Goodman & A. Gilman, *The pharmacological basis of therapeutics* (5th ed.). New York: Macmillan.

Pettinati, H., & Bonner, K. (1984). Cognitive functioning in depressed geriatric patients with a history of ECT. *American Journal of Psychiatry, 141,* 49–52.

Physicians' desk reference. (1973). Oradell, NJ: Medical Economics.

Physicians' desk reference. (1978). Oradell, NJ: Medical Economics.

Physicians' desk reference. (1995). Montvale, NJ: Medical Economics.

Physicians' desk reference. (1996). Montvale, NJ: Medical Economics.

Pitner, J. K., Mintzer, J. E., Pennypacker, L. C., & Jackson, C. W. (1995). Efficacy and adverse effects of clozapine in four elderly psychotic patients. *Journal of Clinical Psychiatry, 56*(5), 180–185.

Plotkin, R., & Rigling, K. (1979). Invisible manacles: Drugging mentally retarded people. *Stanford Law Review, 31,* 637–678.

Podrabinek, A. (1979). Punitive medicine: A summary. In H. Fireside, *Soviet psychoprisons.* New York: Norton.

Pohl, R., & Gershon, S. (1981). Nomifensine: A new antidepressant. *Psychiatric Annals, 11,* 391–395.

Polatin, P., & Fieve, R. R. (1971). Patient rejection of lithium carbonate prophylaxis. *Journal of the American Medical Association, 218,* 864–866.

Pope, H., Keck, P., & McElroy, S. (1986). Frequency and presentation of neuroleptic malignant syndrome in a large psychiatric hospital. *American Journal of Psychiatry, 143,* 1227–1223.

Popova, E. N. (1967). On the effect of some neuropharmacological agents on the structure of neurons of various cyto-architectonic formations. *Journal für Hirnforschung, 9,* 71–89.

Post, L. (1994). Risperidone (letter). *Hospital and Community Psychiatry, 45,* 1147.

Potter, J. W. (1995, April 19). Corrected Judgment and Court's Motion Pursuant to Civil Rule 60.01 and Notice. Fentress et al. v Shea Communications et al. No 90CI0633 Jefferson Circuit Court, Division One, Louisville, KY.

John W. Potter, Judge v. Eli Lilly and Company (95-SC-580-MR). Appeal from Court of Appeals; Opinion by Justice Wintersheimer, reversing, rendered May 23, 1996. *43 K.L.S.5,* pp. 33–35.

Pourcher, E., Cohen, H., Cohen, D., Baruch, P., & Bouchard, R. H. (1993). Organic brain dysfunction and cognitive deficits in young schizophrenic patients with tardive dyskinesia. *Brain and Cognition, 23*(1), 81–87.

Prien, R. F., Balter, M. B., & Caffey, E. M. (1978). Hospital surveys of prescribing practices with psychotherapeutic drugs. *Archives of General Psychiatry, 35*, 1271–1275.

Prien, R. F., Caffey, E. M., & Klett, J. C. (1972). Comparison of lithium and chlorpromazine in the treatment of mania. *Archives of General Psychiatry, 26*, 146–153.

Prien, R. F., Caffey, E. M., & Klett, J. C. (1974). Factors associated with treatment success in lithium carbonate prophylaxis. *Archives of General Psychiatry, 31*, 189–192.

Prison drug bill vetoed by Brown (1977, September 30). *San Francisco Chronicle*, p. 15.

Public Citizen Health Research Group. (1990). Prozac: Benefits and risks of a new antidepressant. *Health Letter, 6*(6), 1–3.

Public Citizen Health Research Group (1991, May 23). Re: Citizens Petition for revision of fluoxetine (Prozac) labeling. Letter to David Kessler, Commissioner, Food and Drug Administration. Washington, DC: Public Citizen.

Pund, E. (1993, January 30). Claiming they were drugged, inmates press for documents. *The Press-Enterprise* [California], p. B-4.

Putnam, F. W. (1990). Foreword. In D. M. Donovan & D. McIntyre, *Healing the hurt child*. New York: Norton.

Quitkin, F., Rifkin, A., & Klein, D. F. (1975). Very high dosage vs. standard dosage fluphenazine in schizophrenia. *Archives of General Psychiatry, 32*, 1276–1281.

Raitasuo, R., Vataja, R., & Elomaa, E. (1994). Risperidone-induced neuroleptic malignant syndrome in young patient. *Lancet, 344*, 1705.

Rall, T. W. (1990). Hypnotics and sedatives; Ethanol. In A. Gilman, T. Rall, A. Nies, & P. Taylor (Eds.), *The pharmacological basis of therapeutics* (8th ed., pp. 345–382). New York: McGraw-Hill.

Randrup, A., & Munkva, I. (1970). Correlation between specific effects of amphetamines on the brain and on behavior. In E. H. Ellinwood & S. Cohen (Eds.), *Current concepts on amphetamine abuse: Proceedings of a workshop, Duke University Medical Center, June 5–6, 1970*. Rockville, MD: National Institute of Mental Health.

Rane, A., Tomson, G., & Bjarke, B. (1978). Effects of maternal lithium therapy in a newborn infant. *Journal of Pediatrics, 93*, 296–297.

Reccoppa, L., Welch, W. A., & Ware, M. R. (1990, November). Acute dystonia and fluoxetine. *Journal of Clinical Psychiatry, 51*, 487.

Regier, D. A., & Leshner, A. I. (1992, February). Request for applications: Cooperative agreement for a multi-site, multimodel treatment study of attention-deficit hyperactivity Disorder (ADHD)/Attention-Deficit Disorder (ADD). MH-92-03. Washington, DC: Department of Health and Human Services; Public Health Service; Alcohol, Drug Abuse and Mental Health Administration; and NIMH.

Reisberg, B., & Gershon, S. (1979). Side effects associated with lithium therapy. *Archives of General Psychiatry, 36,* 879–887.

Remick, R. A. (1978). Acute brain syndrome associated with ECT and lithium. *Canadian Psychiatric Association Journal, 23,* 129–130.

Ricaurte, G. A., Fuller, R. W., Perry, K. W., & Seiden, L. S. (1983). Fluoxetine increases long-lasting neostriatal dopamine depletion after administration of d-methamphetamine and d-amphetamine. *Neuropharmacology, 22,* 1165–1169.

Richardson, G., & Partridge, L. (1993). Clozaril withdrawal syndrome. *Psychiatric Bulletin, 17,* 374–375.

Rifkin, A. (1988). ECT versus tricyclic antidepressants in depression: A review of evidence. *Journal of Clinical Psychiatry, 49*(1), 3–7.

Rifkin, A., Quitkin, F., & Klein, D. F. (1975, May). Akinesia: A poorly recognized drug-induced extrapyramidal behavioral disorder. *Archives of General Psychiatry, 32,* 672–674.

Robitscher, J. (1980). *The powers of psychiatry.* Boston: Houghton Mifflin.

Rodgers, J. E. (1992). *Psychosurgery: Damaging the brain to save the mind.* New York: HarperCollins.

Rogers, J. M. (1971, September). Drug abuse—Just what the doctor ordered. *Psychology Today,* pp. 16–24.

Roizin, L., True, C., & Knight, M. (1959). Structural effects of tranquilizers. *Research Publications of the Association for Research in Nervous and Mental Disease, 37,* 285–324.

Romasenko, V. A., & Jacobson, I. S. (1969). Morpho-histochemical study of the action of trifluoperazine on the brain of white rats. *Acta Neuropathologica (Berlin), 12,* 23–32.

Romme, M., & Escher, S. (1993). *Accepting voices.* London: MIND Publications.

Rosebush, P., & Stewart, T. (1989). A prospective analysis of 24 episodes of neuroleptic malignant syndrome. *American Journal of Psychiatry, 146,* 717–725.

Rosenbaum, A. H. (1979). Pharmacotherapy of tardive dyskinesia. *Psychiatric Annals, 9,* 205–210.

Rosenbaum, A., Maruta, T., Duane, D., Auger, R., Martin, D., & Brenengen, E. (1980). Tardive dyskinesia in depressed patients: Successful therapy with antidepressants and lithium. *Psychosomatics, 21,* 715–719.

Rosenbaum, J. E., Woods, S. W., Groves, J. E., & Klerman, G. (1984). Emergence of hostility during alprazolam treatment. *American Journal of Psychiatry, 141,* 792–793.

Rosenhan, D. L. (1973, January 19). On being sane in insane places. *Science,* p. 1.

Rossoff, I. S. (1974). *Handbook of veterinary drugs.* New York: Springer.

Rupniak, N. M. J., Jenner, P., & Marsden, C. D. (1983). The effect of chronic neuroleptic administration on cerebral dopamine receptor function. *Life Sciences, 32,* 2289–2311.

Sabshin, M. (1992, March 10). To aid understanding of mental disorders (letter). *New York Times,* p. A24.

Sabuncu, N., Sabacin, S., Saygill, R., Kumral, K., & Ornek, T. (1977). Cortical atrophy caused by long-term therapy with antidepressive and neuroleptic drugs: A clinical and experimental study. In L. Roizin, H. Shiraki, & N. Grčević (Eds.), *Neurotoxicology* (pp. 149–158). New York: Raven.

Sachdev, P., & Kruk, J. (1994). Clinical characteristics and predisposing factors in acute drug-induced akathisia. *Archives of General Psychiatry, 51,* 963–974.

Sackeim, H., Prudic, J., Devanand, D., Kiersky, J., Fitzsimons, L., Moody, B., McElhiney, M., Coleman, E., & Settembrino, J. (1993). Effects of stimulus intensity and electrode placement on the efficacy and cognitive effects of electroconvulsive therapy. *New England Journal of Medicine, 328,* 839–846.

Saltz, G. L., Woerner, M. G., Kane, J. M., Lieberman, J. A., Alvir, J. M. J., Bergmann, K. J., Blank, K., Koblenzer, J., & Kahaner, K. (1991). Prospective study of tardive dyskinesia incidence in the elderly. *Journal of the American Medical Association, 266,* 2402–2406.

Salyer, K., Holmstrom, R., & Noshpitz, J. (1991). Learning disabilities as a childhood manifestation of severe psychopathology. *American Journal of Orthopsychiatry, 61,* 230–240.

Salzman, C. (1992). Behavioral side effects of benzodiazepines. In J. M. Kane & J. A. Lieberman (Eds.), *Adverse effects of psychotropic drugs* (pp. 139–152). New York: Guilford.

Salzman, C., Kochansky, G. E., Shader, R. I., Porrino, L. J., Hartzman, J. S., & Swett, Jr., C. P. (1974). Chlordiazepoxide-induced hostility in a small group setting. *Archives of General Psychiatry, 31*, 401–405.

Scanlon, L. (1995, April 20). Secret deal struck at trial not to appeal Prozac verdict. Move halted evidence on 2nd drug, judge thinks. *Courier-Journal* (Louisville, KY), p. B1.

Schatzberg, A., & Cole, J. (1991). *Manual of clinical psychopharmacology* (2nd ed.). Washington, DC: American Psychiatric Press.

Schatzberg, A., & Nemeroff, C. (1995). *American Psychiatric Press textbook of psychopharmacology*. Washington, DC: American Psychiatric Association.

Scher, J. (1966). Patterns and profiles of addiction and drug abuse. *Archives of General Psychiatry, 15*, 539–551.

Schiorring, E. (1977). Changes in individual and social behavior induced by amphetamine and related compounds in monkeys and man. In E. H. Ellinwood, Jr., & M. M. Kilbey (Eds.), *Cocaine and other stimulants* (pp. 481–522). New York: Plenum.

Schlagenhauf, G., Tupin, J., & White, R. B. (1966). The use of lithium carbonate in treatment of manic psychoses. *American Journal of Psychiatry, 123*, 201–207.

Schmauss, C., & Krieg, J-C. (1987). Enlargement of cerebral fluid spaces in long-term benzodiazepine abusers. *Psychological Medicine, 17*, 869–873.

Schmidt, C. J. (1987). Neurotoxicity of the psychedelic amphetamine, methylenedioxymethamphetamine. *Journal of Pharmacology and Experimental Therapeutics, 240*, 1–7.

Schrag, P., & Divoky, D. (1974). *The myth of the hyperactive child*. New York: Dell.

Schou, M. (1957). Biology and pharmacology of the lithium ion. *Pharmacology Review, 9*, 17–58.

Schou, M. (1968). Lithium in psychiatry—A review. In D. H. Efron (Ed.), *Pharmacology: A review of progress 1957–1967* (Public Health Service Publication N. 1836). Washington, DC: U.S. Government Printing Office.

Schou, M. (1976). Pharmacology and toxicology of lithium. *Annual Review of Pharmacology and Toxicology, 16*, 231–243.

Schou, M., Amdisen, A., & Thomsen, K. (1968). The effect of lithium on the normal mind. In P. Baudis, E. Peterova, S. V. Plzen (Eds.),

De Psychiatria Progrediente, Volume II. Amsterdam-London: North-Holland.

Schou, M., & Baastrup, P. C. (1973). Personal and social implications of lithium maintenance and treatment. In T.A. Ban (Ed.), *Psychopharmacology, sexual disorders and drug abuse.* Amsterdam-London: North-Holland.

Schulz, S. C., Koller, M. M., Kishore, P. R., Hamer, R. M., Gehl, J. J., & Friedel, R. O. (1983). Ventricular enlargement in teenage patients with schizophrenic spectrum disorder. *American Journal of Psychiatry, 14,* 1591–1595.

Schwartz, J. (1994a, June 3). Researchers cleared in drug trial deaths: NIH advisory panel's report on hepatitis studies at odds with findings by FDA. *Washington Post,* p. A10.

Schwartz, J. (1994b, October 28). FDA moves to improve safety of new drug trials. *Washington Post,* p. A10.

Sellinger, O. Z., & Azcurra, J. M. (1970). The breakdown of polysomes and the stimulation of protein synthesis in cerebral mechanisms of defense against seizures. In A. Lajtha (Ed.), *Protein metabolism of the nervous system* (pp. 519–532). New York: Plenum.

Semla, T., Palla, K., Poddig, B., & Brauner, D. (1994). Effects of the Omnibus Reconciliation Act 87 on antipsychotic prescribing in nursing home residents. *Journal of American Geriatrics Society, 42,* 648–652.

Seppala, T., Saario, I., & Mattila, M. J. (1976). Two weeks treatment with chlorpromazine, thioridazine, sulpiride, or bromazepam: Actions and interactions with alcohol on psychomotor skills related to driving. *Modern Problems in Pharmacopsychiatry, 11,* 85–90.

Serfaty, M., & Masterton, G. (1993). Fatal poisonings attributed to benzodiazepines in Britain during the 1980s. *British Journal of Psychiatry, 163,* 386–393.

Settle, E. C., & Settle, G. P. (1984). A case of mania associated with fluoxetine. *American Journal of Psychiatry, 141,* 280–281.

Shader, R., & DiMascio, A. (1977). *Psychotropic drug side effects.* Huntington, NY: Krieber.

Shah, D. (1973, July 7). Manic-depressives: Hope in a drug. *National Observer,* p. 4.

Sharkey, J. (1994). *Bedlam: Greed, profiteering, and fraud in a mental health system gone crazy.* New York: St. Martin's Press.

Shaw, E., Stokes, P., Mann, J., & Manevitz, A. (1987). Effects of lithium carbonate on the memory and motor speed of bipolar outpatients. *Journal of Abnormal Psychology, 96*, 64–69.

Sheard, M. H., Marini, J. L., Bridges, C. I., & Wagner, E. (1976). The effects of lithium on impulsive aggressive behavior in man. *American Journal of Psychiatry, 133*, 1409–1412.

Shelton, R. C., Karson, C. N., Doran, A. R., Pickar, D., Bigelow, L. B., & Weinberger, D. R. (1988). Cerebral structural pathology in schizophrenia: Evidence for selective prefrontal cortical defect. *American Journal of Psychiatry, 145*, 154–163.

Shenon, P. (1985, August 22). Lilly pleads guilty to Oraflex charges. *New York Times*, p. A16.

Sheppard, G., Gruzelier, J., Manchanda, R., Hirsch, S. R., Wise, R., Frackowiak, R., & Jones, T. (1983). O positron emission tomography scanning of predominantly never-treated acute schizophrenic patients. *Lancet, 24*, 1448–1452.

Sherman, C. (1995, July). Prozac for kids: 'Landmark' study affirms drug's use. *Clinical Psychiatry News*, p. 1.

Sherman, D. (1987, January/February). Efficacy of antipsychotic agents for behavioral problems. *The Consultant Pharmacist*, 9–12.

Shopsin, B., & Gershon, S. (1975). Cogwheel rigidity related to lithium maintenance. *American Journal of Psychiatry, 132*, 536–538.

Shopsin, B., Kim, S. S., & Gershon, S. (1971). A controlled study of lithium vs. chlorpromazine in acute schizophrenics. *British Journal of Psychiatry, 119*, 435–440.

Shulman, S. R., Hewitt, P., & Manocchia, M. (1995). Studies and inquiries into the FDA regulatory process: An historical review. *Drug Information Journal, 29*, 385–413.

Silver, J., Yudofsky, S., & Hurowitz, G. (1994). Psychopharmacology and electroconvulsive therapy. In R. Hales, S. Yudofsky, & J. Talbott (Eds.), *The American Psychiatric Press handbook of psychiatry* (2nd ed.). Washington, DC: American Psychiatric Press.

Simonson, M. (1964). Phenothiazine depressive reaction. *Journal of Neuropsychiatry, 5*, 259–265.

Simpson, G. M. (1977). Neurotoxicity of major tranquilizers. In L. Roizin, H. Shiraki, & N. Grčević (Eds.), *Neurotoxicology*. New York: Raven.

Singer, S., Colette, R., & Boland, R. (1995). Two cases of risperidone-induced neuroleptic malignant syndrome [one of the two cases] (letter). *American Journal of Psychiatry, 152*, 1234.

Singh, M. M. (1976). Dysphoric response to neuroleptic treatment in schizophrenia and its prognostic significance. *Diseases of the Nervous System, 37,* 191–196.

Skrzycki, C. (1996, February 18). Slowing the flow of federal rules: New conservative climate chills agencies' activism. *Washington Post,* p. A1.

Slater, I. H., Jones, G. T., & Moore, R. A. (1978). Inhibition of rem sleep by fluoxetine, a specific inhibitor of serotonin uptake. *Neuropharmacology, 17,* 383–389.

Slikker, W., Brocco, M., & Killam, K. (1976). Comparison of effects of lithium chloride and chlorpromazine on normal and isolate monkeys. *Proceedings of the Western Pharmacology Society, 19,* 424–427.

Small, J. G., & Kellams, J. J. (1974). Early hospital experience with fluphenazine decanoate. *Diseases of the Nervous System, 35,* 453–456.

Small, J. G., Kellams, J. J., Milstein, V., & Small, I. F. (1980). Complications with electroconvulsive treatment combined with lithium. *Biological Psychiatry, 15,* 103–112.

Small, J. G., Milstein, V., Perez, H. C., Small, I. F., & Moore, D. F. (1972). EEG and neurophysiological studies of lithium in normal volunteers. *Biological Psychiatry, 5,* 65–77.

Smith, B. D. (1993, August 1). Relaxed, firm dads save school events. *New York Times (Education life supplement),* p. 5.

SmithKline & French Laboratories. (1964). *Ten years' experience with Thorazine* (5th ed.). Philadelphia: SmithKline & French.

Smith, J. M., Kuchorski, M. A., Oswald, W. T., & Waterman, M. A. (1979). A systematic investigation of tardive dyskinesia inpatients. *American Journal of Psychiatry, 136,* 918–922.

Smith, M. (1995, March 7). Eight in Texas die after shock therapy in 15-month period. *Houston Chronicle,* p. 1A.

Smith, S. F., & Smith, H. B. (1973). The effect of prolonged lithium administration on activity, reactivity, and endurance in the rat. *Psychopharmacologia, 30,* 83–88.

Snodgrass, V. (1973). Debate over benefits and ethics of psychosurgery involves public. *Journal of the American Medical Association, 225,* 913–920.

Soldatos, C. R., Sakkas, P. N., Bergiannaki, J. D., & Stefanis, C. N. (1986). Behavioral side effects of triazolam in psychiatric inpatients: Report of five cases. *Drug Intelligence and Clinical Pharmacy, 20,* 294–297.

Sommers-Flanagan, J., & Sommers-Flanagan, R. (1996). Efficacy of anti-depressant medication with depressed youth: What psychologists should know. *Professional Psychology: Research and Practice, 27,* 145–153.

Sovner, R., DiMascio, A., Berkowitz, D., & Randolph, P. (1978). Tardive dyskinesia and informed consent. *Psychosomatics, 19,* 172–177.

Spiegel, C. (1991, March 25). Restraints, drugging rife in nursing homes. *Los Angeles Times,* p. A18.

Spohn, H. E., & Coyne, L. (1993). The effect of attention/information processing impairment of tardive dyskinesia and neuroleptics in chronic schizophrenics. *Brain and Cognition, 23*(1), 28–39.

Spotts, J. V., & Spotts, C. A. (Eds.). (1980). *Use and abuse of amphetamine and its substitutes* (DHEW Publication No. ADM 80-941). Rockville, MD: National Institute on Drug Abuse.

Squire, L., & Slater, P. (1983). Electroconvulsive therapy and complaints of memory dysfunction: A prospective three-year follow-up study. *British Journal of Psychiatry, 142,* 1–8.

Stark, P., & Hardison, C. (1985). A review of multicenter controlled studies of fluoxetine vs. imipramine and placebo in outpatients with major depressive disorder. *Journal of Clinical Psychiatry, 46*(3, section 2), 53–85.

State of California, Department of Mental Health, Statistics and Data Analysis Section, July 20, 1989 (untitled, unpublished report).

Sternbach, H. (1991). The serotonin syndrome. *American Journal of Psychiatry, 148,* 705.

Strayhorn, J. M., Jr., & Nash, J. L. (1977). Severe neurotoxicity despite "therapeutic" serum lithium levels. *Diseases of the Nervous System, 38,* 107–111.

Strothers, J. K., Wilson, D. W., & Royston, W. (1973). Lithium toxicity in newborn. *British Medical Journal, 3,* 233–234.

Struve, F. A., & Willner, A. E. (1983). Cognitive dysfunction and tardive dyskinesia. *British Journal of Psychiatry, 143,* 597–600.

Stuss, D., & Benson, D. (1987). The frontal lobes and control of cognition and memory. In E. Perecman (Ed.), *The frontal lobes revisited* (pp. 141–158). New York: IRBN.

Suddath, R., Christison, G., Torrey, E., Casanova, M., & Weinberger, D. (1990). Anatomical abnormalities in the brain of monozygotic twins discordant for schizophrenia. *New England Journal of Medicine, 322,* 789–794.

Sullivan, W. (1996). Personal communication to Peter R. Breggin from the Executive Director of the Vermont Protection & Advocacy Agency, Montpelier, VT, with data from the Vermont Hospital Discharge dataset.

Supersensitivity psychosis thought to often follow withdrawal of neuroleptics after extended use. (1983, September 1). *Psychiatric News*, p. 39.

Suppes, T., Baldessarini, R., Faedda, G., & Tohen, M. (1991). Risk of recurrence following discontinuation of lithium treatment in bipolar disorder. *Archives of General Psychiatry, 48*, 1082–1088.

Survey shows most psychiatrists are poor at diagnosing dystonia. (1992, May). *Clinical Psychiatry News*, p. 19.

Swanson, Jr., C. L., Price, W. A., & McEvoy, J. P. (1995). Effects of concomitant risperidone and lithium treatment. *American Journal of Psychiatry, 152*(7), 1096.

Swanson, J. M., Cantwell, D., Lerner, M., McBurnett, K., Pfiffner, L., & Kotkin, R. (1992). Treatment of ADHD: Beyond medication. *Beyond Behavior, 4*(1), 13–22.

Swartz, M., & Jones, P. (1994). Hyperlithemia correction and persistent delirium. *Journal of Clinical Pharmacology, 34*, 865–870.

Szasz, T. S. (1957). Some observations on the use of tranquilizing drugs. *Archives of Neurology and Psychiatry, 77*, 86–92.

Talbott, J. A., Hales, R. E., & Yudofsky, S. C. (Eds.). (1988). *Textbook of psychiatry*. Washington, DC: American Psychiatric Press.

Tanaka, Y., Hazama, H., Kawahara, R., & Kobayashi, K. (1981). Computerized tomography of the brain in schizophrenic patients. *Acta Psychiatrica Scandinavica, 63*, 191–197.

Tecce, J. J., Cole, J. O., & Savignano-Bowman, J. (1975). Chlorpromazine effects on brain activity (contingent negative variation) and reaction time in normal women. *Psychopharmacologia, 43*, 293–295.

Teicher, M. H., Glod, C. A., & Cole, J. O. (1990). Emergence of intense suicidal preoccupations during fluoxetine treatment. *American Journal of Psychiatry, 147*, 207–210.

Teicher, M. H., Glod, C. A., & Cole, J. O. (1993). Antidepressant drugs and the emergence of suicidal tendencies. *Drug Safety, 8*(3), 186–212.

Teller, D. N., & Denber, H. C. B. (1970). Mescaline and phenothiazines: Recent studies on subcellular localization and effects upon membranes. In A. Lajtha (Ed.), *Protein metabolism of the nervous system* (pp. 685–698). New York: Plenum.

Temple, R. (1987, December 28). Memorandum: Fluoxetine label. From the director, Office of Drug Research and Review, to the director, Division of Neuropharmacological Drug Products. Internal document, Department of Health and Human Services, Public Health Service, Food and Drug Administration, Center for Drug Evaluation and Research. Obtained through the Freedom of Information Act.

Temple, R. (1991, December 31). Approval of Sertraline, NDA 19-839. Memorandum to Paul Leber. Internal document of the Department of Health and Human Services, Public Health Service, Food and Drug Administration, Center for Drug Evaluation and Research. Obtained through the Freedom of Information Act.

Templer, D. I. (1992). ECT and permanent brain damage. In D. I. Templer, L. C. Hartlage, & W. G. Cannon (Eds.), *Preventable brain damage* (pp. 72–79). New York: Springer.

Templer, D. I., Hartlage, L. C., & Cannon, W. G. (1992). (Eds.), *Preventable brain damage.* New York: Springer.

Templer, D. I., & Veleber, D. M. (1982). Can ECT permanently harm the brain? *Clinical Neuropsychology, 4*(2), 62–66.

Tepper, S. J., & Haas, J. F. (1979). Prevalence of tardive dyskinesia. *Journal of Clinical Psychiatry, 40*, 508–516.

Thomas, S. F. (1990, October 24). Give attention deficit disorders their due. *Education Week*, p. 1.

Thompson, L. (1994, March). The cure that killed: Several patients die in clinical trial of drug for hepatitis-B at National Institutes of Health. *Discovery*, p. 56.

Tow, P. (1955). *Personality changes following frontal leucotomy.* London: Oxford University Press.

Tower, D. B., & McEachern, D. (1949). Acetylcholine and neuronal activity. I. Cholinesterase patterns and acetylcholine in the cerebrospinal fluids of patients with craniocerebral trauma. *Canadian Journal of Research, 27*(Sect. E), 105–119.

Treatment seen for drug-related growth problem. (1980, May 16). *Psychiatric News*, p. 28.

Trial court's authority to investigate and determine the correctness and veracity of judgments. (1996, May 30). Hon. John W. Potter, Judge v. Eli Lilly and Company (95-SC-580-MR). Appeal from Court of Appeals; Opinion by Justice Wintersheimer, reversing, rendered May 23, 1996. *43 K.L.S.5,* pp. 33–35.

Tricyclics overtaking barbiturates in overdoses. (1981, October). *Clinical Psychiatry News*, p. 1.

Turner, J. (1971, October). A critical assessment of drug marketing practices. *Journal of Drug Issues*, 301–311.

Turner, S. M., Jacob, R. G., Beidel, D. C., & Griffin, S. (1985). A second case of mania associated with fluoxetine. *American Journal of Psychiatry, 142*, 274–275.

Tuteur, W. (1957). Effect of chlorpromazine and reserpine on budgets of mental hospitals. *American Journal of Psychiatry, 113*, 657–659.

Umbarger, C., Dalsimer, J., Morrison, A., & Breggin, P. (1962). *College students in a mental hospital*. New York: Grune & Stratton.

Ungerstedt, V., & Ljungberg, T. (1977). Behavioral patterns related to dopamine neurotransmission: Effect of acute and chronic antipsychotic drugs. *Advances in Biochemical Psychopharmacology, 16*, 193–199.

Using antipsychotics: Side effect profiles, special concerns in the elderly. (1989, April). *Psychiatric Times*, Supplement, 4 pages.

USP DI (1995). Drug Information for the Health Care Professional (Fifteenth edition). Rockville, MD: United States Pharmacopeial Convention.

van der Kroef, C. (1979, September 8). Reactions to triazolam. *Lancet, 2*, 526.

van der Kroef, C. (1991, July 6). Triazolam. *Lancet, 338*, 56.

van Putten, T. (1974). Why do schizophrenic patients refuse to take their drugs? *Archives of General Psychiatry, 31*, 67–72.

van Putten, T. (1975a). Why do patients with manic-depressive illness stop their lithium? *Comprehensive Psychiatry, 16*, 179–183.

van Putten, T. (1975b). The many faces of akathisia. *Comprehensive Psychiatry, 16*, 43–47.

van Putten, T., & Marder, S. (1987). Behavioral toxicity of antipsychotic drugs. *Journal of Clinical Psychiatry, 48*(Supp.), 13–19.

van Putten, T., & May, P. (1978). Akinetic depression in schizophrenia. *Archives of General Psychiatry, 35*, 1101–1107.

van Putten, T., May, P. R. A., & Marder, S. R. (1980). Subjective responses to thiothixene and chlorpromazine. *Psychopharmacology Bulletin, 16*(3), 36–38.

van Putten, T., Mutalipassi, L., & Malkin, M. (1974). Phenothiazine-induced decompensation. *Archives of General Psychiatry, 30*, 102–105.

van Sweden, B. (1984). Neuroleptic neurotoxicity: Electroclinical aspects. *Acta Neurologica Scandinavica, 69,* 137–146.

Varchaver, M. [American Lawyer News Service] (1995, September 25). Prozac verdict was a sure thing. *Fulton County Daily Report* (Atlanta).

Vatz, R. E. (1993, March 1). Attention-deficit disorder mythology. *Wall Street Journal,* p. A15.

Vick, N. A. (1976). *Griker's neurology* (7th ed.). Springfield, IL: Thomas.

Volkow, N. D., Ding, Y-S., Fowler, J. S., Wang, G-J., Logan, J., Gatley, J. S., Dewey, S., Ashby, C., Lieberman, J., Hitzemann, R., & Wolf, A. P. (1995). Is methylphenidate like cocaine? *Archives of General Psychiatry, 52,* 456–463.

Wade, J. B., Taylor, M. A., Kasprisin, A., Rosenberg, S., & Fiducia, D. (1987). Tardive dyskinesia and cognitive impairment. *Biological Psychiatry, 22,* 393–395.

Waddington, J. L., & Youssef, H. A. (1986). Late onset involuntary movements in chronic schizophrenia: Relationships of "tardive" dyskinesia to intellectual impairment and negative symptoms. *British Journal of Psychiatry, 149,* 616–620.

Waddington, J. L., & Youssef, H. A. (1986). An unusual cluster of tardive dyskinesia in schizophrenia: Association with cognitive dysfunction and negative symptoms. *American Journal of Psychiatry, 143*(9), 1162–1165.

Waddington, J., & Youssef, H. (1988). Tardive dyskinesia in bipolar affective disorder: Aging, cognitive function, course of illness, and exposure to neuroleptics and lithium. *American Journal of Psychiatry, 145,* 613–616.

Wagemaker, H., Lippman, S., & Bryant, D. R. (1979, November/December). Lithium response of a patient diagnosed as a paranoid schizophrenic. *Psychiatric Opinion,* p. 45.

Walkenstein, E. (1972). *Beyond the couch.* New York: Crown.

Wamsley, J. K., Byerley, W. F., McCabe, R. T., McConnell, E. J., Dawson, T. M., & Grosser, B. I. (1987). Receptor alterations associated with serotonergic agents: An autographic analysis. *Journal of Clinical Psychiatry, 48*(3), (Suppl.), 19–85.

Warren, C. (1988). Electroconvulsive therapy, self, and family relations. *Research in the Sociology of Health Care, 7,* 283–300.

Wegner, F. (1985). Postmarketing surveillance (PMS) and geriatric drug use. In S. Moore & T. Teal (Eds.), *Geriatric drug use: Clinical and social perspectives* (pp. 95–97). New York: Pergamon.

Weinberger, D. R. (1984). Computed tomography (CT) findings in schizophrenia: Speculation on the meaning of it all. *Journal of Psychiatric Research, 18,* 477–490.

Weinberger, D. R., Cannon-Spoor, E., Potkin, S. G., & Wyatt, R. J. (1980). Poor premorbid adjustment and CT scan abnormalities in chronic schizophrenia. *American Journal of Psychiatry, 137,* 1410–1414.

Weinberger, D. R., De Lisi, L. E., Perman, G. P., Targum, S., & Wyatt, R. J. (1982). Computed tomography in schizophreniform disorder and other acute psychiatric disorders. *Archives of General Psychiatry, 39,* 778–783.

Weinberger, D. R., & Kleinman, J. E. (1986). Observations on the brain in schizophrenia. *American Psychiatric Association Annual Review, 5,* 42–67.

Weinberger, D. R., Torrey, E. F., Neophytides, H. N., & Wyatt, R. J. (1979). Lateral ventricular enlargement in chronic schizophrenia. *Archives of General Psychiatry, 36,* 735–739.

Weiner, R., Rogers, H., Davidson, J., & Squire, L. (1986). Effects of stimulus parameters on cognitive side effects. *Annals of the New York Academy of Medicine, 462,* 353–356.

Weiner, R. D., Whanger, A. D., Erwin, C. W., & William, W. P. (1980). Prolonged confusional state and EEG seizure activity following concurrent ECT and lithium use. *American Journal of Psychiatry, 137,* 1452–1453.

Weiner, W., & Luby, E. (1983). Tardive akathisia. *Journal of Clinical Psychiatry, 44,* 417–419.

Weingartner, H., Rudorfer, M., & Linnoila, M. (1985). Cognitive effects of lithium treatment on normal volunteers. *Psychopharmacology, 86,* 472–474.

Weller, M., & Kornhuber, J. (1993). Does clozapine cause neuroleptic malignant syndrome? *American Journal of Psychiatry, 54,* 70–71.

Wells, A. B., & Mendelson, M. (1978). Antidepressants. In M. Goldberg & G. Egelston, *Mind-influencing drugs.* Littleton, MA: PSG Publishing Co.

Welsh, P. (1995, June 11). The case for going public. *Washington Post,* p. 1.

Wender, P. H. (1973). *The hyperactive child.* New York: Crown.

Wender, P. H., & Eisenberg, L. (1975). Minimal brain dysfunction in children. In S. Arieti (Ed.), *American handbook of psychiatry* (Vol. II). New York: Basic Books.

Westlin, W. (1991). "Dear doctor" letter to the medical profession from Sandoz Pharmaceuticals accompanied by revised label dated April 15, 1991.

Whalen, C. K., & Henker, B. (1991). Social impact of stimulant treatment for hyperactive children. *Journal of Learning Disabilities, 24,* 231–241.

White, F. J., & Wang, R. Y. (1983). Differential effects of classical and atypical antipsychotic drugs on A9 and A10 dopamine neurons. *Science, 221,* 1054–1056.

Wildi, E., Linder, A., & Costoulas, G. (1967). Schizophrenia and involutional cerebral senility. *Psychiatry and Neurology, 154,* 1–26.

Wilson, A., Schild, H. O., & Modell, W. (1975). *Applied pharmacology* (11th ed.). New York: Churchill Livingstone.

Wilson, I. C., Garbutt, J. C., Lanier, C. F., Moylan, J., Nelson, W., & Prange, Jr., A. J. (1983). Is there a tardive dysmentia? *Schizophrenia Bulletin, 9,* 187–192.

Winslow, R. (1990, May 14). Wonder drug: Sandoz Corp.'s Clozaril treats schizophrenia but can kill patients. *Wall Street Journal,* p. 1.

Wirth, J. (1991, July 19). Deposition. Aubrey vs. The Johns Hopkins Hospital et al. HCA No. 90-0254. In the health claims arbitration office: Baltimore, MD.

Wise, B. (1989, April 21). *Increased frequency report (IFR): Alprazolam and rage.* Rockville, MD: FDA Division of Epidemiology and Surveillance. Obtained through the Freedom of Information Act.

Wise, B. (1989, September 19). *Reports of hostility after exposure to triazolobenzodiazepines* (working paper). Rockville, MD: FDA Division of Epidemiology & Surveillance. Obtained through the Freedom of Information Act.

Wittrig, J., & Coopwood, W. E. (1970). Lithium versus chlorpromazine for manics: Initiative and productivity versus tranquilization and hospitalization. *Diseases of the Nervous System, 31,* 486–489.

Wojcik, J. D., Gelenberg, A. J., LaBrie, R. A., & Mieske, M. (1980). Prevalence of tardive dyskinesia in an outpatient population. *Comprehensive Psychiatry, 21,* 370–380.

Wolf, M. E., & Brown, P. (1987). Overcoming institutional and community resistance to a tardive dyskinesia management program. *Hospital and Community Psychiatry, 38,* 65–68.

Wolf, M. E., Ryan, J. J., & Mosnaim, A. D. (1982). Organicity and tardive dyskinesia. *Psychosomatics, 23,* 475–480.

Wolfe, C. (1995, June 13). Court asked to muzzle Prozac judge. *Indianapolis Star*, p. B1.

Wolkin, A., Jaeger, J., Brodie, J. D., Wolf, A., Fowler, J., Rotrosen, J., Gomez-Mont, F., & Cancro, R. (1985). Low frontal glucose utilization in chronic schizophrenia: A replication study. *American Journal of Psychiatry, 145,* 251–253.

Wolkin, A., Angrist, B., Wolf, A., Brodie, J. D., Wolkin, B., Jaeger, J., Cancro, R., & Rotrosen, J. (1988). Persistent cerebral metabolic abnormalities in chronic schizophrenia determined by positron emission tomography. *American Journal of Psychiatry, 142,* 564–571.

Wong, D. T., & Bymaster, F. P. (1981, April). Subsensitivity of serotonin receptors after long-term treatment of rats with fluoxetine. *Research Communications in Chemical Pathology and Pharmacology, 32,* 41–51.

Wong, D. T., Reid, L. R., Bymaster, F. P., & Threlkeld, P. G. (1985). Chronic effects of fluoxetine, a selective inhibitor of serotonin uptake, on neurotransmitter receptors. *Journal of Neural Transmission, 64,* 251–269.

Wooden, K. (1976). *Weeping in the playtime of others.* New York: McGraw-Hill.

Wysowski, D. K., & Barash, D. (1991, October). Adverse behavioral reactions attributed to triazolam in the Food and Drug Administration's spontaneous reporting system. *Archives of Internal Medicine, 151,* 2003–2008.

Wysowski, D. K., & Barash, D. (1992, July). Use of spontaneous reporting system data. *Archives of Internal Medicine, 152,* 1528–1529.

Yassa, R., Iskandar, H., & Ally, J. (1988). The prevalence of tardive dyskinesia in fluphenazine-treated patients. *Journal of Clinical Psychopharmacology, 8,* 17S–20S.

Yassa, R., & Jones, B. (1985). Complications of tardive dyskinesia: A review. *Psychosomatics, 26,* 305–313.

Yassa, R., Nastase, C., Camille, Y., & Belzile, L. (1988). Tardive dyskinesia in a psychogeriatric population. In M. E. Wolf & A. D. Mosnaim (Eds.), *Tardive dyskinesia: Biological mechanisms and clinical aspects* (pp. 123–134). Washington, DC: American Psychiatric Press.

Yassa, R., Nastase, C., Dupont, D., & Thibeau, M. (1992). Tardive dyskinesia in elderly psychiatric patients: A 5-year study. *American Journal of Psychiatry, 149*(9), 1206–1211.

Zametkin, A. J., Nordahl, T. E., Gross, M., King, A. C., Semple, W. E., Rumsey, J., Hamburger, S., & Cohen, R. M. (1990). Cerebral glucose metabolism in adults with hyperactivity of childhood onset. *New England Journal of Medicine, 323,* 1361–1366.

Zander, T. K. (1977, July/August). Prolixin decanoate: A review of the research. *Mental Law Reporter,* pp. 37–42.

Zec, R. F., & Weinberger, D. R. (1986). Relationship between CT scan findings and neuropsychological performance in chronic schizophrenia. *Psychiatric Clinics of North America, 9,* 49–61.

Zoloft Summary Basis of Approval. (1988, April 13). Also includes Memorandum of Thomas P. Laughren, Supervisory Overview of NDA 19-839 (sertraline), August 9, 1991. Obtained through the Freedom of Information Act.

Index

and serotonergic neurotransmission, 5,
    7–8, 98–99
stimulant actions of, 79–94
and suicidal behavior. *See* Suicidal be-
    havior, in fluoxetine therapy
and violent behavior. *See* Violent be-
    havior, in fluoxetine therapy
withdrawal symptoms from, 100–101
Fluphenazine, 17, 66, 126
and akathisia, 30, 32, 45
and extrapyramidal reactions, 39–40
and suicidal behavior, 33
Flurazepam, 185, 188–189, 195, 198,
    202
Fluvoxamine, 77, 94
Food and Drug Administration, 73
on benzodiazepine therapy, 193
    data from spontaneous reporting sys-
        tem, 195–200
    warning label in, 200–202
drug approval process, 208–233
    design of studies in, 209–210
    efficacy studies in, 209–210
    evaluation of clinical data in, 215–
        218
    failures in, 224–230
    on fluoxetine, 227–228
    limitations of clinical trials in, 212–
        218
    neglected areas in, 218–219
    on neuroleptics, 224–227
    New Drug Application in, 214–215
    ongoing monitoring in, 210–211,
        220–224
    phases in, 209
    profit motive affecting, 219–220
    safety studies in, 211–215
    on sertraline, 228–230
    warning label in, 210, 211
on electroshock therapy, 132–133, 154
on fluoxetine, 78, 79–80, 82, 85–86,
    211
    and akathisia, 97
    approval process in, 227–228
    data from spontaneous reporting sys-
        tem, 88–89

and dyskinesia, 97
    efficacy studies on, 228
    and stimulant syndrome, 88
    and violent behavior, 88–89
    and withdrawal symptoms, 100–101
on neuroleptics, 75
    approval process in, 224–227
    and neuroleptic malignant syndrome,
        224–225
    and tardive dyskinesia, 225–227
    warnings on, 74, 225–227
    spontaneous reporting system, 220–
        224
on benzodiazepine therapy, 195–200
on fluoxetine, 88–89
on stimulant drugs, 106
Frontal lobe
    clozapine affecting, 73
    positron emission tomography of,
        63–64
    syndrome of, 15–16

G

Gender
    in attention-deficit hyperactivity disor-
        der, 175
    in electroshock therapy, 129–132, 136–
        137, 139
Generalized brain dysfunction, 3–4, 9
    clinical evidence of, 56
Germany, fluoxetine in, 92–94
Great Britain
    benzodiazepines in, 201–203
    fluoxetine in, 92–94
    methylphenidate in, 175
Growth and development, methylpheni-
        date affecting, 173

H

Halcion. *See* Triazolam
Haldol. *See* Haloperidol
Hallucinations, 6, 19
Haloperidol, 7, 16, 17, 126
    and akathisia, 31, 32

Haloperidol *(Continued)*
  and deactivation syndrome, 19
  and dopaminergic neurotransmission, 5,
    8
  and dysphoria, 32
  and extrapyramidal reactions, 39–40
  and parkinsonism, 29
Helplessness, iatrogenic, and denial, 5,
    11–12
  in electroshock therapy, 152–153
  in lithium therapy, 123
  in tardive dyskinesia, 43
Hostile behavior in benzodiazepine ther-
    apy, 188, 192–193, 195–198
Huntington's chorea, 38, 55
Hysteria, differentiated from dystonia, 28,
    45

I

Imipramine, 84, 101–102
  interaction with fluoxetine, 95
Impulsive behavior
  in attention-deficit hyperactivity disor-
    der, 160
  in benzodiazepine therapy, 187
  in fluoxetine therapy, 82, 90
Indifference. *See* Apathy and indiffer-
    ence
Insulin, Humalog form of, 231
Iproniazid, 107
Isoniazid, antidepressant effect of, 108

L

Legal issues
  in benzodiazepine therapy, 193
  in electroshock therapy, 153–155
  in fluoxetine therapy, 84–85, 88
  in safety of drugs, 211, 219–220
  in warning label of drugs, 211
Lethargic encephalitis, 29, 50–51, 67–69
Lewy body type dementia, 41
Limbic system, 59, 73
Lithium therapy, 8, 111–126, 128
  in acute mania, 123–124

  assessment of, 122–126
  cognitive function in, 113–120
  creativity in, 118–120
  denial of disorders in, 116, 123
  disabling effects of, 113–118, 122
  drinking water theory on, 126
  drug interactions in, 121
  electroencephalography in, 121
  and electroshock therapy, 121
  mechanism of effect, 122–123
  in normal volunteers, effects of, 4,
    113–117, 123
  in recurrence of manic episodes, 124
  specificity of action, 111–112, 123
  subduing effects of, 112–113
  substitutes for, 126–128
  withdrawal from, 125–126
Lobotomy-like effect, 4
  in electroshock therapy, 153
  in lithium therapy, 114–115, 118
  in neuroleptic therapy, 14–24, 59, 73

M

Magnetic resonance imaging of brain,
    62–63, 65, 70
  in attention-deficit hyperactivity disor-
    der, 172
  in electroshock therapy, 131, 148
  in neuroleptic therapy, 62–63, 65
  in tardive dyskinesia, 63
Mania, 5, 103
  anticonvulsant drugs in, 127
  antidepressant drugs in, 128
  in benzodiazepine therapy, 189–190
  in fluoxetine therapy, 86–87, 91, 99–
    100
  lithium therapy in, 111–126, 128. *See
    also* Lithium therapy
  in lithium withdrawal, 125–126
  neuroleptic therapy in, 123, 126
MEDWatch program, 212–213, 220, 222
Mellaril. *See* Thioridazine
Memory
  in benzodiazepine therapy, 185
  in electroshock therapy, 142–144